Caring in Context

Drawing on ethnographic research conducted by an American nurse, *Caring in Context* is an exploration of how most of the world experiences cancer, and how nurses bear witness and respond to the suffering of others when they have little means to help—or for complex reasons, choose not to.

This compelling book centers on nurses in a government cancer hospital in South India and examines key contexts that influence nursing practice and the delivery of healthcare, including hierarchical legacies of colonialism and the caste system, resource scarcity, power and perceived powerlessness, and gender inequities. These themes are illustrated through intersecting narratives, such as the story of Hameeda, an orphaned teenager with sarcoma who lives at the hospital until she becomes paralyzed, and Sister Meena, a nurse who strives to provide better care but encounters overwhelming structural obstacles and is chastised by her superiors for doing too much.

Offering a critical re-examination of the realities faced by clinicians, patients, and family members who struggle to deliver and receive cancer care, *Caring in Context*'s unique perspective and accessible style will appeal to a wide and interdisciplinary audience, from practitioners, academics, and advocates to anyone interested in the complex context of the human experience.

Virginia LeBaron is the Kluge-Schakat Associate Professor of Compassionate Care at the University of Virginia School of Nursing, in Charlottesville, Virginia (USA).

Routledge Research in Nursing and Midwifery

Caring in Context

An Ethnography of Cancer Nursing in India

Virginia LeBaron

Routledge
Taylor & Francis Group

LONDON AND NEW YORK

First published 2024
by Routledge
4 Park Square, Milton Park, Abingdon, Oxon OX14 4RN

and by Routledge
605 Third Avenue, New York, NY 10158

Routledge is an imprint of the Taylor & Francis Group, an informa business

© 2024 Virginia LeBaron

British Library Cataloguing-in-Publication Data
A catalogue record for this book is available from the British Library

ISBN: 978-1-032-53688-0 (hbk)
ISBN: 978-1-032-53860-0 (pbk)
ISBN: 978-1-003-41315-8 (ebk)

DOI: 10.4324/9781003413158

Typeset in Sabon
by codeMantra

For nurses, everywhere

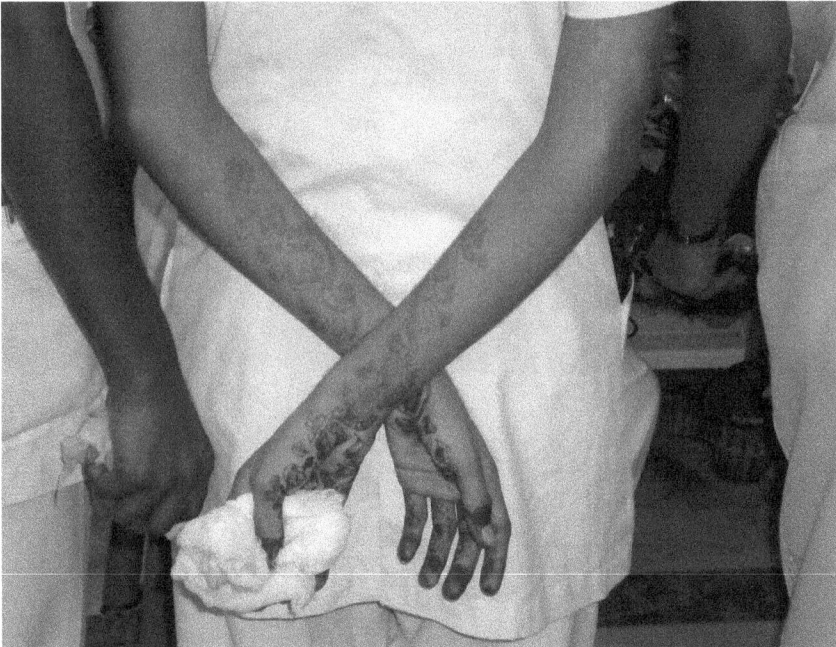

Figure 0.1 Student nurses, one with hands and arms decorated with henna, South Indian Cancer Hospital, Intensive Care Unit.

Contents

Acknowledgments

First and most importantly, I am indebted to the healthcare providers, particularly the nurses, along with patients and family members at the South Indian Cancer Hospital and other nearby health institutions, who trusted me with their stories and welcomed me into their community of care; for their generosity, openness, and warmth, I am deeply humbled and appreciative. I am also grateful to the Fulbright-Nehru Research Fellowship program, the American Cancer Society, the University of Utah College of Nursing, and the University of Virginia School of Nursing whose funding and academic support made this project feasible. I am especially thankful to: Susan Beck for her inspiring creative vision, consistent encouragement, and remarkable talent for seeing both the big picture and the details; Jane Ingham, Ian Magrath, Stuart Brown, and P. Gayatri, who made it all possible from the very beginning; Mark Nichter, for his generous mentorship and uncanny ability to find just the right article, and say just the right thing to help me cope with crises of faith while in the field; my research assistant, R. Vineela, who remains the most organized and efficient individual I know; T.V. Lakshmi, K. Priya, B. Navdeep, V. Aditya, and V. Kiran, who all provided crucial help with translation, transcription, and translation verification; J. Aditya for being an astute spiritual guide and cultural ambassador; Fraser Black, Martha Maurer, Kristin Cloyes, Patricia Berry, Margaret Robertson, Buddy Beck, John Wright, Veronique Poulin, Patricia Tennison, and John Lach, who gave careful reads and constructive feedback on earlier drafts; Doug Ennals, Sara Lewis, John Round, Emily Ogden, Kimberly Acquaviva, Dominique Tobbell, and Tanner Wallace, for delivering bits of well-timed wisdom, humor, and advice; Nate Pierce, Abhipsha Chatterjee, and Sophie Amirsultan, whose connections helped me turn critical corners in the field; Trudy Hale of The Porches and the entire staff of the Virginia Center for the Creative Arts for creating ideal writers' havens that enabled the project to maintain momentum; and to Amber Steen, whose all-encompassing support afforded me the time and space to get this project over the finish line. Also, a very special thank you to Phyllis Deutsch whose incisive review and sound counsel gave this book essential direction and focus, long after her official obligation to the project had ended.

Thank you to everyone at Routledge Press/Taylor & Francis, especially Grace McInnes and Amy Thomson, for their advocacy and patience in shepherding me through the publication process and for helping this project find the ideal publishing home. And, of course, to John, Emmett, and Owen for their support, love, and encouragement—you make it all worthwhile.

List of Featured Participants
(*all pseudonyms)

This is a work of nonfiction. Names and certain details have been changed to protect the identity of individuals, organizations, and institutions.

South Indian Cancer Hospital (SICH)

Palliative Care Team

>   Dr. Madhu (physician)
>   Dr. Darshan (physician)
>   Dr. Amit (physician)
>   Pradeep (nurse)
>   Daya (nurse)
>   Abhipsa (nurse)
>   Sarah (social worker)
>   Radha (ayah, housekeeper)
>   Hameeda (patient)

Home Care Team

>   Jotika (health counselor)
>   Menakshi (nurse)
>   Leah (nurse)

Pediatrics

>   Dr. Rashi (physician)
>   Bishnu (social worker)
>   Vasudha (social worker)
>   Kavita (nurse)
>   Bharati (nurse)

General Wards

>   Dr. Rama (physician)
>   Jasmine (administrative coordinator)

Ward Nurses

  Sister Adishree (Intensive Care Unit, ICU)
  Sister Agnes
  Sister Asha
  Sister Chaaya
  Sister Deepa
  Sister Eliza
  Sister Hema (Head Nurse)
  Sister Lavanya
  Sister Meena
  Sister Nalini (Paying Wards)
  Sister Naveena
  Sister Pooja
  Sister Preeti
  Sister Ruth
  Sister Sonia (ICU)

Pharmacy

  Sima (head pharmacist)
  Jyoti (pharmacist)
  Prerna (pharmacist)

Volunteers

  Kate (U.S.)
  Jennifer (Australia)
  Marcus (Germany)
  Dr. Varun (U.S.)

Life

  Joanie (flatmate)
  Ruma (flatmate)
  Esha (translator)
  Mayank (translator)
  Hasan (watchman's son)
  Noora (watchman's daughter)
  Fathima (cook)
  Lakshmi (housekeeper)
  Paul (friend)

PART I
Introduction

Introduction

In the end, this is a story about resources. And power. And whom we see as worth saving—and whom we let suffer.

Imagine: you are a 42-year-old woman whose mother died of breast cancer when you were a teenager. You live in a middle-class, suburban neighborhood in the U.S., or maybe Canada, or perhaps Australia. Because of your increased risk of developing breast cancer, each year your health insurance pays for you to have the most technologically up-to-date type of mammogram to screen for any suspicious breast masses. This time, the radiologist sees something—it is very small, but the doctors are concerned, and they send you for a biopsy that confirms an early stage, aggressive type of breast cancer. You are referred for surgery and radiation and chemotherapy. Your nurse has been well educated and enjoys her job; in fact, she received specialized training in cancer care and is certified in how to safely administer chemotherapy. You undergo six months of treatment, and while it is not easy, you are given medications to manage nausea and pain and are able to continue working. After you complete therapy you have regular visits with your oncologist, who carefully checks to make sure there is no evidence that the cancer has returned. Five years later, you are declared cancer-free.

Now, consider an alternative scenario: you are a 42-year-old woman living in India, or perhaps Nepal, or maybe Tanzania. You live in a rural village, far from a general doctor, further from a hospital, and further still from an oncologist and specialized cancer treatment center. A year ago, you noticed an unusual lump in your breast, but you did not say anything because you are afraid and embarrassed. The lump has now grown to the size of an orange and has burst through your skin. You can no longer ignore it as the pain is excruciating and people in your village have begun to avoid you because there is a terrible smell coming from the wound. A local doctor eventually examines you and says, "There is nothing for you here. Go to the big city. Go to the government hospital. They will help you." You take a two-day bus ride with your son to a government hospital in the capital city. It is a difficult ride because you are in so much pain. You know the government hospital will be crowded and under-resourced, but you do not have money to pay for a

DOI: 10.4324/9781003413158-2

private hospital. When you arrive at the hospital, you must wait another four days to see a doctor because there are so many other patients also waiting to be seen. You do not have any relatives who live in the city to stay with, so you and your son sleep outdoors on the hospital grounds. When you are finally seen in the clinic, your son is quickly told you have advanced breast cancer and there is no cure, but they can try some chemotherapy. You are admitted to the female ward, which is overflowing with patients. There is one nurse on duty. She is overwhelmed because there are over 50 patients on the ward, and she has not received any formal training in caring for patients with cancer or how to safely administer chemotherapy. Unfortunately, this hospital—like most others in the city—does not routinely stock morphine so despite your horrible pain, the nurse can only give you acetaminophen (Tylenol) and ibuprofen (Motrin), which does nothing. After your chemotherapy is complete, you take the two-day bus trip back to your village. You are nauseous and cannot eat or sleep because you are in so much pain. You are too weak to return to the hospital for any more treatment, and even if you felt better, you could not go as you have no money left to pay for another trip. A month later you die, struggling to breath and in unbearable pain.[1]

The Growing Global Cancer Burden

The second scenario is how the majority of the world experiences cancer.[2] When most people think about global health, it is highly publicized infectious diseases—like Ebola and more recently COVID-19—that typically come to mind. While combatting existing and emerging epidemics and pandemics must clearly be a priority, the less sensational reality is that as the global population grows, and people live longer, the world is buckling under the steady strain of noncommunicable (noninfectious) diseases. Noncommunicable diseases, such as cancer, cause 75% of deaths globally, with almost

---

1 These case examples are intended to illustrate the stark disparities in cancer treatment and outcomes that often exist between a high- and low- and middle-income country. The second case highlights key factors that can result in late diagnoses and higher cancer mortality rates in low- and middle-income countries, including poverty, stigma, limited knowledge of cancer, and lack of access to cancer screening and prevention services. However, it is critical to acknowledge that serious disparities also exist within higher resourced countries. For example, within the U.S., the outcome for the patient in the first case is likely to be significantly worse if they lack health insurance, belong to a minoritized or historically oppressed group, or live in a medically underserved area. Of note, The US Department of Health and Human Services, National Institutes of Health, National Cancer Institute National Cancer Plan (2023) includes "eliminate disparities" as one of its eight strategic goals.
2 In 2020, of the nearly ten million cancer-related deaths worldwide, 70% occurred in low- and middle-income countries. See (1) World Health Organization (WHO)/International Agency for Research on Cancer: Data visualization tools for exploring the global cancer burden in 2020; (2) American Cancer Society, Global Cancer Burden (2023).

80% occurring in low- and middle-income countries (LMICs).[3] Around the world, cancer is the second leading cause of death (after heart disease) and kills more people each year than AIDS, malaria, and tuberculosis combined.[4] This doesn't often make the headlines.

What is particularly disturbing about the exploding global cancer crisis is the inequity of its distribution and impact. By 2040, the number of new cancer cases diagnosed each year is expected to increase by almost 50% globally, with a staggering 64–95% relative increase in the developing world.[5] In other words, the most devastating effects of the world's growing cancer burden will be felt most acutely in countries least resourced to cope with its impact. In much of the world, a diagnosis of cancer remains a death sentence and too many patients struggle to obtain access to screening, treatment, and basic symptom management.[6] The harsh reality is that a patient's chance of dying from cancer depends largely on where they happen to live. For example, nearly 90% of cervical cancer deaths—a highly preventable cancer—occur in LMICs[7]; in 2020, death rates from cervical cancer in India were almost five times higher than that of the U.S.[8]

3 The reasons for this are multifaceted but are primarily due to a combination of a rapidly aging global population and more people around the globe adopting a lifestyle characterized by unhealthy diets, tobacco use, and lack of exercise. For further discussions related to the global impact of noncommunicable diseases, see: (1) Global Burden of Disease 2019 Cancer Risk Factors Collaborators. *The global burden of cancer attributable to risk factors, 2010–2019: A systematic analysis for the Global Burden of Disease Study. Lancet* 2022; 400; 563–591; (2) Daniels, M., Donilon, T., & Bollyky, T. J. The emerging global health crisis: Noncommunicable diseases in low- and middle-income countries (December 5, 2014). Council on Foreign Relations Independent Task Force Report No. 72. (3) Partridge, E. E., Mayer-Davis, E. J., Sacco, R. L., & Balch, A. J. (2011). Creating a 21st Century global health agenda: The General Assembly of the United Nations high level meeting on non-communicable diseases. *CA: A Cancer Journal for Clinicians*,61, 209–211; (4) American Cancer Society, The Cancer Atlas, Global Cancer Burden https://canceratlas.cancer.org/the-burden/the-burden-of-cancer/; and World Health Organization Non-Communicable Diseases FactSheet, 2022.
4 See American Cancer Society, Global Cancer Facts & Figures , 4th Edition.
5 See Sung, H., Ferlay, J., Siegel, R.L., Laversanne, M., Soerjomataram, I., Jemal, A., & Bray, F. (2021). Global cancer statistics 2020: GLOBOCAN estimates of incidence and mortality worldwide for 36 cancers in 185 countries. *CA: A cancer Journal for Clinicians*, 71(3), 209–249.
6 See (1) Lamas, D., & Rosenbaum, L. (2012). Painful inequities: Palliative care in developing countries. *The New England Journal of Medicine* 366, 199–201; (2) The National Academies of Sciences Engineering & Medicine. Cancer care in low-resource areas: Cancer treatment, palliative care, and survivorship care: Proceedings of a Workshop, 2017.
7 See (1) WHO Cervical Cancer Factsheet, 2022; (2) American Cancer Society, Global Cancer Facts & Figures , 4th Edition; (3) Hull et al. (2020). Cervical cancer in low- and middle-income countries. *Oncology letters*, 20(3), 2058–2074.
8 In 2020, India's age-standardized cervical cancer mortality rate was 11.4 compared to 2.1 in the U.S. See the excellent and user-friendly International Agency for Research on Cancer (IARC) interactive database on global cancer statistics.

This book describes the nine months I lived in a large South Indian city conducting ethnographic[9] research at a government cancer hospital as a Fulbright Fellow. I went to India to understand how advanced cancer is managed in settings where core resources, such as essential pain medicines, are often unavailable, and how nurses, as frontline care providers, cope with this reality. The project evolved from years of prior global health work[10] with the goal to make the reality of nursing in a country such as India personal and real and to raise awareness about how most of the world experiences cancer. I wanted to give context to the statistics and a voice to nurses who practice in settings where the demands are staggering and the rewards are few. Nurses are the largest healthcare workforce globally (there are about 27 million of us[11]), and they will increasingly be called upon to care for the world's rapidly growing number of cancer patients. Understanding their work, fears, and challenges—how and when they advocate for patients, and why and when they don't—is not just of academic or humanitarian interest, it is in our own individual best interest as potential future patients.

Palliative Care and Pain Relief as a Human Right

I am a cancer nurse; this has been the core of my professional identity for over two decades. More specifically, I am an oncology palliative care nurse, which means I specialize in the care of cancer patients who are seriously and terminally ill. By now, many have heard the term palliative care, even if they are not entirely sure what it means. The "best" definition of palliative care depends on who you ask, but in essence, the goal of palliative care is to alleviate suffering and provide comprehensive support—physical, emotional, social, and spiritual—to patients, and their families, facing life-threatening illness. Ensuring patients receive optimal pain management is particularly important and considered a foundational element of quality palliative care.[12] Ideally, palliative care is delivered by an interdisciplinary team, including nurses, physicians, social workers, chaplains, and volunteers, who are trained to provide care compatible with a patient's wishes and values. This book focuses on cancer, but palliative care is relevant for patients suffering

---

9 Ethnography is a type of qualitative research with its roots in the discipline of anthropology. The broad goal of ethnographic research is to understand cultural and social groups through immersive fieldwork that includes spending time observing and talking with people in their natural environment.
10 From 2004 to 2014, I worked with a European-based nonprofit, nongovernmental organization committed to partnering collaboratively and longitudinally with clinical partners in LMICs to strengthen the delivery of cancer care. See Chapter 11 for more details about my engagement with this organization and how it influenced this project.
11 See World Health Organization, Key Facts, Nursing and Midwifery, 2022.
12 See World Health Organization (WHO) Palliative Care Key Facts (2020) for a brief overview of palliative care from a global perspective.

from all types of difficult illnesses, including heart failure, HIV/AIDS, respiratory diseases, neurological disorders, and dementia. Palliative care is not synonymous with hospice, but they are closely related and share many overlapping goals.[13]

In 2014, the World Health Assembly (WHA, the voting body of the World Health Organization, WHO, comprised of delegations from all WHO Member States) officially recognized palliative care as a critical component of national health systems.[14] While there have been improvements in palliative care development across the globe since the WHA resolution, and many outstanding examples of palliative care capacity building and community outreach exist in LMICs,[15] the unfortunate reality is that outside of North America, Western Europe, and Australia, access to palliative care remains limited.[16]

---

13 Terminology can vary depending on the country and health system, but hospice typically refers to care provided to patients (and their families) in the last months or weeks of life. In the U.S., the benchmark Medicare hospice benefit requires eligible patients to have an estimated prognosis of six months or less and agree to forego curative therapies. Palliative care generally has a broader interpretation focused on symptom management regardless of prognosis, and many patients who receive palliative care are still receiving life-prolonging therapies, such as chemotherapy.

14 See 67th World Health Assembly, Strengthening of palliative care as a component of comprehensive care throughout the life course, WHA67.19, May 2014

15 Noteworthy palliative care initiatives include pioneering and exemplary community-based programs and training through Pallium India, Hospice Africa Uganda, and the African Palliative Care Association. Hospice Africa Uganda has been particularly recognized for their unique morphine distribution program, allowing nurses to distribute liquid morphine to rural patients; see Uganda: Delivering analgesia in rural Africa, opioid availability and nurse prescribing, *JPSM*, 2007. The Indian state of Kerala has been at the forefront of palliative care development with the creation of the organization Pallium India in 2003 and the Trivandrum Institute of Palliative Sciences in 2006, which has trained a multitude of palliative care providers and was designated a WHO Collaborating Center in 2012. One of the founders of Pallium India, Dr. M.R. Rajagopal, is considered by many in the field to be the leading champion of palliative care in India; his substantial contributions to palliative care development (and beyond) have been recognized by multiple professional bodies and organizations, including Human Rights Watch and The American Academy of Hospice and Palliative Medicine. One of Dr. Rajagopal's greatest achievements was his contribution in convincing the Parliament of India to amend the draconian Narcotic Drugs and Psychotropic Substances (NDPS) Act of 1985; the Amendment was passed in 2014 and significantly improved access to pain relief for patients in need by removing numerous barriers, including fear of harsh punishment for clinicians who prescribe opioids. A documentary about his life and work, "Hippocratic: 18 Experiments in Gently Shaking the World," was released by Moonshine Agency, Australia, on World Palliative Care Day in 2017.

16 The Worldwide Hospice Palliative Care Alliance (WHPCA) publishes a Global Atlas of Palliative Care which provides detailed maps describing the level of palliative care development efforts around the world. The WHPCA 2020 report reveals that outside of North America, Western Europe, and Australia, palliative care development remains severely limited, despite the reality that 76% of the need for palliative care exists in LMICs. More specifically, a 2017 survey of 198 countries found that palliative care at the highest level of development is available for only 14% of the global population, the majority in high-resourced European countries. The bottom line is that the current pace of palliative care development will not

The lack of access to palliative care in LMICs is particularly egregious given the high percentage of patients who are first diagnosed with advanced cancer and in desperate need of pain relief.[17]

Many patients with cancer fear pain more than they do death.[18] When I was a young volunteer at a local community hospital in Pennsylvania, I vividly recall patients with cancer suffering with poorly managed pain: an elderly man riddled with prostate cancer, slick with sweat, hobbling to the bathroom; a young father whose cancer had wrapped around his spine, writhing in agony, twisting his bedsheets into damp, tangled knots, begging to die; a cachectic mother in the last stages of cervical cancer, crying and hopping from foot to foot to try to ease her pain. These images, from over 30 years ago, are forever burned into my psyche.

But it doesn't have to be this way—not in the U.S., not in India, not in any other country. We have effective treatments to lessen cancer pain, and one of the most effective treatments is with a class of medications that have existed for millennia—opioids. Morphine is the most common and well known of the opioids and is considered the gold standard medication to manage difficult cancer pain. In fact, morphine is classified by the WHO and the International Association for Hospice and Palliative Care as an "essential

---

be enough to meet the projected need, as an 87% increase in serious health-related suffering is predicted by 2060. For more discussion related to this topic, see Clark, D., Baur, N., Clelland, D., Garralda, E., López-Fidalgo, J., Connor, S., & Centeno, C. (2020 April). Mapping Levels of Palliative Care Development in 198 Countries: The Situation in 2017. *Journal of Pain and Symptom Management*, 59(4), 794–807.e4. https://doi.org/10.1016/j.jpainsymman.2019.11.009.

17 Estimates of cancer pain incidence vary, but according to the WHO (Palliative Care Key Facts, 2020), 80% of cancer patients experience moderate to severe pain at the end of their lives. A 2016 systematic review and meta-analysis (van den Beuken-van Everdignen, M. H., et al. (2016). Update on the prevalence of pain in patients with cancer: Systematic review and meta-analysis. *Journal of Pain and Symptom Management* (51, 1070–1090) reported global pain prevalence rates of 55% for patients undergoing treatment and 66% for patients with advanced, terminal disease. Moderate to severe pain (a score of ≥5 on a 0–10 numeric pain scale, with 0 meaning no pain, 10 meaning the worst pain) was reported by 38.0% of all patients. One survey study by Doyle et al. (2018) of 1,600 patients with cancer at four Regional Cancer Centers in India found close to 90% of patients reported pain in the last seven days; 60% reported severe pain; and almost 70% did not receive pain treatment in accordance with WHO recommendations.

18 See: Lemay, K., Wilson, K. G., & Buenger, U., et al. (2011). Fear of pain in patients with advanced cancer or in patients with chronic noncancer pain. *The Clinical Journal of Pain*, 27(2), 116–124; Meier, E. A., Gallegos, J. V., Thomas, L. P. M., Depp, C. A., Irwin, S. A., & Jeste, D. V. (2016). Defining a good death (successful dying): Literature review and a call for research and public dialogue. The American Journal of Geriatric Psychiatry, 24(4), 261–271; Steinhauser, K. E., Christakis, N. A., Clipp, E. C., McNeilly, M., McIntyre, L., & Tulsky, J. A. (2000). Factors considered important at the end of life by patients, family, physicians, and other care providers. *JAMA*, 284(19), 2476–2482; Steinhauser, K. E., Clipp, E. C., McNeilly, M., Christakis, N. A., McIntyre, L. M., & Tulsky, J. A. (2000). In search of a good death: Observations of patients, families, and providers. *Annals of Internal Medicine*, 132(10), 825–832.

medication," which means it is a medication that every country must have in adequate amounts to meet the basic health needs of its population.[19]

Despite this mandate, access to opioids and pain relief remains problematic throughout the world and is particularly dire in almost all LMICs, where opioids can simply be absent from a country, hospital, or pharmacy.[20] The reasons for this are complex and multifactorial, but are largely the result of outdated and unbalanced policies that prioritize strict regulation of controlled substances over access for medicinal purposes. Shockingly, a handful of high-income countries (primarily the U.S., Canada, Australia, New Zealand, and Western Europe)—home to *less than 20%* of the world's population—have historically *consumed over 90%* of the world's morphine supply used for the management of pain and suffering.[21] Consequently, millions of patients with cancer in LMICs suffer and die in avoidable pain. This persistent disparity is viewed by many as a violation of human rights and a global social justice call-to-action.[22]

19 See De Lima, L., Krakauer, E. L., Lorenz, K., Praill, D., MacDonald, N., & Doyle, D. (2007). Ensuring palliative medicine availability: The development of the IAHPC list of essential medicines for palliative care. *Journal of Pain and Symptom Management*, 33, 521–526; World Health Organization, http://www.who.int/topics/essential_medicines/en/

20 The term "opioid availability" is often used interchangeably with "opioid accessibility," but there is an important distinction. In higher income countries, such as the U.S., opioid issues have historically involved those of accessibility—the proper medications are available, but they do not reach the patient due to barriers of access, cost, or health care provider fears related to prescribing or administering the drug. It gets more complicated in lower income countries where the same barriers that affect accessibility often exist, but there is an additional problem of opioid availability—the medication is simply absent from the country, hospital, or pharmacy. A tremendous amount of research and advocacy related to opioid availability in LMICs has been undertaken. As examples, see: Cherny, N. I., Cleary, J., Scholten, W., Radbruch, L., & Torode, J. (2013). The Global Opioid Policy Initiative (GOPI) project to evaluate the availability and accessibility of opioids for the management of cancer pain in Africa, Asia, Latin America and the Caribbean, and the Middle East: Introduction and methodology. *Annals of Oncology*, 24(suppl_11), xi7–xi13; Maurer, M. A., Gilson, A. M., Husain, S. A., & Cleary, J. F. (2013). Examining influences on the availability of and access to opioids for pain management and palliative care. *Journal of Pain & Palliative Care Pharmacotherapy*, 27(3), 255–260.

21 See the 2016 report from the International Narcotics Control Board, 'Availability of Internationally Controlled Drugs: Ensuring Adequate Access for Medicinal and Scientific Purposes, Indispensable, Adequately Available, and Not Unduly Restricted available at: https://www.unodc.org/documents/drug-prevention-and-treatment/INCB_Access_Supplement-AR15_availability_English.pdf; and also International Narcotics Control Board (INCB). Supplement to the annual report of the Board for 2022 on the availability of internationally controlled substances: No patient left behind: Progress in ensuring adequate access to internationally controlled substances for medical and scientific purposes. March 2023. Available at: https://www.incb.org/documents/Publications/AnnualReports/AR2022/Supplement/E_INCB_2022_1_Supp_1_eng.pdf

22 Brennan, F., Carr, D. B., & Cousins, M. (2007). Pain management: A fundamental human right. *Anesthesia & Analgesia*, 105, 205–221; Human Rights Watch; Global state of pain treatment: Access to palliative care as a human right; 2011; Human Rights Watch, Unbearable pain: India's obligation to ensure palliative care, 2009; www.hrw.org.

The sad bottom line is this: your chance of dying from advanced cancer, and dying in pain, are exponentially higher if you are one of the six billion people who happen to live in a lower income country—a country where access to cancer care is limited, and tragically, so is palliative care and basic pain relief.[23]

The Dual Epidemics of Untreated Pain and the Opioid Epidemic

The year I left to conduct research in India—2011—is the same year the Centers for Disease Control and Prevention (CDC) sounded the alarm that the U.S. was in the throes of an "opioid epidemic"—with unprecedented numbers of Americans dying from overdoses attributed to prescription opioid medications.[24] Abruptly, there was a major shift in thinking about pain management in the U.S.; one characterized by increased scrutiny of pain advocacy organizations and their funding sources; heightened concern about diversion and misuse of prescription pain medications; and a renewed skepticism about the benefits and appropriateness of opioid therapy for patients in pain. It is true that prescription opioid medications carry risks, and healthcare providers have an obligation to educate patients and their families, while taking precautions to minimize the misuse of these powerful drugs. It is also

23 See   https://data.worldbank.org/income-level/low-and-middle-income;   and   Knaul,   F. M., Farmer, P. E., & Krakauer, E. L., et al. (2018). Alleviating the access abyss in palliative care and pain relief – An imperative of universal health coverage: The Lancet Commission report, *Lancet*; Available at http://www.thelancet.com/pdfs/journals/lancet/PIIS0140-6736(17)32513-8.pdf;
24 See Centers for Disease Control and Prevention (CDC). Prescription painkiller overdoses at epidemic levels 2011 available at https://www.cdc.gov/media/releases/2011/p1101_flu_pain_killer_overdose.html. Many have attributed the U.S. "opioid epidemic" to indiscriminate and irresponsible opioid prescribing practices, fueled by aggressive and misleading marketing campaigns by large pharmaceutical companies that coincided with an influx of heroin trafficking in middle America. Sam Quinone's 2015 book, *Dreamland: The True Tale of America's Opiate Epidemic*, and Beth Macy's 2018 *Dopesick: Dealers, Doctors and the Drug Company that Addicted America* both explore the role of aggressive marketing of Oxycontin in contributing to the opioid epidemic and its devastating impact on rural America. An important note about both of these non-fiction books is that while they present compelling and important portraits related to the harms associated with the misuse and abuse of prescription opioids, an argument can be made that unequal attention is given to the epidemic of untreated pain for patients with legitimate medical need. See also Meldrum, M. (2016). The ongoing opioid prescription epidemic: Historical context. *American Journal of Public Health*, 106(8), 1365–1366, for a succinct historical overview that focuses on chronic pain and the opioid epidemic in the U.S. and Monnat's book review of "Dreamland: The true tale of America's opiate epidemic." *Journal of Research in Rural Education*, 31(4), 1–3. It is important to also note that opioid fatality statistics can be complicated by diverse state and local practices related to how death certificates are issued as well as disparate reporting mechanisms that can, for example, combine fatalities from illegally obtained "street" opioids—such as illicitly manufactured synthetic fentanyl—with prescription opioids obtained through legitimate means.

equally true that opioids are inexpensive, low-tech, and highly effective in treating the vast majority of cancer pain. Opioids are not the right medication for every patient, but for many patients suffering with terminal illness, particularly in low-resource settings, they are simply the most effective, and sometimes the only, therapy we have to offer.

Five years after their initial warning, the CDC released controversial opioid prescribing guidelines which recommended, among other things, prescribing caps and prescriptions of limited duration.[25] Importantly, the CDC guidelines explicitly stated they were not intended for patients with cancer or for people at the end of life. Despite this critical caveat, and the fact that the CDC guidelines were later revised in 2022,[26] they nonetheless have had a chilling effect, making it more difficult for patients with legitimate medical need to obtain prescriptions for opioid therapy from clinicians and access the medication from pharmacies.[27] As this pendulum continues to swing, it is expected that tighter opioid regulations in the U.S. will likely have a ripple effect in the developing world, creating even more barriers for the millions of patients with advanced cancer and other serious illnesses who already struggle to obtain basic pain relief.[28]

25 Centers for Disease Control and Prevention (CDC) Guideline for Prescribing Opioids for Chronic Pain, 2016.

26 The CDC updated the guidelines in 2022 (see CDC Updated Clinical Practice Guidelines for Prescribing Opioids for Pain) to more clearly address the role prescription opioids play in ensuring pain control for those with legitimate medical need. However, much of the impact from the 2016 CDC guidelines has lingered.

27 There are anecdotal data and a growing body of empirical evidence that patients in the U.S. with legitimate pain needs, including patients with cancer, are experiencing significant difficulty accessing opioids. For example, the University Health System with which I am affiliated sends regular emails to employees regarding supply and medication shortages; reported shortages have included opioids such as morphine, hydromorphone, and fentanyl (all common opioid medications for treating difficult pain); these shortages were attributed in part to manufacturing disruptions in Puerto Rico after Hurricane Maria in 2017, but also due to new manufacturing limitations imposed by the Drug Enforcement Administration (DEA). Compounding the problem, many patients with cancer now face increased stigma for taking prescription opioid medications, and minoritized populations already at high risk for under-treated pain can encounter even more barriers. See Enzinger, et al. (2023). Racial and ethnic disparities in opioid access, *Journal of Clinical Oncology*; 5ASCO Policy Statement of Opioid Therapy: Protecting access to treatment for cancer related pain, 2016; Paice, J. (2018). Cancer pain management and the opioid crisis in America: How to preserve hard-earned gains in improving the quality of cancer pain management, *Cancer*; Kwekkeboom, K., Serlin, R. C., Ward, S. E., LeBlanc, T. W., Ogunseitan, A., & Cleary, J. (2021 June 1). Revisiting patient-related barriers to cancer pain management in the context of the US opioid crisis. *Pain, 162*(6), 1840–1847.

28 See Matlock, D. D. (2015). The pain pendulum swinging again. *Journal of Palliative Medicine, 18*(9), 734–735; and Lohman, et al., "Advancing palliative care over two decades: health system integration, access to essential medicines, and pediatrics," for an excellent historical overview of key palliative care milestones from 2000–2020, including a discussion of how the "opioid epidemic" in the U.S. has negatively impacted global efforts to ensure access to essential pain medications.

Since 2004, I have been collaborating with local physicians, nurses, and global health colleagues, primarily in South Asia, to advocate for improved opioid availability and access to quality palliative care and pain management. Dedicated individuals in these countries have worked for years to change governmental regulations and policies to help those suffering with terrible, painful illnesses.[29] Back from India in 2012, having witnessed profound suffering due, in part, to opioid fears, shortages, and crippling bureaucracy, I found myself sitting on opioid epidemic panels and workgroup committees in the U.S., defending the need to ensure access to these very same medications. It was disorienting. At these meetings, I was often a lone voice, urging the vocal majority to remember patients with legitimate medical need for pain relief. Not everyone seemed particularly interested in a message of balance.[30] Given the national dialogue and stigma surrounding opioids, and what is at stake for patients in pain, the message of this book has an element of urgency I did not initially anticipate. By presenting the other side of the opioid epidemic—the epidemic of patients in pain—I hope we will think critically about how we approach pain management and not add additional burden and suffering to where it already exists.

About This Book

While the subject matter of this book will most likely appeal to nurses and other clinicians, particularly those who practice or teach in the areas of

29 Many individuals have been working for decades to improve opioid availability in LMICs. As one example, The Pain & Policy Studies Group (PPSG), formerly at the University of Wisconsin and now housed within Indiana University, Walther Global Palliative Care & Supportive Oncology, led the Pain Policy Fellowship Program which matches clinician champions and government officials from LMICs with mentors to advocate for balanced opioid policies and regulations. This pioneering work has led to groundbreaking advances in access to morphine within many countries, such as Nepal; see Paudel, B. D., Ryan, K. M., Brown, M. S., Krakauer, E. L., Rajagopal, M. R., Maurer, M. A., & Cleary, J. F. (2015). Opioid availability and palliative care in Nepal: Influence of an international pain policy fellowship. *Journal of Pain and Symptom Management, 49*(1), 110–116. Among other key resources, PPSG has maintained a database of country-level opioid consumption data based on data reported annually to the International Narcotics Control Board regarding the amount of opioids used for medicinal and scientific purposes.

30 The "Principle of Balance" is a core message advocated by the WHO and leading medical and scientific groups related to opioid policy. The Principle of Balance aims to achieve balanced access to opioids – mitigating risk and reducing harm while concurrently ensuring patients with medical need can access pain relief without undue barriers; see Integrating Palliative Care and Symptom Relief into Primary Health Care, WHO, 2018; and Pain Management & the Opioid Epidemic: Balancing Societal and Individual Benefits 7 Risks, National Academies of Sciences, Engineering and Medicine, 2017. Unfortunately, despite this recommendation, regulation and control often is prioritized over balanced access. However, there are some country-level examples where the Principle of Balance has been implemented effectively; see Bhadelia, A., et al. (2019). Solving the global crisis in access to pain relief: Lessons from country actions. *American Journal of Public Health*.

oncology, palliative care, or global health, *Caring in Context* is intentionally written to be accessible to general readers with an interest in cancer care, health equity, social justice, and the culture and context of India. I also wrote this book to serve as an example ethnography to help others, especially my fellow nurses, who may be considering or already engaged in similar work. This book does not attempt to hide my missteps in the field or my own humbling self-discoveries as a person of privilege[31] coming face to face with human suffering in an unfamiliar country and culture; I learned that I am not as good a person as I hoped and that I, too, am capable of ignoring suffering. Students or instructors of qualitative methods and ethnography may find Chapter 11 ("Notes on Methods") especially helpful to facilitate dialogue about ethical dilemmas in the field. In fact, for some academic readers, it may be helpful to read Chapter 11 after this Introduction and before beginning the main text of the book.

A particular ethical dilemma—discussed later in Chapter 11 but one that warrants earlier mention—relates to the tension between my training as a nurse and my role as researcher. Readers may wonder why I did not intervene when witnessing troubling or distressing healthcare interactions or procedures, or what guided my rules of engagement while in the field. Frankly, this was a source of significant distress and anxiety during my fieldwork and at times I felt complicit when observing inappropriate or harmful care. In specific and limited instances, I did intervene, primarily by suggesting alternative courses of action or by performing simple tasks that anyone without medical training would likely do as a fellow human (such as helping a patient sit up after a physical exam). I reminded myself frequently that I had not been invited to the fieldsite to provide direct clinical care, nor was I being asked to do so by my colleagues (with limited exceptions, discussed in Chapters 3 and 7), and in fact, I was not officially authorized or licensed to practice nursing in India. I was also keenly aware that despite my commitment to deep understanding, I still did not have the entire picture, nor the full context with all of the information. I was a visitor and a guest who happened to be a nurse. For all of these reasons, my overall approach was one of noninterference.

As an instructor of qualitative research methods for PhD nursing students, I discovered there are very few full-length ethnographies about nurses *by* nurses.[32] This is unfortunate as nurses and emerging nurse scientists need examples of how their powerful stories can be amplified using this methodology to shape critical conversations about their practice and be a vehicle for positive

---

31 See Chapter 11 ("Methods") for a fuller discussion about my positionality and its influence related to this research.

32 There are numerous, excellent healthcare focused ethnographies (see Appendix), but few examples of nurse-led ethnographies published as full-length books; there are even fewer ethnographies *about* nurses *by* nurses. In my research preparing this book, I found only one full-length book ethnography about cancer nurses by a nurse (The Cancer Unit: An Ethnography by Carol Germain published in 1979).

change. *Caring in Context* aims to give voice to nurses in LMICs, where the majority of the world's population lives, and will die, and offers a critical examination of the realities of cancer care in highly resource-constrained settings. Importantly, this book also challenges beliefs and assumptions about the moral obligations of nursing practice and asks readers to reconsider the ethics of expecting nurses to care for others when no one is caring for them.

* * *

Although there are uncomfortable scenes described in the following pages, the intent is not to single out India or South Indian Cancer Hospital[33] (SICH, the primary fieldsite) as alone in their struggles. This research could have been conducted in any number of hospitals or countries (including the U.S.), and India is certainly not the only country with challenges related to the delivery of palliative care, opioid availability, or nursing care of cancer patients. This book simply provides one look at the complex challenges that many healthcare institutions around the world encounter, and a specific look at these challenges in a resource-constrained setting. An important goal of this book is not only to present difficult moments, but also to capture moments of joy and beauty, and to challenge us to think more deeply about "why?" and "how could things be different?" The world clearly has no shortage of overwhelming problems, many with no solution in sight. In contrast, the problem of people around the world dying in avoidable pain is, to a large extent, *fixable*. We can actually *do* something about it. We have medications that work, and they are inexpensive and highly effective and not technologically complicated. But, as this book illustrates, getting the right amounts of the right medication to the right place is only part of the solution. We must care enough and have enough societal courage to probe the cultural underbelly that encourages us as humans to label others as less than and not worthy of relief. This, it seems, is the real and more intractable challenge.

This is a work of nonfiction. The events, places, conversations, and people described are real and were experienced during fieldwork conducted in South India from September 2011 through June 2012. While it is true that my memories of India have softened with time, the core of what you will read was written in the moment. Like some sort of literary juggernaut, this book practically flung itself at me and compelled itself to be written on scraps of paper on trains and busses and autorickshaws. Real-time observations were scratched into small notebooks I carried in a beat-up blue satchel (or, as I discovered later, sent to myself via text messages) and written out in full prose after long days in the hospital, late in to the evening on an old, stained white table while my roommates sang along to Bollywood music in the next room, or early in the morning before the prayer calls sounded and the heat of the day fell oppressively over the city. Interviews were audio-recorded

---

33 A pseudonym; names of people, places, and institutions have been changed to protect identities.

(with permission) and informal conversations written as verbatim as possible immediately afterwards so I would not forget crucial details or specific phrasing. I was absolutely rigid in this; with the exception of a handful of days, I recorded everything that happened the same day and I wrote every day—a lot. Things were coming at me so fast, and I instinctively knew I had a fleeting opportunity to capture it all, like morning fog visible now, but that will be gone the next day. By the time I left India, I had written roughly 700 pages of single-spaced text. Never in my life have I written so much, or so furiously. I know I am not the first person to discover India has a unique way of pushing a person to extremes. Clearly in this final book, I could not include everything and deciding what to keep and what must go has been an arduous and painstaking task. In the end, I chose the events, interactions, and observations that seemed most representative of the people and places I had the privilege to know while in India and that may have the greatest potential to raise awareness and spark dialogue about opportunities for productive change.[34]

India is dauntingly complex. This book records events that took place in a specific hospital, in a specific location, at a specific point in time in a vast, diverse, and dynamic country. To understand the larger picture, I made a concerted effort to observe at other government and private hospitals in India, to talk with people about their experiences working in other hospitals and how they compared to SICH, and to seek out additional sources (e.g., books, popular culture, memoirs, scholarly and newspaper articles, other experts) to help corroborate themes emerging in the project. I spent hundreds of hours with nurses in the hospital and in the community, talking with them about the challenges and rewards of their work and observing their interactions with patients, family members, and other healthcare providers. To honor confidentiality, names and identifying details have been changed or omitted, and in some circumstances, situations have been amalgamated or reordered for clarity, brevity, or ethical considerations. I have striven to represent those who shared their stories and lives with me with integrity and honesty, and to be a responsible steward of their experiences. All inaccuracies and misperceptions are mine alone.

While there is an obvious emphasis on health care, this is not solely a book about nurses, doctors, patients, and family members who struggle to provide and receive cancer care in difficult circumstances. It is also my story, at least in part, as an American nurse living in India, and the people I encountered in

---

34 This approach was inspired, at least in part, by a powerful talk I heard given by Dr. Robert Twycross, largely considered one of the gurus of palliative care, at the Indian Association of Palliative Care conference in Kolkata, 2012. During his address, Dr. Twycross stated, "let the anger in compassion be a catalyst for change." In other words, let our discomfort and anger related to the disparities and inequities in palliative and end-of-life care be a motivating, powerful force for action.

my day-to-day life. It is the story of my roommates, Joanie and Ruma, two young, independent, professional Indian women, pushing back against the powerful current of traditional societal norms. It is the story of the housekeeper, Lakshmi, and the cook, Fatima, who cleaned our apartment and cooked our food, and the complicated social dynamics and constant negotiations that accompanied their employment. It is the story of the watchman's family who lived in the garage of our apartment building, and whose young children ran errands for us instead of attending school. It is the story of other Westerners I met, like Kate, a volunteer in the pediatric ward, and how they processed and coped with what they saw in the hospital.

By default, this book is also about gender. Because most nurses in India (and around the world) are female,[35] this book cannot escape documenting what it is like to be a woman in India—which in my experience was challenging and at times unsettling. In a society where women are often not valued, perceived as a burden, expected to perform an incredible amount of household labor, and subject to discrimination, sexual harassment and worse,[36] it is essential to consider how gender influenced the role of the nurse and the care provided to patients. In the beginning, I naively and seriously underestimated the role of gender, not only in my research and for the nurses I worked with, but also in my daily life. Gender was the factor that permeated everything. It influenced who was an acceptable translator and how I conducted interviews. It determined when nurses arrived at the hospital and whether female patients received treatment. It dictated the seat I could buy on a bus and the line I stood in to purchase movie tickets. I quickly discovered that there was little, if any, context for platonic relationships between men and women,[37]

---

35 Of the 107 total nurses at SICH during my fieldwork, only 2 were male—and they both worked in palliative care. According to the "Sustain and Retain in 2022 and Beyond: The Global Nursing Workforce and the COVID-19 Pandemic" published by the International Council of Nurses and the International Centre on Nurse Migration, 90% of nurses worldwide are female.

36 In 2018, India was reported by the Thomson Reuters Foundation to the most dangerous place in the world to be a woman due to the high risk of sexual violence and slave labor; see also the Pew Research Center Report, How Indians View Gender Roles in Family and Society, 2022; and the 2017 documentary "A Suitable Girl" which follows three young Indian women in their marriage journey; the documentary resonated strongly with my experiences in India. During my fieldwork, I was groped numerous times; I was lucky, as most of these experiences were more aggravating than frightening, but they were all traumatizing and served to reinforce the reality of gender inequality and vulnerability.

37 Kate, a hospital volunteer who was born in India and raised primarily in the U.S., shared this story with me during my fieldwork: *I have a good friend [in India], 23 years old, from a sophisticated family. I brought her here to the hospital [South Indian Cancer Hospital] to visit the pediatric ward. She is usually so bubbly and friendly. But here she was quiet and reserved, not making eye contact with people. I asked her why. She told me it's the first time she has talked to a man who is not related to her... Many of the women here, after they get married they don't sleep with their husbands for months. They don't know what's going on [makes a sweeping, vague gesture over her lower abdomen]. Their whole lives they have been*

and social gestures I performed automatically—smiling, making eye contact, engaging in conversation—all had the potential to be wildly misconstrued. Having so much of my everyday existence defined and influenced by my gender registered as a close second, right after confronting the gritty realities of abject poverty and suffering, as to what I found most different, and difficult, about adapting to life in India.

A Different Way of Nursing

The hospital where I conducted my research, SICH, is a 300-bed government cancer center located in Dandaka, a city of over eight million people.[38] The building is a large, three-story, nondescript beige concrete structure separated by an open gate and two relaxed security guards from a frighteningly busy intersection and the cacophony of street-side vendors, small medical supply and pharmacy shops, and a pulsing crowd of people. As a government hospital, and the only public cancer treatment center in the entire State,[39] SICH serves predominantly an impoverished and illiterate population of patients, many of whom travel from hundreds of kilometers away to seek treatment. Even though care is provided largely free of charge, or at highly subsidized rates, SICH is perceived as a place of last resort due to the negative reputation of government sector hospitals. Even desperately poor patients often go first to private, corporate hospitals, believing they will receive better care.[40] There, unscrupulous physicians may let families deplete their limited financial assets by paying out of pocket for tests and treatments they may not need, cannot afford, and often do not understand. "Always look at a woman's arms," one SICH physician advised during my early days of fieldwork. "If she is not wearing gold bangles—and even the poorest women have them as a marker of marriage—she has sold them to pay for medical treatment. The sign of absolute destitution," the doctor told me matter-of-factly.

Thousands of patients present to SICH each year; like a tumor itself, overburdened by its own implausible growth, the hospital overflows with patients and families who set up makeshift camps in the cramped corridors and surrounding hospital grounds. In the absence of access to early detection screenings and treatment, compounded by fear, poverty, and stigma, patients arrive at SICH in the late stages of cancer with symptoms rarely seen in higher resourced settings—massive, fungating tumors; blindness due

---

told not to interact with men, they've spent a lifetime being told to ignore men, to be afraid of them, and then all of sudden they are thrust together in marriage and expected to have sex. There's no warm-up, no gradual getting to know men.

38 Dandaka is a pseudonym and this was the estimated population during my fieldwork; 2023 population estimates are closer to ten million.

39 This was true at the time of my fieldwork.

40 See Balarajan, Y., Selvaraj, S., & Subramanian, S. V. (2011 Feb 5). Health care and equity in India. *Lancet, 377*(9764), 505–515.

to retinoblastoma; total paralysis from spinal cord compression. It seems inevitable that the overwhelming nature of it all would make even the most committed individual withdrawal. In hindsight, it's amazing how many people continued to try, given the dire circumstances under which they were expected to provide care. Water taps frequently ran dry, the electricity would cut unpredictably, there were rarely enough beds, and nurses had no supplies to protect themselves from the hazards of giving chemotherapy or patients who may have hepatitis, tuberculosis, or HIV. The physical, emotional, and social needs of patients were like a tsunami, relentless and crushing. For the nurses who did try, there was little, if any, recognition for their efforts, and for almost all of them a second full-time job awaited as soon as they exited the hospital, returning home to face a never-ending cycle of domestic obligations.

The majority of nurses I met during my fieldwork were from modest or poor economic backgrounds themselves. Without the disposable income to hire cooks and maids (extremely common in India, even for average middle-class families[41]), nurses' days began hours before they started their shift at the hospital—preparing food for large extended families, caring for their in-laws, husband, and children, and ensuring an orderly household. With few exceptions, the nurses I met were married young, some as young as 15 or 16, to men their parents chose for them. Nurses asked me repeatedly how marriages are arranged in the U.S.—and were incredulous when I told them they are not. Most of the nurses were Christians, some Hindus, and a few Muslims.[42] Many had not wanted to become nurses, but were pressured into the profession by their families, seeking the stable employment and consistent income offered by a government position. Three distinct groups of nurses existed within the hospital, each with its own power, reputation, and role—government nurses, contract nurses, and nurses who worked in pediatrics and palliative care. Understanding the complex dynamics between these three groups was an important part of my fieldwork, as it greatly influenced the care provided to patients. Only a handful of nurses at SICH—six out of 107 nurses during my fieldwork—had earned a Bachelor's degree in nursing. The vast majority practiced with General Nursing and Midwifery diplomas.[43]

---

41 It is very common, and socially expected, for middle- and upper-class Indians (and foreigners) to hire a cook and a housekeeper (and often a driver) who generally come daily. The cost is nominal by Western standards. In fact, it can be viewed as problematic if you can afford to hire domestic help and don't—as then you are denying employment to a bloated labor market.

42 This may surprise some readers; the reasons for this are further discussed within the book.

43 Educational preparation for nurses in India generally falls in to three categories: Bachelor of Science (BSc), a four-year degree granting program that requires one's intermediate studies be focused in the biological sciences; General Nurse and Midwifery (GNM), a three-and-a-half-year diploma certificate program that does not require a specific focus for intermediate studies; and the Auxiliary Nurse and Midwifery (ANM), an 18-month training

I was, at first, a novelty in the hospital, and then, as I became known, more of a tolerated freak. Not only did I stand out physically with white skin, short, frizzy blond hair, blue eyes, but socially—unmarried, childless, a doctoral student—I was positively alien. I vividly remember being stopped abruptly by a family member who asked me in broken English who I was and what I was doing at the hospital. As I tried to explain, I could see his dark, brown eyes taking me in, not unkindly or licentiously, but earnestly attempting to process this essentially un-processable information. Finally, his verdict: "you are so strange looking, this is why I ask."

I like to think I am fairly tough, but SICH tested my mettle in unexpected ways. Based on previous international nursing work, I knew to expect patients in pain with advanced tumors. I did not, however, expect them to be treated harshly, especially by my fellow nurses. I witnessed patients and family members, illiterate, frightened, poor, and desperate, being ignored and severely admonished for unclear transgressions. Family members who provided the bulk of care to their hospitalized relatives were unceremoniously shooed off the wards when doctors arrived to conduct hospital rounds, forfeiting the chance to ask questions or get medical updates. The wards had large iron grate doors that were sometimes latched shut during physician rounds, and as I walked through the hospital hallways in the morning, I would see family members gripping the bars, peering in, trapped outside.

I slowly came to understand that there were strong cultural norms underpinning these interactions: that these sharp exchanges were expected by, and familiar to, both parties and generally perceived as the only effective way to get things done. What I found terribly distressing was seemingly accepted as normal by everyone else. Sometimes, these patterns of communicating (or failing to) seemed warranted as crowds swelled to claustrophobic proportions and nurses struggled to provide even the most basic of care in any semblance of a safe manner. Other times, the behavior seemed unnecessarily cruel, like continuing to bully someone who is already sobbing. Then, just as quickly, I would witness a nurse or doctor or pharmacist or social worker behave with heartbreaking compassion and kindness, extending themselves selflessly.

One of the most challenging aspects of writing this book was letting go of my preconceived notions about the role of a nurse. My fieldwork in India presented me with a view of the profession so radically different from what I knew that I was forced to critically reexamine basic assumptions about what

---

program that allows the individual to perform limited nursing tasks. GNM is roughly equivalent to an Associate's Degree (AD) in nursing in the U.S.; ANM is roughly equivalent to a Licensed Practical Nurse (LPN) in the U.S. The majority of nurses at SICH practiced with a GNM. For a more comprehensive overview of global nursing education and training, see the landmark "2020 State of the World's Nursing: Investing in education, jobs and leadership" report published by the WHO.

it means to be a nurse and care for those who are ill and dying. In the U.S., nurses are trained, socialized, and expected to be staunch advocates for the patient and supporters of the patient's family. We are taught that it is our ethical duty to question physician orders, to be the voice for those who cannot speak for themselves, and that our input matters. We are generally rewarded for treating patients equitably, being accountable, critical thinking, and for participating in professional development activities (that are often paid for by our employer). As the reader will discover, this was not the norm in India; throughout the book, I try to explore and better understand why this may be.

Looking Back

Living in India was a smorgasbord of sensory overload. At first, the constant intensity was downright terrifying. After acclimating, it became cumulatively exhausting. Just as colleagues at the hospital told me, within hours of each other, that I was getting both fat and looked too thin, friends in the U.S., upon seeing pictures, commented that I looked the most alive they'd ever seen and that I had never looked so tired. It was true: I felt simultaneously exhilarated and profoundly fatigued—everything making me feel most alive in India seemed dangerously close to doing me in. Pain seemed to simmer right below a fragile veneer of beauty, and every day I was confronted by the unfamiliar and situations over which I had no control and little ability to help. This personal powerlessness ranged from the irritating (being asked repeatedly about my marital status, my religious beliefs, what I ate for breakfast, my salary), to the physical (when I was groped on public transportation, in a yoga class, and on the streets), and to gut-wrenching images that haunt me still (disfigured children weaving amid traffic pleading for money; patients with horrific wounds caused by the consequences of untreated cancer; mangled dogs limping miserably along busy highways).

But I also vividly remember the color and the light—a glimpse of a bright pink sari disappearing down a narrow dusty alley, the flashing strings of neon lights strung with care along the roof of an autorickshaw, the intricate, bright rangoli designs etched at the entrance of a small village hut, the fractured rainbow light from a stained-glass window of a Jodhpur hotel coloring the wall in shifting yellows, blues, and reds. I remember the joyous enthusiasm for small things: a sparkly bangle, new pens, small Dixie-sized cups of steaming milky chai. There was the pregnant sense of possibility, just below the surface, the sense that anything could happen, at any moment. Coming back to the U.S. was jarring, not only because it was so quiet and orderly, but because it was so damn predictable. While it was less likely that I would witness something shocking, it was also far, far less likely I would stumble across something surprising, beautiful, and amazing.

Time has passed since I lived in India, and my life has more or less returned to normal. I try not to take things for granted, like reliable electricity, clean tap water, and being able to wear skinny jeans without causing a scene, but I'm sure I do. When I think back to India now, it is with a wistful sense of wonder and disbelief, almost like the protective cloud of new-mother amnesia after they have given birth. I'd like to think I am a better person for having lived in India. It is certainly more convenient than trying to explain the opposite. There is no doubt that living and traveling in India exposed me to alternative perspectives and ways of life that would be impossible to comprehend without the sensory experience of actually *being* in India. I am more attuned to the consequences of social inequity and abject poverty; I have seen, at least a little, how much of the world actually lives. However, the reality is that at the end of each difficult day at the hospital, I went back to my simple, yet comfortable, apartment, where I wasn't worried if I would have food to eat, or enough clean water, or a bed to sleep in. But my time in India has also increased my worries about humanity. I remain concerned that deeply embedded notions of who is valued, and who is not, ultimately thwart well-intended development efforts. I worry about a global society that can tolerate such unbearable suffering, or that has resigned itself to what it believes to be an insurmountable and inevitable reality.

These issues are, of course, not unique to India, but they seem pronounced in a country with such a sheer volume of people, kaleidoscope of cultural diversity, and stark disparities between the haves and have-nots.

Despite these myriad challenges, I believe there is hope for the patients who seek care at hospitals like SICH. The reason is simple: it is people like Jasmine and Dr. Madhu and Dr. Rashi and nurses like Pradeep and Sister Meena. People who attempt to care against all odds, who continue to return to work, day after day, knowing the difficulties that await. People who have not given up. Perhaps the greatest lesson of India is that kernels of kindness exist even in the most desperate of circumstances and that in the darkest of situations life can still shine through.

Organization of the Book

This book is written in a first-person narrative, a style not without controversy for this type of project.[44] However, this was an intentional choice with the goal to immerse the reader as fully as possible within the culture of India and SICH, and to help make the book readable and accessible to an audience beyond academia. Events are presented primarily chronologically. This was also a very conscious decision intended to illustrate interactions and conversations over time, the evolution of relationships in the field, and the progression of patient illness. The reader may wonder why some situations, such as difficult wound care, or particular interactions between nurses and patients are presented more than once but in slightly different contexts. This was done

---

44 See Matthew Desmond's eloquent discussion of the pros and cons of narrative voice in ethnographic fieldwork, Evicted: Poverty and Profit in the American City, pp. 334–335.

not to be repetitive, but to justify the themes discussed in the conclusion, and to emphasize their basis in patterns of events versus isolated occurrences. The narrative arc of the book is also supported by my own growth and relationship with the staff and nurses, evolving from suspicion and distrust to a shared camaraderie and recognition of the shared struggles faced as nurses and women.

This book is organized into five parts: Part I, the Introduction (what you are reading now), which provides essential foundational context for the project; Parts II–IV, organized by the locations and institutions that contributed most to the research (SICH, the Community, and Other Hospitals); and Part V, the Conclusion, which describes the end of my fieldwork, provides essential interpretation of the preceding narratives and key themes, and discusses important methodological details. Chapter 10 is especially critical to contextualize the fieldwork findings and is intended to be a required accompaniment to the experiences described. A summary of policy recommendations across levels of the social-ecological model (individual, interpersonal, organizational, and system/government) are offered based on the fieldwork findings and presented within the Appendix. The SICH section is the most comprehensive in describing clinical care, as it was the primary fieldsite where I spent the majority of my time.

Within each part of the book, chapters present specific experiences and individuals related to the care of patients with cancer, based on in-depth interviews, informal interactions, and observations conducted in the field. Each chapter begins with one or two direct quotes excerpted from interviews of individuals affiliated with SICH that help frame the subject matter of the chapter. Interspersed are selected details related to personal experiences navigating the hospital and everyday life in India. My worlds in India were not separate—my life outside of the hospital continually collided with life inside the hospital; pretending otherwise seems disingenuous and misses an opportunity to make important connections about how critical themes related to gender, class, and status intersect and overlap. I also included these details as a way to provide a more balanced view of the hospital and India in general. Although much of what I observed and was told during my fieldwork was difficult and grim, there were also moments of tremendous joy and connection I felt important to capture and describe.

A final note about the glossary and footnotes. Potentially unfamiliar medical terms not explained within the text are included in the glossary. The footnotes in this book are important and provide key contextual details and excerpts from field notes, as well as supporting citations and recommended resources; the reader is strongly encouraged to read them.

Why Now and What Has Changed?

This book has been a long time in the making. Unexpected publishing twists and turns, the desire to let some time elapse to help further protect identities, and the inevitable vicissitudes of life, all caused delays. In the interim, the world underwent seismic change since my initial fieldwork and numerous iterations and revisions of this book. Most notably, the COVID-19 pandemic upended society and healthcare delivery, with its impact felt most acutely in lower-resourced countries. References in this book to nursing practices, such as the continual wearing of facial masks, that seemed unusual or even unnecessary in 2012, now seem prescient. Similar to how I did not anticipate the degree to which debates and controversies surrounding opioids in the U.S. would be relevant to this book, I also did not anticipate how the pandemic would catalyze global conversations about the conditions in which nurses practice and the stressors of their work. Perhaps this book assumes additional importance in the post-pandemic era as another opportunity to shine light on the hard realities of nursing practice and caring for other humans in exceedingly difficult circumstances.

My last visit to India and SICH was pre-COVID in 2015; it is critical to contextualize this research prior to the pandemic and to acknowledge it does not account for the impact of COVID on the delivery of care at SICH and similar settings. Likewise, it is important to acknowledge that facts and figures cited within the book—such as currency conversions, discussions of nurses' salaries, or statements about available health services—were accurate, to the best of my knowledge, at the time of my fieldwork; changes that may have occurred since my fieldwork are not fully reflected. The Afterword in Chapter 10 provides a brief summary of updates as this book went to press.

Concluding Thoughts

Ultimately, this book is about how the world's poorest and most vulnerable patients experience cancer, and how humans bear witness and respond to the suffering of others when they have little means to help—or for complex reasons, choose not to. The title, *Caring in Context*, is meant to reflect the reality that there are multiple and complex contexts constantly at play that influence nursing practice and the delivery of healthcare in India and everywhere—resource allocation, gender dynamics, stigma, to name just a few. Isabel Wilkerson argues in *Caste: The Origins of Our Discontents* that the overarching and foundational context is that of caste, the fixed and unconsciously embedded value we assign to someone's worth. In the following pages, there are many instances where caste manifests as the predominant context and where the rigidity of social ranking, power, and status impacted patient care in harmful and destructive ways. Addressing this head-on seems to be the only path forward if we are truly committed to sustainable change and improving the lives of *all* patients and their families.

References

African Palliative Care Association. Available at: https://www.africanpalliativecare.org
American Cancer Society, Global Cancer Facts & Figures, 4th Edition. Atlanta: American Cancer Society, Inc. 2022. Available at: https://www.cancer.org/content/

dam/cancer-org/research/cancer-facts-and-statistics/global-cancer-facts-and-figures/global-cancer-facts-and-figures-4th-edition.pdf

American Cancer Society, Global Cancer Burden; available at: https://www.cancer.org/about-us/our-global-health-work/global-cancer-burden.html

American Cancer Society, The Cancer Atlas, Global Cancer Burden. Available at: https://canceratlas.cancer.org/the-burden/the-burden-of-cancer/

American Society of Clinical Oncology (ASCO). ASCO policy statement of opioid therapy: Protecting access to treatment for cancer related pain, 2016. Available at: https://old-prod.asco.org/sites/new-www.asco.org/files/content-files/advocacy-and-policy/documents/2016-ASCO-Policy-Statement-Opioid-Therapy.pdf

Balarajan, Y., Selvaraj, S., & Subramanian, S. V. (2011). Health care and equity in India. *The Lancet*, *377*(9764), 505–515.

Bhadelia, A., De Lima, L., Arreola-Ornelas, H., Kwete, X. J., Rodriguez, N. M., & Knaul, F. M. (2019). Solving the global crisis in access to pain relief: Lessons from country actions. *American Journal of Public Health*, *109*(1), 58–60.

Brennan, F., Carr, D. B., & Cousins, M. (2007). Pain management: A fundamental human right. *Anesthesia & Analgesia*, *105*(1), 205–221.

Buchan, J., Catton, H., & Shaffer, F. (2022). International Council of Nurses and the International Centre on Nurse Migration. *Sustain and retain in 2022 and beyond: The global nursing workforce and the COVID-19 pandemic*. Available at: https://www.icn.ch/system/files/2022-01/Sustain%20and%20Retain%20in%202022%20and%20Beyond-%20The%20global%20nursing%20workforce%20and%20the%20COVID-19%20pandemic.pdf

Centers for Disease Control and Prevention (CDC). (2011). Prescription pain-killer overdoses at epidemic levels. Available at: https://www.cdc.gov/media/releases/2011/p1101_flu_pain_killer_overdose.html

Centers for Disease Control and Prevention. (2016). CDC Guideline for Prescribing Opioids for Chronic Pain – United States. Available at: https://www.cdc.gov/mmwr/volumes/65/rr/rr6501e1.htm

Centers for Disease Control and Prevention. (2022). CDC Clinical Practice Guideline for Prescribing Opioids for Pain – United States. Available at: https://www.cdc.gov/mmwr/volumes/71/rr/rr7103a1.htm?s_cid=rr7103a1.htm_w

Cherny, N. I., Cleary, J., Scholten, W., Radbruch, L., & Torode, J. (2013). The Global Opioid Policy Initiative (GOPI) project to evaluate the availability and accessibility of opioids for the management of cancer pain in Africa, Asia, Latin America and the Caribbean, and the Middle East: Introduction and methodology. *Annals of Oncology*, *24*, xi7–xi13.

Clark, D., Baur, N., Clelland, D., Garralda, E., López-Fidalgo, J., Connor, S., & Centeno, C. (2020). Mapping levels of palliative care development in 198 countries: The situation in 2017. *Journal of Pain and Symptom Management*, *59*(4), 794–807.

Daniels, M., Donilon, T., & Bollyky, T. J. (December 5, 2014). The emerging global health crisis: Noncommunicable diseases in low- and middle-income countries. Council on Foreign Relations Independent Task Force Report No. 72. Available at: http://dx.doi.org/10.2139/ssrn.2685111

De Lima, L., Krakauer, E. L., Lorenz, K., Praill, D., MacDonald, N., & Doyle, D. (2007). Ensuring palliative medicine availability: The development of the IAHPC list of essential medicines for palliative care. *Journal of Pain and Symptom Management*, *33*(5), 521–526.

Desmond, M. (2016). *Evicted: Poverty and profit in the American city*. Crown Publishers: New York.

Doyle, K. E., El Nakib, S. K., Rajagopal, M. R., Babu, S., Joshi, G., Kumarasamy, V., … & Palat, G. (2018). Predictors and prevalence of pain and its management in four regional cancer hospitals in India. *Journal of Global Oncology*, 4, 1–9.

Enzinger, A. C., Ghosh, K., Keating, N. L., Cutler, D. M., Clark, C. R., Florez, N., … & Wright, A. A. (2023). Racial and ethnic disparities in opioid access and urine drug screening among older patients with poor-prognosis cancer near the end of life. *Journal of Clinical Oncology*, JCO-22, Volume 41, Number 14.

Evans, J., Sahgal, N., Salazar, A. M., Starr, K. J., & Corichi, M., Pew Research, Center. (2022). How Indians view gender roles in family and society. Available at: https://www.pewresearch.org/religion/2022/03/02/how-indians-view-gender-roles-in-families-and-society/

Germain, C. (1979). *The Cancer Unit: An Ethnography*. Nursing Resources. Wakefield, Massachusetts.

Global Burden of Disease 2019 Cancer Risk Factors Collaborators. (2022). The global burden of cancer attributable to risk factors, 2010–19: A systematic analysis for the Global Burden of Disease Study 2019. *Lancet*, 400, 563–591. Available at: https://doi.org/10.1016/S0140-6736(22)01438-6

Goldsmith, B., Beresford, M., Thomson Reuters Foundation. (2018). India most dangerous country for women with sexual violence rife – global poll. Available at: https://www.reuters.com/article/women-dangerous-poll-idINKBN1JM076

Hospice Africa Uganda. Available at: https://www.hospice-africa.org/uganda/

Hull, R., Mbele, M., Makhafola, T., Hicks, C., Wang, S. M., Reis, R. M., … & Dlamini, Z. (2020). Cervical cancer in low and middle–income countries. *Oncology Letters*, 20(3), 2058–2074.

Human Rights Watch. (2011). Global state of pain treatment: Access to palliative care as a human right. Available at: https://www.hrw.org/report/2011/06/02/global-state-pain-treatment/access-medicines-and-palliative-care

Human Rights Watch. (2009). Unbearable pain: India's obligation to ensure palliative care. Available at: https://www.hrw.org/report/2009/10/28/unbearable-pain/indias-obligation-ensure-palliative-care

International Agency for Research on Cancer (IARC). (2020). Cancer today: Data visualization tools for exploring the global cancer burden in 2020. Available at: https://gco.iarc.fr/today/home

Jagwe, J., & Merriman, A. (2007). Uganda: Delivering analgesia in rural Africa: Opioid availability and nurse prescribing. *Journal of Pain and Symptom Management*, 33(5), 547–551.

Khurana S., Mundhra, S. (2017). A Suitable Girl (documentary). Available at: https://www.imdb.com/title/tt6604050/

Knaul, F. M., Farmer, P. E., Krakauer, E. L., De Lima, L., Bhadelia, A., Kwete, X. J., … & Zimmerman, C. (2018). Alleviating the access abyss in palliative care and pain relief—an imperative of universal health coverage: The Lancet Commission report. *The Lancet*, 391(10128), 1391–1454. Available at: http://www.thelancet.com/pdfs/journals/lancet/PIIS0140-6736(17)32513-8.pdf

Kwekkeboom, K., Serlin, R. C., Ward, S. E., LeBlanc, T. W., Ogunseitan, A., & Cleary, J. (2021). Revisiting patient-related barriers to cancer pain management in the context of the US opioid crisis. *Pain*, 162(6), 1840.

Lamas, D., & Rosenbaum, L. (2012). Painful inequities: Palliative care in developing countries. *The New England Journal of Medicine*, *366*, 199–201.

Lemay, K., Wilson, K. G., & Buenger, U., et al. (2011). Fear of pain in patients with advanced cancer or in patients with chronic noncancer pain. *The Clinical Journal of Pain*, *27*(2), 116–124.

Lohman, D., Cleary, J., Connor, S., De Lima, L., Downing, J., Marston, J., … & Pettus, K. (2022). Advancing global palliative care over two decades: Health system integration, access to essential medicines, and pediatrics. *Journal of Pain and Symptom Management*, *64*(1), 58–69.

Macy, B. (2018). *Dopesick: Dealers, doctors and the drug company that addicted America*. Little, Brown & Company (NOT Bloomsbury), New York.

Matlock, D. D. (2015). The pain pendulum swinging again. *Journal of Palliative Medicine*, *18*(9), 734–735.

Meldrum, M. L. (2016). The ongoing opioid prescription epidemic: Historical context. *American Journal of Public Health*, *106*(8), 1365.

Monnat, S. M. (2016). Dreamland: The true tale of America's opiate epidemic. *Journal of Research in Rural Education (Online)*, *31*(4), 1.

Maurer, M. A., Gilson, A. M., Husain, S. A., & Cleary, J. F. (2013). Examining influences on the availability of and access to opioids for pain management and palliative care. *Journal of Pain & Palliative Care Pharmacotherapy*, *27*(3), 255–260.

Meier, E. A., Gallegos, J. V., Thomas, L. P. M., Depp, C. A., Irwin, S. A., & Jeste, D. V. (2016). Defining a good death (successful dying): Literature review and a call for research and public dialogue. *The American Journal of Geriatric Psychiatry*, *24*(4), 261–271.

Moonshine Agency, Australia. (2017). Documentary: "Hippocratic: 18 Experiments in Gently Shaking the World". Available at: https://hippocraticfilm.com/

National Academies of Sciences, Engineering, and Medicine. (2017). *Cancer care in low-resource areas: Cancer treatment, palliative care, and survivorship care: Proceedings of a workshop*. Washington, DC: The National Academies Press. https://doi.org/10.17226/24743.

National Academies of Sciences, Engineering, and Medicine. (2017). *Pain Management and the Opioid Epidemic: Balancing Societal and Individual Benefits and Risks of Prescription Opioid Use*. Washington, DC: The National Academies Press. https://doi.org/10.17226/24781.

Paice, J. A. (2018). Cancer pain management and the opioid crisis in America: How to preserve hard-earned gains in improving the quality of cancer pain management. *Cancer*, *124*(12), 2491–2497.

Pallium India. (2023). Available at: https://palliumindia.org/

Pallium India. (2012). Does anger have a place in our work? Anger in compassion: Dr. Robert Twycross addresses IAPCON 2012. Available at: https://palliumindia.org/2012/03/does-anger-have-a-place-in-our-work

Paudel, B. D., Ryan, K. M., Brown, M. S., Krakauer, E. L., Rajagopal, M. R., Maurer, M. A., & Cleary, J. F. (2015). Opioid availability and palliative care in Nepal: Influence of an international pain policy fellowship. *Journal of Pain and Symptom Management*, *49*(1), 110–116.

Partridge, E. E., Mayer-Davis, E. J., Sacco, R. L., & Balch, A. J. (2011). Creating a 21st Century global health agenda: The General Assembly of the United Nations high level meeting on non-communicable diseases. *CA: A Cancer Journal for Clinicians*, *61*(4), 209–211. Available at doi: 10.3322/caac.20120.

Quinones, S. (2015). *Dreamland: The true tale of America's opiate epidemic.* Blooms-bury Press, New York.

Steinhauser, K. E., Christakis, N. A., Clipp, E. C., McNeilly, M., McIntyre, L., & Tulsky, J. A. (2000). Factors considered important at the end of life by patients, family, physicians, and other care providers. *JAMA, 284*(19), 2476–2482.

Steinhauser, K. E., Clipp, E. C., McNeilly, M., Christakis, N. A., McIntyre, L. M., & Tulsky, J. A. (2000). In search of a good death: Observations of patients, families, and providers. *Annals of Internal Medicine, 132*(10), 825–832.

Sung, H., Ferlay, J., Siegel, R. L., Laversanne, M., Soerjomataram, I., Jemal, A., & Bray, F. (2021). Global cancer statistics 2020: GLOBOCAN estimates of incidence and mortality worldwide for 36 cancers in 185 countries. *CA: A Cancer Journal for Clinicians, 71*(3), 209–249.

The Pain & Policy Studies Group, Indiana University, Walther Global Palliative Care & Supportive Oncology. (2023). Available at: https://walthercenter.iu.edu/about/index.html

The U.S. Department of Health and Human Services, National Institutes of Health, National Cancer Institute. National Cancer Plan. (April 2023). Available at: https://nationalcancerplan.cancer.gov/national-cancer-plan.pdf

The World Bank. (2023). Low and middle-income country data. Available at: https://data.worldbank.org/income-level/low-and-middle-income

67th World Health Assembly. (May 2014). Strengthening of palliative care as a component of comprehensive care throughout the life course. WHA67.19. Available at: https://apps.who.int/gb/ebwha/pdf_files/WHA67/A67_R19-en.pdf

World Health Organization, Non-Communicable Diseases Fact Sheet. (2022). Available at: https://www.who.int/news-room/fact-sheets/detail/noncommunicable-diseases

World Health Organization (WHO), International Agency for Research on Cancer (IARC). (2020). Data visualization tools for exploring the global cancer burden; available at: https://gco.iarc.fr/today/home

World Health Organization. (2022). Cervical Cancer Factsheet. Available at: https://www.who.int/news-room/fact-sheets/detail/cervical-cancer

World Health Organization (2020). Palliative Care Key Facts. Available at: https://www.who.int/news-room/fact-sheets/detail/palliative-care

World Health Organization (WHO). (2018). Integrating palliative care and symptom relief into primary health care: A WHO guide for planner, implementers, and managers. Available at: https://apps.who.int/iris/bitstream/handle/10665/274559/9789241514477-eng.pdf?ua=1

World Health Organization (WHO). (2022). Key Facts, Nursing and Midwifery. Available at: https://www.who.int/news-room/fact-sheets/detail/nursing-and-midwifery

World Health Organization (WHO). (2020). State of the world's nursing 2020: Investing in education, jobs and leadership. Available at: https://www.who.int/publications/i/item/9789240003279

Worldwide Hospice Palliative Care Alliance (WHPCA). (2020). Global Atlas of Palliative Care, 2nd Edition. Available at: http://www.thewhpca.org/resources/global-atlas-on-end-of-life-care

United Nations, International Narcotics Control Board. (2016). Report: Availability of Internationally Controlled Drugs: Ensuring Adequate Access for Medicinal and Scientific Purposes, Indispensable, Adequately Available, and Not Unduly Restricted. Available at: https://www.unodc.org/documents/drug-prevention-and-treatment/INCB_Access_Supplement-AR15_availability_English.pdf

United Nations, International Narcotics Control Board. (2023). Supplement to the Annual Report of the Board for 2022 on the Availability of Internationally Controlled Substances: No Patient Left Behind: Progress in Ensuring Adequate Access to Internationally Controlled Substances for Medical and Scientific Purposes. March 2023. Available at: https://www.incb.org/documents/Publications/Annual-Reports/AR2022/Supplement/E_INCB_2022_1_Supp_1_eng.pdf

Van Den Beuken-Van, M. H., Hochstenbach, L. M., Joosten, E. A., Tjan-Heijnen, V. C., & Janssen, D. J. (2016). Update on prevalence of pain in patients with cancer: Systematic review and meta-analysis. *Journal of Pain and Symptom Management*, *51*(6), 1070–1090.

Wilkerson, I. (2023). Caste: The origins of our discontents. New York: Random House.

PART II
South Indian Cancer Hospital

1   In the Struggle

Except in palliative care, no nurses here even touch a wound, they don't do any dressing changes. There are 2 dressers in the hospital, they come, do the dressing, they go. That's all. And even that is not 100% good. They just apply some Betadine, put a pad. There are patients who have had dressing changes downstairs, and then they come here, to us, with maggots...so the whole burden falls on us. And the work we do is good.

Pradeep, palliative care nurse

The palliative care clinic at South Indian Cancer Hospital (SICH) teems with patients. I enter the small room and see a 40-year-old man with a large, soiled bandage across his left jaw and a tube dangling from his nose lying on one of the cots. His face and eyes look painfully swollen, but his legs and arms are thin. A strong, foul odor permeates the room, and most staff are wearing thin paper masks that cover their mouth and nose.[1]

"Maggots," Pradeep says to me as I glance at the cot, partly obscured by the portable curtain partition.

The patient's wife in a tangerine-colored sari tentatively enters, followed by the patient's mother and brother. Daya, another one of the palliative care nurses, sees them and immediately reacts. A heated dialogue erupts between Daya and the patient's wife, who begins to cry. Pradeep listens intensely, but does not intervene. Daya is clearly upset, angry even. Her words are tense and harsh, loud and staccato. The wife continues to weep as Daya berates her. I haven't yet seen what is under the bandage, but I don't have to—a quick look tells me this is very, very bad.

"Settle, down. Enough of this," Pradeep eventually says, and the wife scurries out of the clinic.

Daya is frustrated because the family will not do the wound care properly. "We have told them. They only do the most peripheral of care and then it

---

1 A reminder to the reader that this fieldwork took place prior to the COVID-19 pandemic. During my fieldwork, many staff and nurses wore thin paper masks; the reasons for this were sometimes unclear, but often to cope with difficult odors.

DOI: 10.4324/9781003413158-4

becomes very bad. And the wife doesn't want to deal with this now. She is saying the mother will do it, but she will not," Pradeep explains. Daya nods in agreement as she prepares the materials for the dressing change. "For 1 year," Daya adds.

My heart aches—for Daya and Pradeep because it is gruesome to clean these malignant wounds, and as a nurse I understand the frustration when instructions are not followed and a small problem morphs in to a much bigger one. But I also ache for this family. It takes a strong constitution to handle these types of wounds; I know many health care providers who could not do it.

"Why do you think that is? That she doesn't want to do it?" I probe. "It looks like a very bad wound," I add gently.

Pradeep hesitates. I am not sure he has considered this question before.

"She doesn't want to be involved, she doesn't want to do it," he repeats.

"Sometimes we have a similar problem in the U.S.," I say. "Some people cannot handle bad wounds, or the level of care a patient needs. It is very challenging."

"Yes," agrees Pradeep. "But we are not always there, they must do it," he says practically.

He is, of course, correct. No one can say to this impoverished family who lives far from the capital city of Dandaka.[2] "We'll send a home care team out to see you" or "Why don't you hire someone to help you at home?"

Daya brusquely prepares the items for the dressing change. She ties her dupatta[3] behind her back and gets to work; Pradeep assists, and I hold the flashlight. The bandage is removed to reveal the worst wound I have ever seen: a massive grapefruit sized erosion that looks like what I imagine happens when an explosive detonates near someone's face. The patient's entire mandible bone is exposed, like a sliver of moon, and the soft flesh of his pink tongue pulsates below a mass of gray rotting tissue that appears weirdly ashy and fluffy, like a wasp's nest.

Daya applies Terpint (a medicinal turpentine oil) with a syringe and the wound begins to writhe. Despite 16 years as a nurse, I struggle to suppress my strong urge to gag. Daya and Pradeep take turns picking out maggots with tweezers that squirm to the surface. The row with the patient's wife forgotten, at least for now, Daya gently applies a gauze bandage over the patient's eyes; I am not sure if this is to prevent him from seeing the maggots that are being extracted from his diseased face or simply because it is the one

---

2 Dandaka, like all other names in this book, is a pseudonym. I intentionally do not name the Indian State where my fieldwork occurred or discuss in detail the politics, geography, or history of the region in order to help protect identities. This decision is discussed further within Chapters 10 and 11.

3 A decorative scarf worn draped across the shoulders and neck as part of an Indian woman's salwar kameez suit, a long tunic covering loose trousers. Traditionally, the dupatta is a symbol of female modesty as it can be used as a veil and/or to cover the chest.

compassionate gesture that can be offered in the midst of this tremendous suffering.

After about 20 maggots have been removed, Pradeep irrigates the wound with saline. The patient lies remarkably still as the salt water is squirted into the gaping wound and then drains as a milky brown liquid from the tube dangling from his nose. The wife, who has now returned, hovers close by, timidly peering behind the curtain. Daya hands her a mortar and pestle and tells her to crush some Metrogel and Sucralfate tablets. Both powders are then sprinkled in the wound to reduce odor and bleeding, and then the large hole is repacked with fresh gauze.

Daya softens as she reaffixes the tape that holds the drain attached to the patient's nose in place. The patient is turned, and a gush of brown liquid is violently expelled from the tube into a waiting bucket. The other bucket, full of irrigated saline, Terpint solution, and dead maggots is whisked away by the patient's wife and then brought back empty.

***

Daya is like a storm burst—an unpredictable downpour followed by a gentle, quiet rain. And I can't say I blame her. These wounds, grotesque, complicated, and fetid, are an overwhelming assault to the senses. This is only my second week and it's hard to keep track of all the patients who come to have maggots extracted from their cancerous wounds.

The palliative care department at SICH was established in 2006 under the highly capable leadership of Dr. Madhu, who was trained first as an anesthesiologist and then later as a palliative care specialist. She was recruited to help establish palliative care at SICH, and now it is the only formal program in all of Dandaka and the State, with one of the largest and most consistent supplies of morphine in India.[4] Patients are referred by their primary oncologist for end-of-life care and pain management, and the team sees approximately 60 patients a day in the outpatient clinic, which consists of four rooms—two smaller spaces for staff and equipment and two larger front offices for seeing patients, one primarily for physicians, the other for nurses. Privacy is limited: there is no separate exam room, and only one rickety cloth curtain that is

---

4 This was accurate at the time of my fieldwork. Dr. Madhu explained that SICH's pharmacy actually stocked oral morphine starting in 2003, but it was procured through the antiquated and complicated Narcotic Drugs and Psychotropic Substances (NDPS) State regulations which made the supply highly erratic and infrequently used. During Madhu's first few years at SICH, even though the demand for morphine was increasing as more patients were being referred to palliative care, supply was still erratic, absent, or insufficient. After my fieldwork concluded, in 2014, a landmark amendment to the NDPS was passed by the Indian Parliament that officially recognized the medical and scientific use of opioids and denotes Essential Narcotic Drugs. See https://palliumindia.org/2020/04/ndps-amendment-act-2014-2

occasionally hauled out of the back room to shield others from witnessing particularly disturbing sights or procedures.

Multiple interactions are happening simultaneously and it's difficult to know where to focus my attention. Patients, family members, and staff mill about, interrupting, interjecting, overhearing, answering cell phones, lingering, thrusting forth medical charts, standing in a tight huddle around the tables where the doctors and nurses sit. Curious bystanders peer into doorways, pop their heads through the shuttered windows of the clinic, and create a logjam in the hallway outside the entrance. It's still early morning, and I am already perspiring profusely; the building smells like a combination of bleach and sweat.

Paper documentation is everywhere, and I am struck by its sheer volume: inpatient's medical charts; in the foot-high stacks of legal-sized ledgers used to record and log prescriptions, procedures, dispensed morphine tablets, admissions, and supply inventories; in smaller green pamphlet-type books that function as patient medication diaries. Tattered colored folders with papers spilling out of them are crammed into a floor-to-ceiling high bookshelf that leans precariously to one side.

Dr. Darshan, one of the palliative care doctors sitting at the table in the clinic room, glances at a blue folder in front of him and calls out a patient's name, staring straight ahead. He has been working as a physician in the palliative care department for almost three years, after a brief stint in a corporate hospital. "*Chowdhury!*" Dr. Darshan calls again from his chair, barely audible above the din. When no one appears, he calmly moves on to the next folder. It is now close to 10:30 am and the crowd outside the clinic door has exploded. Some of the sickest patients sit on a narrow bench in the corridor; others sit and crouch on the cement floor. Dr. Darshan is unfazed.

Sitting across from Dr. Darshan at the same table is Dr. Amit, another palliative care physician. He is presented with an elderly female patient who sits on a metal stool placed by the table; her son stands by her side. Dr. Amit talks primarily with the patient's son and makes little eye contact. He pulls a copy of the patient's CAT scan from a white sleeve, holds it above his head toward the light to review, squinting at the images. He does not lay hands upon the patient to examine her, and when his cell phone rings in the middle of the consultation he answers it.

Dr. Darshan's next patient has appeared and seven people are now crowded around the table—the two actual patients, sitting less than two feet apart, the two doctors, sitting in chairs on opposite sides of the table, myself, and two family members standing alongside each patient. It's quite loud and I have trouble hearing what is being said at the table. Dr. Amit writes what appears to be a prescription on a square shaped piece of white paper, gives it to the patient's son, and then sits back in his chair waiting for the next patient. The entire interaction takes about five minutes.

In the adjacent nurses' room behind the rickety exam curtain, Daya is again working to extract maggots out of a woman's infected facial tumor, while Radha, the ayah,[5] assists by shining a flashlight onto the patient's face. The woman's face is ravaged by tumor, her painfully swollen lips split open like spoiled fruit. Apparently, the palliative care team plucked two small buckets of maggots yesterday from the woman's wound. The woman holds a cloth over her eyes and lies unbelievably still as Daya inserts metal tweezers deep into the woman's flesh, which separates easily with each probe.

***

Dr. Rashi, one of the pediatric oncologists, frequently eats lunch in the back room of the palliative care clinic. She is a large woman—in stature and personality, with a kind, moonlike face and a booming, infectious laugh, her long wavy hair pulled into a soft knot at the nape of her neck. She is intrigued by my research project, as she is a member of the hospital ethics committee, which reviewed and approved the study. I am interested in her career path, which involved oncology training in the U.S. and then a return to practice in India, an uncommon occurrence.

"I am not sure the nurses care much about the suffering around them," she says, removing the lid from her tiffin, a circular metal container, of rice. "The general ward nurses don't do much hands-on nursing care." She opens other small tins containing roti (flat tortilla like bread) and curries, spicy vegetable, and meat sauces that complement the rice.

"On the wards the nurses stand behind a desk, call out people's names, the patients come forward, and they administer the chemotherapy. They probably give 30–40 chemotherapy treatments in an hour." She scoops one of the curries on top of a heap of white rice and offers me some, using the tin lid of her tiffin as a makeshift plate. With her right hand, she mixes and mashes together the rice and curry.

"In my 5 years of working here, I have never had a nurse come to me or another physician and advocate for the patient, saying 'this patient is in pain, this patient needs such and such.'" Dr. Rashi kneads the rice and curry into neat balls, which she scoops into the palm of her right hand and adeptly pops in her mouth. I try to imitate this traditional way of eating an Indian meal, but am not particularly successful. Dr. Rashi reaches for the communal water bottle on the table, and I notice how she tilts both her head and the water bottle back, allowing a carefully controlled stream of water into her mouth without her lips ever touching the bottle.

"Why do you think that is?" I ask.

"I'm not exactly sure. Maybe it is a way to distance themselves from the situation. Maybe they just don't care and have no empathy. I think it

---

5 Ayahs (also sometimes referred to as sweepers) are female workers delegated with low-status tasks related to sanitation and hygiene (in the hospital setting) or childrearing and housekeeping (in the home setting). Along with ward boys (orderlies) at SICH, ayahs were designated as Class IV employees, the lowest level of government workers.

is the way they are trained: to make beds, to follow doctors' orders as best they can; they are not trained to be the patient's champion. It might be that there's just too much work for them to do. Just take the pediatric ward, which is supposed to be one of the better-equipped wards in the hospital. We have 1 nurse on duty in the afternoon, and 1 nurse in the night and an average of 50 children. So, what symptoms can the nurse ask about, and what is she going to do? If she gives the patients' injections on time, the antibiotics go in on time, that itself is a lot. If a patient tells her at 8:30 in the night that he's having pain, there's not much the nurse can do. If she calls a physician, there's only 1 physician on-call for the 350 patients in the hospital and for him it's not a priority. He's dealing with the shortness of breaths, the blood transfusions, the medication reactions, and this and that, so for somebody with a known history of cancer, someone who is terminally ill, with pain, he'll say, 'let's wait until tomorrow morning.' So the evening and night nurses, I think, they just can't do anything even if they assess symptoms, so, they'll stop asking after a point. In the morning the nurses are busy giving the chemotherapies so I think that they don't come up with these questions. I feel that they don't even notice that a patient has pain or that they are not moved by it. Have they rationalized it? I don't know. Have they internalized the whole thing and said, 'I'm not going to do anything about it, it's not my job to worry about the patient's pain, it's the physician's job.' I don't know."

I nod and she continues. "This is very different from my experience in North Carolina where nurses are expected to serve in this role," she says, re-ferring to her oncology fellowship training in the U.S. "And even if the nurses did advocate here and say, 'Mr. so-and-so has pain, he needs pain medicine,' what do we do when he has no money and can't buy it? It is better not to look too deep because the problems are too big and cannot be solved by the nurse, or the doctor. No food, no place to live, no money."

She sighs and looks directly at me. "I shut down too," she admits. "I don't go in to details, I don't ask a lot of questions. I don't want to know. I look at the bloodwork, the liver function, the kidney tests. I write the orders for chemotherapy, but I do not ask many questions about social history, the patient's personal situation, because there is nothing I can do. Maybe I could hold the patient's hand for a few minutes, and he may feel better for a bit, but there is no guarantee that I will be available to hold his hand again, the next time he needs something. Maybe the nurses feel the same way."

Dr. Rashi tacos some rice into a roti, chews, swallows. "So, your project really interests me, Virginia. Why are we this way? How do we emotionally connect with patients? Do we see their suffering?"

By now, other members of the team have entered the small room and are preparing their own lunches. The conversation quickly switches to rapid Hindi. I sit back, digesting.

***

A 65-year-old woman with advanced rectal cancer is lying on the bed in the nurse/procedure room of the palliative care clinic. She is shielded partly by the folding curtain, but the room is still crowded and buzzing with activity. Her daughter and son-in-law stand by her as she clutches her abdomen and moans. The patient reaches out to grab her son-in-law's shirt, but he pulls away, avoiding her grasp.

Daya undoes the bulky gauze dressing covering the patient's belly. Immediately, an overpowering smell permeates the room, causing Sarah, a social worker, to abruptly stand up from the consultation table midsentence, blurt out something loudly I do not understand, and retreat to the back room. I am offered a small paper mask to cover my nose and mouth.

The patient grimaces and writhes on the bed as multiple people try to start an intravenous (IV) line, to no avail. Radha swabs the patient's forearm with some antiseptic and squeezes to simulate a tourniquet. Eventually, the team gives up on establishing IV access and refocuses attention to her abdomen.

"It looks like she is in pain," I say to Radha and Sarah, who has since reemerged from the back room. "Do you ever give morphine subcutaneously when you can't start an IV?" I ask cautiously. I am told she is not in pain.

The patient's belly is a gelatinous mass of protruding tumor caked with feces and blood. Kate, a Dandaka-born, American-raised, young woman who is visiting family and volunteering at SICH for a few months, stands beside me. She draws her breath in sharply and whispers, "What *is* that?" Before I can answer, Dr. Madhu appears to assess the situation. "That is gangrenous tumor and a colorectal-cutaneous fistula," she explains.

Kate looks at me for translation. "Basically, it's dead, infected cancer tissue and a fistula is an abnormal tunnel between two body structures that shouldn't be connected. Her large intestine, her colon, has made a tunnel to her skin," I say very quietly. Kate's eyes widen. "Did the cancer cause that?" she whispers back. "Yes," I say.

Dr. Madhu instructs Daya to clean the wound and apply a fresh bandage; the patient will be sent directly to hospice. It is a new hospice, though, only a month old and Madhu worries that the staff is poorly trained and ill-equipped. But there is no other option, as it is the only hospice in Dandaka, a city of eight million people.[6] Daya spends over an hour tending to the wound. With each movement or adjustment, the patient winces; she calls out repeatedly in Hindi: *please stop, please stop, please stop*. I am again assured the patient is not in pain.

At one point, the patient's son hands Daya an egg. At first I think it is meant as a token of gratitude for the care, but then Daya breaks the egg into a metal emesis basin and mixes in karaya powder to make a paste that will help soothe the irritated skin around the tumor site. Daya spreads the paste evenly around the patient's abdomen and then covers it with cut up pieces of

6 This was the approximate population of the city during my fieldwork.

plastic from the discarded packages of exam gloves. Then she places gauze bandages over the entire area and attempts to contain the leaking stool with an ostomy bag set on top of the bulky gauze. Without a secure seal, I'm not sure how effective the set-up will be in containing fecal drainage and odor, but Daya has done her best, given the extent of the wound and the limited supplies.

After Daya finishes with the abdominal wound, the patient is turned on her side to assess her buttocks for bedsores. The patient cries out in agony. I look up and count the number of people in the small procedure room: 16.

Then the power cuts.

* * *

Dr. Madhu tells me the scenario I witnessed with the rectal cancer patient is common. "By the time patients get to SICH, their cancer is very advanced, there is very little we can do. They have often gone to large, private hospitals where they are told they can be cured, that there is treatment for them, and then they spend all of their money, or their state government insurance benefit is used up,[7] and they have nothing left. Then they come here."

---

7 The Madada (pseudonym) Health Care (MHS) Insurance Scheme (plan) is a reimbursement program administered by the State and provides fixed payments to hospitals and physicians to cover the costs of treating certain diagnoses for patients whose income is below a certain level. MHS reimbursement is based on the physician's treatment plan and the pre-agreed amount of coverage for that service—50,000 rupees for a course of radiation, for example. Almost all patients (over 95%) who come to SICH qualify for MHS. At the time of this fieldwork, MHS covered palliative care services at a (total) rate of 3,000 rupees (about $60 USD). Additional information about MHS, from my fieldnotes:

> I talk with Sanjay, one of the hospital insurance case managers in charge of keeping track of MHS. He explains that the State-wide plan started 4 years ago and helps cover some health care costs for the very poor. His job is to help submit applications and claims and keep the MHS records straight for the palliative care department. He shows me a sophisticated-looking internet-based database used to log information, submit applications, and pull statistics. In contrast, next to his computer, a floor-to-ceiling wooden bookshelf strains with piles of colored patient files stacked haphazardly. I ask him how many patients at SICH are on the MHS insurance program. "100%," he says. "So every patient?" I ask. "Maybe 95%," he adjusts the figure. He tells me it takes at most a day—or a day and a half—to get the MHS application approved by the State. He scans in the application and submits it electronically. "Who qualifies to receive the MHS plan?" I ask. Sanjay explains that patients are eligible for MHS based on prior eligibility of a "ration" card that the State issues to families who are extremely poor. In contrast to MHS approval, which is surprisingly expeditious, I am told it can take "a long time" to get a ration card. "Here, this is what a ration card looks like," he says, pulling a laminated ration card with a color picture of the qualified family—five people standing solemnly together— out of a drawer to show me. Sanjay goes on to explain that MHS reimbursement is based on the physician's treatment plan and the pre-agreed amount of coverage for that service—50,000 rupees for a course of radiation, for example. "Now MHS covers palliative care," he says proudly. "They give 3,000 rupees (about $60 USD) for palliative care." What happens if the person needs more care than that?" I ask. "In rare exceptions, the amount can be

"Other nurses won't deal with this," Madhu explains. "I have so much respect for our palliative care nurses, they really get in there and take care of these wounds that no one else wants to touch."

Daya sits down next to me after she has finished talking with the family of the patient with rectal cancer about wound care. She explained that they will need to cut up bits of old saris, boil them for sterilization, and use them for the dressings.

"I have a list for you," she announces suddenly.

"A list?"

"Yes, a list of all my concerns. I want to tell you."

"About nursing?"

"Yes," she says. "But my English, it is not good enough. So, I will write."

I can see the urgency on her face.

"Five years I am here, it is very hard, this work. Many times, I say, 'why? Why do you do this?' It makes me very sad, some days." I am desperate to know more about what Daya is saying, but the language barrier is too great.[8]

---

increased. But if patients don't have a ration card or qualify for MHS they are expected to pay out of pocket," Sanjay says. "What happened before you had MHS?" I ask. Sanjay shrugs. "Well, this is a government hospital, so costs are nominal, but some patients had to sell all their property to pay for treatment. They would say—'I sold this; I sold this.'" On the bottom of the MHS application form is a statement that reads, "I further state that I am not covered by any other institution/reimbursement scheme by Govt." and indicates a place for the signature or left thumbprint of the patient. Sanjay pulls out an inkpad, presses his thumb against the damp blue surface and affixes it firmly to this space. "Isn't that for the patient?" Sanjay isn't at all offended by my question. He smiles and shrugs again and simply says, "India. This is India. In India, everything is for money," and he rubs his thumb against his index and middle finger in the universal sign for cash. "Corruption, bribes, it is very bad here."

What a physician shared with me about his opinions regarding the MHS plan: "And another thing that happened about 3 or 4 years ago, the State instituted this health insurance scheme. It is an ideal scheme because it helps pay for treatment for people who don't have any resources to pay, for example, for their gallbladder to be removed. If they go to a hospital, it may cost, say Rs 2000. They may not have that. But, with the MHS scheme, they can have that done and that scheme pays for that anywhere, at any hospital, wherever you choose. Sounds fine. But is it fine? I don't think so. The reason being is that the scheme doesn't cover any primary care. If you had proper primary care, you might not even need that surgery. But they pay for the surgery. So, what happened was all these corporate hospitals jumped in, and started doing hysterectomies, bypass surgeries, whatever they can get paid for, they do it. Some people question does the patient really need this surgery? But it didn't matter, because they get paid for it, and the patient who is not really educated, even if they are educated, how much do they know about medical things? If a doctor tells you, 'you need bypass surgery,' the first thing the patient thinks is—'Can I afford that?' And if somebody says you don't have to worry about that because the government is going to pay for it, then the patient doesn't care. He doesn't think to sit and ask the question—'Do I need the surgery?'"

8 A combination of Hindi, two regional languages, and English were all spoken at the fieldsite; proficiency in English generally stratified along socioeconomic and educational lines. I relied on a designated translator for my formal interviews, and during informal interactions in the

I try to explain that I want to talk with her more, that I will find a translator, but I'm not sure she understands.

* * *

Pradeep tends to an elderly woman whose pain has not been well controlled on morphine. He holds up a fentanyl patch, a sticky piece of plastic impregnated with a drug similar to morphine that is absorbed through the skin. The patient is among the more comfortable looking patients I have seen.

"You know these?" he asks.

"Yes, I do, we use them a lot," I say. "Do you have them often here?"

"Sometimes yes, sometimes no," he answers. "Today, yes, some were donated. They are expensive."

Pradeep asks me where he should apply the patch, but I have the strong sense he already knows and is only asking my opinion to be polite. I am surprised this patient who looks very comfortable is receiving a fentanyl patch when the woman with the rectal cancer and gangrenous bowel is writhing in pain on the bed behind us. She looks so miserable, I try once more.

"Pradeep, do you think that patient needs more pain medication?" I motion to the patient with rectal cancer.

"No," he says confidently, "she is not in pain. She is more uneasy about her wound and her disease." I hope he is right.

I sit on a hard metal stool, making available for a patient or family member the more comfortable wooden chair with a back. Most of the patients who shuffle into the palliative care clinic are so incredibly sick looking: emaciated, sullen, depressed—it seems the least I can do.

Abruptly, I am scolded by Sarah and Daya.

"That chair is not for patients!" they tell me animatedly, pointing to the wooden chair I have purposely left empty. They gesture toward the hard metal stool. "*That* is the chair for patients!" they say, and insist I move from the metal stool to the wooden chair. I do so reluctantly.

Seated in this new position, a male family member accidently brushes my lower leg. He immediately backs up, flustered and embarrassed, and offers a blessing.

* * *

Saturday is a much quieter day in the palliative care clinic. Pradeep performs a paracentesis on a gaunt man with a hugely swollen abdomen—a procedure most nurses in the U.S. cannot do. He tells me that the man has come from very far away to have the fluid drained.

---

field multiple individuals helped to translate when needed. The smattering of English, nonverbal cues, and a growing familiarity with the languages as my fieldwork progressed all assisted in my understanding of conversations and interactions. However, my lack of fluency was a clear limitation and is further discussed in Chapter 11.

"No one else will do this, so he has to come all the way here," Pradeep says as he expertly inserts the needle into the man's belly and straw-colored fluid drains into a basin underneath the bed.

I see Sarah talk tenderly to a patient's family member and get a complete symptom history. Daya gently explains a medication regimen to an old man wearing a white dhoti[9] who hobbles into the clinic, a large thick wooden stick supporting his weight; she offers him a plastic chair as soon as he enters. Pradeep swings into action when a distressed 35-year-old with metastatic breast cancer is brought to the clinic in a rusty, rickety wheelchair with "CT Scan" stamped in black lettering on the side complaining of severe pain and breathlessness; 10 mg of IV (intravenous) morphine, 2 mg Versed (a valium like drug), Decadron (a steroid), and Zantac (antacid) are quickly given and the woman finally looks comfortable.

Radha brings up the chai and everything stops for five minutes to drink the warm, milky, sweet tea poured from the grubby blue and white thermos into flimsy, plastic, thimble-sized cups: it is a daily ritual that is not missed, no matter what chaos swirls in the clinic. Radha squats on the floor below us in a crab-like posture of servitude that no one else seems to mind, including Radha, but that makes me deeply uncomfortable.

Daya and Sarah tell me that they are especially sympathetic toward patients who have been abandoned and have no one to look after them.

"The doctors are often unaware, but we look after the orphan patients," says Daya.

"Who does?" I ask.

"The team in the department. We give them tea or food that we bring for ourselves. We are looking after 10 to 15 patients now," says Daya. Sarah explains that she collects donations from members of her church to help buy abandoned patients clothes or supplies.

"Remember Pavani?" Daya asks Sarah and Abhipsha.

"Yes, no one can forget her," says Abhipsha, joining the conversation. I am just getting to know Abhipsha, as she recently returned from leave to care for a dying parent in her native village. As a contract nurse without government benefits, she had to take two months of unpaid leave.

Pavani was a patient with cervical cancer from a village over 500 kilometers away. She had five sisters, whom she educated, secured marriages for, and got settled. Pavani didn't have children of her own, but she adopted her sister's son and provided him with a good education as an engineer. When Pavani became ill, for reasons the team did not understand, her family completely abandoned her at SICH. Even when the doctors gave up hope and told Pavani to go home, she refused, explaining there was nobody to take care of her. So, Pavani slept under a tree outside the hospital, because she

---

9 Dhoti: a traditional garment worn by male Hindus, consisting of a piece of material tied around the waist and extending to cover most of the legs.

couldn't have a hospital bed for such a long period of time—they keep the beds for patients receiving chemotherapy. In the morning, Radha would go outside and give her a bath and then bring her up to the palliative care department where the staff would give her food and medicines. "We'd talk with her; that made her feel better. She'd say, 'Ah okay, my relatives are not here, but you will take care of me,'" says Sarah.

"For 6 months, every day! She would spend 1 hour, 2 hours with us, making everybody laugh," Daya says, smiling, remembering.

Pavani's illness continued to worsen, and she began to require almost daily draining of her abdominal fluid. At that point, Sarah called her family, again asking them to come, telling them the time was near. But they still did not come, and Pavani's condition rapidly deteriorated. One morning, Radha took the stretcher outside but it was too late—Pavani had already died on the road under the tree, in front of the hospital. Even after Pavani died, her family did not come for her, and the team had to send her body to the mortuary at Desai General Hospital. "We cannot forget her, still," repeats Sarah, sadly. "What courage she had. That was a horrible death. She led a good life. Her husband was a teacher, they had their own house. But in her time of need, even her adopted son would not come see her," says Sarah.

"It was a waste having so many relatives," Abhipsha adds. "She sent her boy to study engineering, but even he did not come for her."

* * *

After tea, Pradeep patiently instructs a patient's daughter how to change her mother's complicated dressing. At first, the daughter was very anxious, but after Pradeep asked what she is most afraid of—bleeding—and then explained how they could manage it, she relaxed. "So, she's come today to practice one more time with the dressing change. She did perfect last time! Very good last time!" Pradeep smiles warmly, clearly proud of successfully teaching a family member an important skill. "And this is so much better, because they live far away and it must be changed daily and if she doesn't do it then so-and-so will come and charge 100 rupees per dressing change, but now she can do it herself."

Pradeep watches the patient's daughter change the dressing, kindly providing helpful instructions and suggestions along the way. They smile and share a few laughs; the interaction is unhurried and relaxed. The daughter is diligent and careful and listens attentively to all that Pradeep says. What a difference it makes, I think, not to be surrounded by 40 patients, and be able to focus and concentrate on one person.

On the opposite bed, Daya rolls and cuts bandages. A young girl wearing a hijab, sits on the bed helping. She looks up at me and smiles.

"Does she work here?" I quietly ask Pradeep, confused. "No, no, that's Hameeda, a patient," he clarifies. "She's an orphan patient, getting a long treatment for osteosarcoma. She comes and helps us here when she is bored," he explains.

Pradeep is one of the handful of Bachelor's prepared nurses in the hospital; he received his degree in Mumbai and worked for a short period of time in a large, well-known, corporate hospital. Pradeep gets frustrated sometimes due to the lack of understanding about palliative care and the purpose of the palliative care clinic. "Our patients suffer a lot because of misinformation," Pradeep tells me. "Doctors may say to them, 'Nothing is going to happen, everything will be fine. Just go to palliative care and collect the medicines.' But the patient will be bedridden, coming to the palliative care on a stretcher. Do you think it is helpful? No way. His condition is not good. But false hope was given, and tomorrow if something goes wrong we have to face that, not the other doctor. We have to explain to the patient and family, 'this is not the way, this is going to happen.' But they don't agree sometimes. 'Why are you telling me this?' they'll say. 'The doctor we have been seeing, who cost me 2 lakhs[10], told us everything would be okay. Why are you telling us that something is wrong, and he's going to die soon?' They don't believe us."

I tell Pradeep we have the same problem in the U.S., remembering the stress and conflict that too frequently occurred when our palliative care team was asked to see a terminally ill patient who was unaware of their grave prognosis.

All of this is compounded when the palliative care team runs out of morphine and patients have to fill their prescription at another hospital. But this is not easy, and involves time and money. Despite the dozens of corporate hospitals across Dandaka, only two have an even somewhat reliable stock of morphine, and they are often reluctant to dispense their meager supply to individuals who are not patients in their hospital, and who may require large doses. Patients also have to be able to afford transportation back and forth to the corporate hospital *and* be able to afford whatever the corporate hospital charges for the morphine tablets—which is significantly more than SICH. Sometimes patients come from a long distance and they are only able to get a very small supply of tablets. "How can that help them?" asks Pradeep rhetorically. "Nothing! Only morphine for 1 or 2 days. So, in that way we see a lot of suffering, because they will ask, 'What do I do tomorrow? Today I have tablets, but what do I do tomorrow?' That is the main question."

Pradeep fills me in on another strategy they employ: the palliative care department keeps its own emergency supply of morphine, separate from the inventory in the hospital pharmacy. They use this if a patient in excruciating pain needs immediate pain management, cannot travel to another hospital, or afford the cost of buying morphine from a private hospital, or requires more tablets than can be dispensed from another hospital's stock. But it's not a perfect work-around, as sometimes even the emergency stash becomes depleted.

---

10 Lakh: a unit in the South Asian numbering system equal to 100,000, written as 1,00,000.

"Running out of stock, these major things cannot be controlled by a nurse. It is out of our hands," Pradeep says slowly. "Even I am not able to tell you how to express that because it is such a big suffering. We are in the middle."

"In the middle?"

"In the struggle."

Reference

Pallium India. (2014). Narcotic Drugs and Psychotropic Substances (NDPS) Amendment. Available at: https://palliumindia.org/2020/04/ndps-amendment-act-2014-2

2   What We Can Do, We Do

Mistaken for a Spy

Our nurses have learned by experience. They do not get any training in how to deliver chemotherapy. They have no training in how to read protocols. If you see a typical oncology nurse abroad they know how to give chemotherapy, they know everything about sterile technique, they know protocols, they know how to measure and check the correct doses—everybody is checking the dose, the pharmacist checks the dose, the physician checks the dose, 2 nurses check the dose, check the name, this, that. There's nothing like that in place here. Here the nurses are calculating all the chemo doses in their mind. They don't even check if the dose is correct. If I write for 3,500 grams of cyclophosphamide [an improbable and lethal dose of chemotherapy] it is going to be given. How many vials of 1 gram am I going to use? How many grams of 200 am I going to use? Am I going to round it off to a 50 or am I going to round it off to 100? Each nurse does her own thing. Maybe her senior teaches her. And if she's got a good senior she will get a better training. But a lot of it is done in the brain. Will we see those mistakes? I don't know, I don't know. We might be. Since we are in short supply of medicines most of the time I think if anything we give less of a dose than more of a dose. But are they calculating doses incorrectly? They might be. You'd never know. We only think that the patient is not responding to the treatment. Maybe it's because the nurses have given a lower dose and we have no idea about it. There is no way of checking and counterchecks are not in place. For oncology nurses there is no training at all, in the private or in the government sector.

Dr. Rashi, oncologist

Female Ward I has 50 cot-like beds, spaced a few inches apart along either wall. With its high ceilings and open communal space, it has the feel of a cavernous warehouse or airplane hangar. Today the patient census is 65, it can go as high as 100; when that happens, patients double up in beds or sleep on the floor. There are three nurses on duty. Sometimes new admissions are turned away, told to go home, come back tomorrow, or stay somewhere else because the ward is too full.

DOI: 10.4324/9781003413158-5

"How do so few nurses take care of so many patients?" I ask Sister[1] Asha, thinking how I often struggled to care for four or five patients as a staff nurse.

"Family attendants. They are required to have a family member with them to receive treatment," she says simply.

Belying her diminutive stature, Sister Asha is a force to be reckoned with. She is one of a handful of nurses at South Indian Cancer Hospital (SICH) who have a Bachelor's degree and is a Senior Staff Nurse, one incremental, but crucial, step below Head Nurse. I notice her nurses' cap is smaller and prettier—lacy instead of the stiff cardboard white cap the majority of nurses wear. I later learn this is an indication of her Bachelor's education status. All of the nurses on the general wards wear uniforms, white jackets over long white skirts, many of them visibly worn and soiled.

There are three large tables at the front of the massive ward. One serves as the nurse documentation desk, one as the chemotherapy mixing area, and one is primarily reserved for doctors. Multiple ceiling fans whirl slowly high above us. There are no curtains or partitions between beds, and although it is a female ward, there are many males present—ostensibly family members and caregivers of patients. I am astounded by the amount of paperwork; ledgers and notebooks and forms in triplicate, all dutifully filled out by Asha, who is the assigned documentation nurse today and a diligent scribe. Patient charts and files are tossed from table 1 to table 2 to table 3 and then back around again in a seemingly never-ending bureaucratic cycle.

Chemotherapy drugs are carried from the hospital pharmacy ("medical store") to Female Ward I in a battered Styrofoam tub by an elderly ayah wearing a simple blue cloth sari. Small cardboard boxes with vials of Cisplatin, Adriamycin, Etoposide, Taxol, Cytoxan, Vincristine, and Bleomycin[2] are bundled in worn white plastic bags labeled with patient names. Asha tells me there is no formal chemotherapy administration course or certification offered by the hospital; nurses learn on the job, trained by other nurses who also learned on the job.

The table that serves as the chemotherapy mixing area is covered with a white sheet splattered with the unmistakable red stains of Adriamycin and strewn with bottles of IV fluid, uncapped syringes, papers, opened vials, and medical charts. I don't think I am imagining the acrid smell that lingers around the table. Sister Chaaya, a young, sweet-faced nurse, pops the lids off vials of powdered chemotherapy agents, injects saline to mix the powder in to a liquid, then draws up the chemotherapy drug from the vial into a syringe and squirts it in to an IV bottle. It's not clear to me how she knows the proper

---

1 Nurses in India (and other countries as well) are often referred to as "Sisters"; this term comes from the historical context of hospitals serving as charitable institutions staffed by nuns. Nurses on the general wards at SICH used this title.

2 These are all common types of chemotherapies (cytotoxic, cell-killing drugs) used to treat a variety of different cancers.

dose; I don't see her consulting any medical chart nor double-checking any math to ensure the right dilution of the medication. She does not wear gloves, a mask, or a gown to prevent the drug from getting absorbed into her own body, and there is no hood or ventilation system to protect her from inhaling aerosolized particles of chemotherapy. As she mixes the medications, she laughs and talks into her cell phone, which is propped against her ear with her raised shoulder. The plastic IV bottles are scrawled with a black magic marker: "Taxol," "Adriamycin," "Cisplatin," and then handed to a family member to take to the patient's bed. Family members crowd around the desk; some are recruited to help reconstitute the chemotherapy and they take this responsibility very seriously: solemnly rotating the vial back and forth until the saline the nurse has injected into the vial absorbs all of the powdered drug.

I watch Chaaya with her mobile phone crooked to her ear as she continues to mix chemotherapy. Does she understand the risks as she casually handles these drugs? Does she realize these medications are cytotoxic, as in cell-killing? I am tempted to rush over and push her back from the table, "Please, put some gloves on! Don't breathe in this stuff! Refuse to do this! You'll get hurt, this is unsafe!"

And then...?

Once I stop her, mid-syringe pull,...what next? I don't have boxes of gloves to distribute, or chemotherapy gowns, or masks—and even if I did it would be a finite supply. I don't have a way to effectively communicate any of this to her in her native language, not without a translator. Nor any idea how to go about building a ventilation hood or training the entire pharmacy staff how to properly mix the chemotherapy. And if the nurses stop giving chemotherapy, refuse to do it, then *no* patients will get treatment.[3] This is the only government cancer hospital in the entire State. If treatment stops here, these patients get nothing. Is that better?

I turn away, feeling complicit and confused.

* * *

Sister Chaaya, like many nurses, tells me that mixing the chemotherapy is the most stressful part of her job, although she has adjusted to it somewhat over the course of the two years she has been at SICH. When she first came to SICH, Chaaya was overwhelmed by the number of cancer medicines and the different types of cancer. In fact, she shyly tells me she was so frightened

---

3 During my fieldwork, there was a 4–5-day strike when general ward nurses stopped giving chemotherapy; this is discussed later in this chapter. However, the demand was for higher reimbursement from the government for administering chemotherapy, not for personal protective equipment or safer chemotherapy administration protocols. During the strike, physicians gave chemotherapy, still largely assisted by the nurses. After the strike, I did not observe any noticeable changes in how chemotherapy was delivered.

by what she saw of cancer she did not sleep well for an entire year. No one formally trained her, but after about a month of observing senior colleagues, and paying close attention to how the combinations of drugs were ordered by physicians, she felt ready to prepare chemotherapy independently. She confirms that it is a requirement for patients to have a family member present to receive treatment. "Yes, compulsory," Chaaya says, and she goes on to describe in more detail the responsibilities of family members. "When we call the patient's name to give out the medication, if the patient cannot come, the attendants[4] come forward and take the medicines and keep them and give them to the patient. We'll explain to the attendant—'this tablet is for night, this tablet is for morning,' and they'll take the tablets and go. They do the personal activities, like brushing hair, giving the patient a bath, washing their clothes, changing clothes, they take care of all that. And also, if the patient needs a blood transfusion, for example, if blood is not available here, they have to go to other blood banks and obtain the blood. When chemotherapy is given, the patients have problems like vomiting and diarrhea. The attendant should be there to take care of that. If anything happens, if they come and inform us, we will inform the doctors."

Before coming to SICH, Chaaya worked next door at Pillalu Hospital, the large government hospital for women and children. There, she saw more routine surgeries and illnesses, such as asthma, with a much better response rate. "If a patient has a surgery in Pillalu or the general hospital, we feel—'Okay, it is an operation, just a repair and surgery. He has become okay now and he has gone home.' We have that hope. There is no such thing here."

Chaaya particularly remembers a young patient, 25 years old with uncontrolled pain even after being given tramadol (a weak opioid) and Buscopan (an antispasmodic medication to treat stomach cramps) together. He always held his stomach, bent over, walking and crying out—"Amma, *mother*, it is paining. It is paining a lot. It has not come down even with injections. I am not able to sleep." The doctors said to him, "it will be like that for you. You have stomach cancer. You will have pain. We cannot control it. It will be like this for some days. Then, we will operate and remove it. You will have pain." Chaaya shakes her head sadly when I asked if they considered giving morphine to the patient. "The duty doctors will not do that, ever. In the last stage, when there is no hope, the doctors will refer the patient to palliative care, and then the palliative care people will give morphine. They will not give morphine at the start, only at the last stage.[5]"

---

4 Family members are referred to as "attendants," because they are "attending" to the patient in the hospital.

5 This presents a difficult scenario, as many patients in low- and middle-income countries initially present for medical care with advanced stage cancer and significant symptoms. See Brand, N. R., Qu, L. G., Chao, A., & Ilbawi, A. M. (2019). Delays and barriers to cancer care in low- and middle-income countries: A systematic review. *The Oncologist*, 24(12), e1371–e1380.

"Giving the chemotherapy here is *very* stressful," Asha agrees, overhearing our conversation. "We're in so much tension when the patient comes. We'll write the indents,[6] we'll send it to the RMO (Resident Medical Officer), she won't be there, so we do not get the signatures and we have to wait. Meanwhile, the patients come and ask us, 'When are you going to give the medicine? When are you going to give the medicine?' That is very stressful. Sometimes we have to *fight* with the patients. They don't always listen, and they don't understand."

Before I can ask Asha exactly what she means by "fighting with patients," we are interrupted by one of the oncology postgraduates (medical residents, often called PGs) on the ward, a young man named Dr. Raja. He has heard about the American nurse doing research at SICH and tells me he would like to be interviewed for my project. We exchange contact information, but something about the interaction unsettles me.

"Do I need to be concerned about interviewing men for my project?" I ask Dr. Madhu later that afternoon in the palliative care clinic. "I know gender relationships are different here, and I don't want anyone to get the wrong idea."

"No, no," she quickly reassures me. "Everyone here is very professional, they are used to this." The next day I email Dr. Raja to arrange a time for our interview. He decides we should meet over dinner. I decide I should have trusted my gut. I stall.[7]

I notice that all of the patients have peripheral IVs; there are no central intravenous lines that would help ensure safer administration of the chemotherapy. An infusion of Adriamycin is started in a vein on the top of the patient's left hand, a particularly hazardous location. Once it is hung by Asha, she does not go back to check on the patient or assess the IV site.

"Do you worry about extravasation?" I ask Asha, referring to the dreaded complication of chemotherapy administration that involves the leaking of toxic medication out of the veins into the surrounding soft tissue. In its worst form, extravasations can necessitate limb amputations due to the extensive tissue damage. Asha's eyes widen.

"Yes, sometimes this happens," she says in a tone that implies she does not wish to discuss it further.

I ask about allergic reactions, another possibility when giving chemotherapy that requires rapid intervention. Given the layout of the ward, it seems difficult, or impossible, for nurses to detect reactions that may occur in the far corners of the immense and hectic ward.

"We give immediate hydrocortisone and IV fluid," Asha says simply. I jot a few notes in my small notebook as discreetly as possible.

6 An "indent" is a formal inventory request for a supply or medication.
7 I never do formally interview Dr. Raja who becomes an unwelcome and persistent suitor during my fieldwork, until my roommate Joanie intervenes and tells him to back off.

In the afternoon, I sit with Asha and another nurse, Pooja, at the front desk. They both are documenting in separate ledgers. A young family member wearing a bright orange sari and sparkly earrings approaches with a bag of red blood cells. Although I don't understand all that is being said, it seems she is asking when the nurses can start the blood transfusion. Pooja puts her palm lightly on the bag, feels its temperature, and then dismisses the woman with a flick of her wrist. The woman slowly backs away from the desk, but reapproaches a few minutes later: the same thing happens. The third time the woman approaches the desk, Pooja reluctantly opens the patient's medical file and sees an order for "1 packed cells." Asha leans over to inspect the order too; she takes exception that it doesn't clearly state, "*transfuse* 1 bag packed cells." Asha brings this to Pooja's attention, who then again dismisses the woman from the desk, who looks baffled and on the verge of crying.

"What happened? You can't give the transfusion?" I ask, curious.

Asha shows me the order, "Shouldn't it say *transfuse*? What are we supposed to do with an order that says '1 packed cells?'"

I admit that, yes, ideally the physician order should say "transfuse." Asha is clearly bright, and it seems unlikely she doesn't know this; is she being an inflexible stickler for the sake of protocol or trying to prove a point?

"Mmm…but you don't want the bag of blood to expire…," I say slowly, thinking about this woman who has most likely traveled to another hospital in the city to obtain the blood and paid dearly for it.[8] "Maybe you can you call the doctor for clarification?" I suggest gently. I am told the doctor has left and is no longer in the hospital. I look at the woman who continues to stand in front of the nurses, her large doe-like eyes wide and brimming with tears.

Finally, after an awkward few minutes of silence Pooja pushes her chair back from the table, rises, and calls the on-call doctor who says, yes, yes, give the blood transfusion. The woman looks at me, relieved. She waits by the table until Pooja slowly walks over to the medication table to prepare the infusion tubing.

---

8 Even though SICH technically had a blood bank, it did not have a consistent or full inventory of blood products and primarily organized voluntary self-donations prior to planned surgeries. I was told many stories about the severe difficulties obtaining blood products for patients, a common therapy required to combat expected side effects of chemotherapy and treat certain types of cancer. Family members were commonly dispatched to find blood products from elsewhere—a serious investment of time and money—and bring them back to SICH to be administered. One experienced SICH nurse told me: '*One time, another sister and I were going home in an auto[rickshaw]. A small boy, around 8 or 9 years old, asked us to give him a lift in our auto, and we said, yes. 'Where are you going?' We asked. 'To Gandhi Hospital to try to get some blood,' he told us. 'For what purpose?' we asked. He explained that his sister is a patient at South Indian Cancer Hospital, sick with osteosarcoma. 'Where are your parents?' we asked him. 'I don't have a father and my mother is handicapped, that is why I am going to Gandhi Hospital for blood.'* A SICH physician also recounted to me the herculean efforts she made to obtain platelet transfusions for a bleeding patient, including donating blood herself and recruiting her family members to donate on behalf of the patient.

"You see, actually what is happening is we want to be very kind to the patients, but you are observing, no? So many patients. So much stress on us. So, if we want to be kind also, sometimes it is not possible to be like that," Asha says to me.

"Because...?" I probe.

"Because of workload, heavy workload."

***

Pradeep stops me the next morning as I walk by the palliative care clinic on my way to Female Ward I for another day of observation.

"Virginia," he says, somewhat urgently. "There is a problem."

"What? What's wrong?" I ask, concerned.

"The Sisters think you are a spy from the U.S. Government. That you are going to write a report about how badly they are working and all the problems at the hospital."

"What? Really?" I ask.

He bobbles his head vigorously in the ambiguous motion that could mean yes, or no, or sometimes maybe; this time, I fear it is a clear affirmative. I feel my face flush. How did I possibly screw things up so early in the game? I am embarrassed that they are right: I am *technically* from the U.S. Government—my funding is through the Fulbright Program, which is funded through the U.S. Department of State. And based on what I have observed so far, there *are* some legitimate safety concerns. I think back to my earlier meeting with the Nursing Superintendent and her senior assistants—they seemed to understand and be enthusiastic about the project. What happened?

"But I met with the Nursing Superintendent just the other day to explain everything and...," I say defensively.

Pradeep cuts me off.

"They didn't understand you."

I flash back to yesterday on Female Ward I. Did I ask too many questions? Take too many notes? I thought I was being discreet, but clearly, I missed the mark.

This revelation of my perceived status as a spy sent from the U.S. Government creates a flurry of animated discussion between Dr. Madhu, Dr. Amit, and Pradeep. Madhu suggests that the study information sheet should be translated into the local dialect, because it turns out not all of the nurses have as much proficiency in English as I was led to believe,[9] and that a formal

---

9 Prior to entering the field, I made multiple inquiries regarding language proficiency of the general nursing staff. I was repeatedly assured all nurses were fluent in English; however, I quickly discovered this was not the case. Some nurses did not want to admit to being less than fluent in English (as this was a marker of status), and so to normalize language barriers and to ensure I fully understood what was being said, I invited the translator to all formal interviews.

meeting needs to be held for *all* the hospital nurses to let them know about the project and clear up any misunderstandings. This seems so painfully obvious in hindsight, and I am deeply embarrassed. Pradeep and I walk immediately to the Nursing Superintendent's office: she is not there, but a Senior Assistant Nurse is. She is all smiles, compliments my outfit, introduces me to her son and daughter-in-law who are visiting. She certainly doesn't seem upset by me or my project.

While Pradeep talks with her briefly in rapid Hindi, I notice a sign posted in the office: a list of ten rules of etiquette for the nursing staff written out in fancy cursive script:

(1) You should be courteous to all. Be gentle and polite in your talk;
(2) You should greet your seniors;
(3) You should address the seniors with proper title;
(4) Excuse yourself with over-talking a senior person;
(5) Maintain silence whenever and wherever necessary;
(6) Keep your dress neat and tidy;
(7) While on duty never use any form of jewelry;
(8) Obey seniors without arguing;
(9) Be punctual always;
(10) Say "excuse me" even if you hurt others accidently.

The Senior Assistant Nurse sees me reading the sign. "My own handwriting!" she says proudly, smiling. I can't help but smile back.

"It is very nice," I say neutrally.

"Yes," she says, smiling beneath her enormous winged white cap.

* * *

"What did she say?" I ask Pradeep quietly as we walk back to the palliative care clinic.

"She said the Nursing Superintendent wants additional documentation that your study has been approved."

"But I gave her everything I have! The Institutional Review Board approval, the ethics committee letter, a letter from the Indian Government…"

"Yes, yes, but what we can do?" counters Pradeep, echoing a common idiom I will hear frequently over the coming months. Dr. Madhu tells me not to take it personally. "It's just internal politics, Virginia. And you have to remember, they are not used to a nurse doing research. It is the first time."

Within minutes, Dr. Madhu, Dr. Amit, and I are dispatched to the Director's office for additional damage control. We are shown into an air-conditioned office where the SICH Medical Director sits at the end of a long, wooden boardroom table, looking over some papers. He smiles, friendly and encouraging. I show him the project summary and consent form, which, theoretically, he has already seen since he had to sign off on it months ago. Dr. Madhu interjects and explains the misunderstanding by the nurses.

The Director shrugs and doesn't seem terribly concerned. "Sometimes the nurses over-react. They bring their personal problems to work," he says matter-of-factly. "You should go live with one of the nurses in their home so you can understand their domestic situation; it flows into their work situation!" Everyone laughs, but I take his comment seriously.

"You should spend time with nice, cooperative nurses in the beginning; get them to trust you first." I swallow, nod, thinking that's what I thought I was doing.

"But...," the Director pauses. "You could not have picked a better place to do your study," he assures me. "You see, the experience of pain in poor people, is very, very different than the experience of pain in rich people," he says knowingly, taking off his wire-rim glasses, massaging the bridge of his nose with this thumb and index finger and looking straight at me. "There is much, much to see here and you will go home with a wealth of experience. Take full advantage of this opportunity."

"I will," I say, and I mean it.

We return upstairs to the palliative care clinic. While I was meeting with the Director, Pradeep apparently went back to the Nursing Superintendent's office. He delivers the verdict: no meeting with the nurses will take place soon—the upcoming Diwali festival and the regular bandhs[10] (strikes) apparently make scheduling a meeting too complicated. "Maybe next month?," he ventures optimistically. I sigh, thinking of the consequences of this unanticipated delay. Dr. Madhu and Dr. Amit say not to worry, we will have food and invite the nurses to the palliative care department on Monday to smooth everything over.

I email one of my mentors to lament my situation; his answer is simple: *For goodness sake, STOP taking notes in front of them.*
So I do.[11]

* * *

Outside of the hospital, my two Indian flatmates, Joanie and Ruma, are actively preparing for Diwali and invite me along to the Old City to purchase some new items for the apartment. I met Joanie and Ruma through a series of convoluted but fortuitous connections during the early days of my fieldwork, when they were eager to find someone to share the expenses of their

10 Bandh, originally a Hindi word meaning "closed," is a form of protest and civil disobedience used by political activists in South Asian countries such as India and Nepal. During a bandh, a political party or a community declares a general strike and often expects the general public to stay at home and not report to work. Most affected are shopkeepers who are expected to keep their shops closed, as well as public transport operators of buses and cabs who are expected to stay off the road and not carry passengers. During my fieldwork, a separatist movement within the State became active, resulting in episodic riots, protests, and bandhs.

11 After this incident, I did not stop taking notes altogether in the field, but I did stop being so obvious about it. I used strategies such as retreating to the bathroom, one of the few private places in the hospital, to jot down notes or conversations into a much smaller notebook or texting myself key phrases and reminders on my mobile phone, which was discreet and not seen as disruptive.

two-bedroom apartment and I was desperate for a place to live.[12] Both Joanie and Ruma are forging nontraditional paths, as young, single, professional Indian women living alone and far from their natal families. Despite their admitted reluctance to rent a room to an American, which they divulged after I moved in, I am grateful for how graciously they have welcomed me into their home and lives.

Joanie buys me a coconut from a roadside vendor who deftly whacks the top off the furry nut with a machete and pops in a thin, overly flexible green straw so I can drink the sweet liquid from its center. After I finish, Joanie instructs me to hand the coconut back to the man who then slices it completely open and hands it back, so we can scoop out and eat the slippery, white innards. We wander through an impossible labyrinth of crooked and narrow alleyways packed with colorful shops leaning into each other like falling dominos, shops selling fruit, sparkly bangles (rigid bracelets) and decorative bindis,[13] pots and pans, reams of cloth, heaps of brilliant yellow and orange marigolds.

On the way home, the auto[14] chugs its way up a moderately sized hill; it sputters and strains until finally the driver says something in Hindi to Ruma and Joanie. Words are exchanged. Ruma nudges me. "Get out, we have to get out." Confused, I exit the auto. Ruma and Joanie start to walk up the hill, as the auto moves along beside us, markedly less stressed.

"We had to get out so the auto could make it up the hill?" I ask incredulously.

"Yep," Ruma says.

"And look, now he can get up the hill just fine," Joanie says dejectedly, upset that our combined weight was too much for the auto to handle.

"Really?" I say, erupting into laugher. But I am the only one who thinks it is funny.

At home, Diwali preparations continue, which primarily involve Joanie cleaning like a mad woman. She wants the sheets changed, the curtains washed, floors scrubbed, the kitchen reorganized. I'm slightly confused as to why they don't ask Lakshmi, the housekeeper they have gone to great lengths to hire, if she will help with some of this, but I am quickly told the maid doesn't do heavy cleaning.

"Just the other day, we gave her the rupee test," Joanie explains. "Ruma left 10 rupees out and it wasn't stolen." Apparently, though, this is only weak evidence of trustworthiness and Joanie tells me they now will have to up the

---

12　In the beginning of my fieldwork, I had an exceedingly difficult time finding a safe, reasonably priced place to live close to the hospital as most landlords did not want to rent to a single, American woman due to fears related to sexual promiscuity and general impropriety.

13　A common forehead mark (often a red dot) traditionally worn for religious reasons or to indicate a woman is married. Bindis are also worn by women regardless of their marital status for cultural or religious reasons or as a fashionable adornment (sold as press-on stickers).

14　Auto is short for "autorickshaw," open-air, three-wheeled motorized vehicles that serve as taxis in India.

ante. "Now we'll leave more—100 or 200 rupees. It can be an expensive loss, but then at least you know—this person is honest, or not." I ask what happens if the money goes missing. "Well, then we'll just tell her we no longer need her."

Joanie explains that Diwali is a celebration of wealth and success, and it is a very auspicious time to play poker, gamble, or invest in the stock market. "Oh! It is beautiful, Virginia! Beautiful! You will *love* it! Lots of candles and lights and fireworks. And we'll do puja, give offerings to the gods, mostly Lakshmi, the goddess of wealth."

Although this puja comes with some strings attached: once you bring an idol in to your home, it demands constant attention; it is not like a crèche that you bring out at Christmas and then pack away in the attic, forgotten about until the next year. "It's complicated, Virginia," Joanie explains. "If I bring in Ganesh or Lakshmi, flowers need to be offered, incense burned. I cannot forget them!"

* * *

Sister Agnes is an eloquent and soft-spoken nurse who wears wire-rimmed round glasses and smells pleasantly of what I can best identify as a combination of vanilla and soap. We meet in the Early Detection Clinic, where she is rotating through an assignment to assist with colposcopies. When I arrive, Sister Agnes, a gynecologist, and four medical students are behind a partition tending to a woman who is having a pelvic exam performed. After they are finished Agnes greets me, wearing her nursing uniform and a cloth mask that covers her nose and mouth.

I wonder how far the patient had to travel for this test and how she was convinced to have it done.

"Well, there were no patients scheduled, so there was no one for the students to observe. So, they found an attendant, a family member here, and motivated her to come and get the test," she explains. "She was *very* nervous," Agnes volunteers. "*Very* nervous," she reiterates, her body language emphasizing the woman's reluctance, which resonates with a concerning hint of coercion. Agnes assures me that if the test is positive, patients are followed up and that even the poorest people have cell phones and so can be contacted. I try not to think about the possibility that the woman was cajoled in to having a test she did not want for the sake of medical education,[15] and if it is positive, will never know.

---

15 Some nurses expressed concern that medical trainees practiced unnecessary or harmful procedures on vulnerable patients. During one interview, a nurse at SICH told me how she tries to prevent elderly patients with a poor prognosis being taken to surgery: "*Here, PGs [postgraduate, medical residents] experiment with patients for experience. Now, if patient is of a young age, they may live for sometime if they undergo surgery. But older people, 80 or so, they do for experience. I will tell 'no.'*" A related scenario is described in the article by

Agnes cleans up after the procedure and then says she has to complete documentation. She produces two large ledger books: one is an expenditure book, the other an injection inventory log. The injection inventory log is a list of all parenteral medications given and stocked on Female Ward II. Essentially, it is a manual Pyxis[16] system and pharmacy requisition accounting system that requires Agnes to copy information from one log book to the other, and then fill out corresponding pharmacy requisition sheets. Agnes confirms that the hospital pharmacy maintains their own records of the same information.

She dutifully transcribes patient identification numbers from the expenditure book into the injection inventory log ledger. Her soft eyes trace the numbers across the page as she keeps her place by moving her index finger slowly underneath the scrawl. I am saddened to see this smart, caring, and motivated nurse with so much potential reduced to paperwork. After watching her work for a while, I can't help but ask how she feels about it.

She pauses, and lets out a small sigh. "Boring," she says. "It's *boring*."

"I bet," I say sympathetically.

Agnes first worked as a nurse at a well-known private dental hospital. She was rapidly promoted to Junior Administrator and offered a position with an international medical team that performs oral surgeries to those in need. Agnes loved that job, and worked with the organization for almost two years, traveling around the world. Then, she got married and accepted a position at SICH. The dental hospital was very disappointed when Agnes did not return to work there after her international assignment.

"I had to consider my family, my husband, and my in-laws. The decision was not mine to make," Agnes states simply.

Agnes is still documenting when another nurse approaches and says she needs the expenditure ledger. Agnes hands it over. After it disappears, Agnes says, "Well, there's not much else we can do now." We walk to Female Ward II to find the chemotherapy log book which apparently needs some additions, but this ledger has been taken to get the signature of one of the chief oncologists, so it is also currently unavailable. Agnes looks a bit at a loss. I gently ask her if she would be willing to give me a brief tour of the hospital, since I really have only seen one part of the hospital so far—the female oncology wards and the palliative care clinic. She kindly agrees and off we go.

Agnes leads me through an area of the hospital that is significantly darker with lower ceilings that I assume is the older part of the building, but later

---

Mayra et al., where a participant describes the obstetric care of vulnerable women in India: "Everyone looks at her as someone you can perform cases on. They see that this is a case in my logbook … they want to give an episiotomy so one can get an episiotomy repair done and write about it in logbook" (p. 6).

16 A type of automated medication dispensing and inventory system common in many American hospitals.

learn is actually the newer section. We walk through the narrow corridor of the outpatient clinic area on the basement level, which is packed with people lining the hallways, sleeping on mats and sharing chairs. I am shown the pathology department, the blood bank, the radiology wing, and the operating theaters—which are separated from the waiting crowd by a glass door and green curtains. The high-dose radiation waiting area consists of a collection of chairs in an open-air corridor situated amongst crumbling construction.

Behind the radiation rooms, dozens of families and patients have set up temporary camps under a partly sheltered portico. Territories are staked out with blankets and mats laid edge-to-edge on the dirt and the minimal possessions of the displaced—a plate, a mug, a bag of rice. There is a large communal bathroom with a flooded floor that charges 2 rupees to enter. Agnes tells me the patients and families are too poor to travel back and forth for daily radiation treatments, so they spend weeks, sometimes months, living under the portico.

We pass a "Department of Informatics" which surprises me, given the mounds of paper documentation I have seen. I ask Agnes about it; she isn't really clear what the purpose of the department is, and suggests that it was active for a while, but is no longer in operation. Curious, I peek into the open door of the office. Two dusty central processing units are crammed in a corner and a man sits at a desk typing into his mobile phone.

I spend the rest of the day with Agnes on Female Ward II, similar in layout to Female Ward I, but with slightly fewer beds. I watch as Agnes and another more senior nurse sit at the table and dutifully copy and record information from the patient's medical file into a series of oversized ledgers: the Diet Book, Expenditure Book, Admission Book, Chemotherapy Log Book, and Shift Report Book. Later, Agnes shows me a stack of about 20 other ledgers, used to record and log a variety of facts and details, such as medication tablet inventories.

"What happens to all this information, Agnes?" I ask, hoping that it is compiled for a productive purpose, given how much time and effort the nurses devote to it. She shrugs and tells me when a ledger is full, it is sent and stored in the archive room and a fresh ledger is issued.[17]

* * *

Dr. Madhu has organized a Diwali celebration for the pediatric patients who are too sick to go home for the festival. That evening in the hospital parking lot about 50 patients, siblings, parents, and curious neighborhood children gather and are given sparklers to wave and small flower-pot firecrackers are

---

17 I observed an incredible amount of documentation performed by nurses during my fieldwork, a practice with historical roots in the bureaucracy promulgated during British colonialism. The majority of this documentation had minimal relevance to patient care or outcomes.

lit which spin around frenetically on the ground before shooting unpredictably upwards with a whimpering whine. We stand in a circle, the sulfur smell
of unleashed pyrotechnics wafting above us in the cool evening air, and the
glow from sparklers held by small hands illuminating the shiny bald heads of
children receiving chemotherapy. After the celebration, everyone crowds into
the pediatric playroom where small bags of salty snack mix and milk sweets
are distributed. The children laugh and smile, and I am struck by how many
of the children are male.[18]

I do notice, however, one female patient who looks to be about seven years
old. Everything is too big for her: the white plastic chair she sits on, the dark
sunglasses that dwarf her face, her bright yellow and blue dress. Her father
leans over her, tenderly helping her open her bag of snack mix. She slouches
in the chair, as she tentatively eats her milk sweet. Dr. Madhu catches me
looking at the girl, leans over to me and whispers,

"That's Neha," she says. "Two children have recently lost their sight."

"Retinoblastoma?" I ask, referring to a type of eye cancer that most commonly affects young children and can cause loss of vision. Dr. Madhu nods.

Kate is present for the celebration in the pediatric ward, too, and confirms
what I hear from others multiple times during my fieldwork: SICH is the last
stop for every patient, even the poor ones. They all go somewhere else first to
try to get cured and then they have no money left. Kate tells me that's what
happened to Neha's parents: they are destitute now, her father was a teacher,
but is no longer able to work and he sleeps outside, homeless, under the hospital portico, hoping his daughter will get well.

* * *

After the pediatric party, Paul, the one other Fulbright fellow currently in
Dandaka, and I shop for fireworks. All along Road Number One, distribu-
tors have sprung up, hawking their impressive array of pyrotechnics under
expansive tents festooned with colorful electric lights. We stop at Krishna
Crackers where table after table is stacked with boxes of fireworks printed
with crazy names and even crazier pictures: "Classic Bomb!" depicts two
cherubic white children in blue overalls hugging each other. We pile fireworks
into a bucket: Rainbow Torches, Platinum Rain, Red Coconut, Sky Wheel
Rocket, Color Bursts, Parachutes, Coronation Rockets, amazed at the selec-
tion, the cheap prices, and the lack of any obvious safety restrictions.

Later that night on the rooftop terrace of my apartment building, we decide to test out a few of the fireworks. Talk turns to the pervasive hierarchy
of Indian society and how everyone seemingly has their place, so securely,

---

18 I was told during my fieldwork that this was due, at least in part, to families with limited
financial means prioritizing the care of male children, who are traditionally more highly
valued and seen as able to contribute more to a family's prosperity.

so firmly, so absolutely, and we wonder if we, too, will start to see people differently.

"It's already happening to me," Paul admits.

"Really?" I ask, as I embarrassingly think how over the past few weeks each time I see Hasan and Noora, the watchman's children who live under our building,[19] I associate them immediately with the basement and am acutely aware when they come upstairs to help with some task that they are not where they normally are. It alarms and frightens me that soon I may even start to think: where they belong.

"I think part of it is that there are just so many people around you, all the time," Paul says. "Think about buying fireworks tonight. How many people were helping us, following us around the store? Fifteen? Twenty? It's impossible to address everyone politely, 'No, I don't need any help. No, I'm fine, thank you. No, I don't want that.' If you did that, you'd just be engaged in conversation all the time—constantly. So, you have to ignore some of them."

And that doesn't feel good, we both admit.

"Do you think if we lived here long enough, we'd start to behave the same way?" I pour the last bit of wine into Paul's glass. He purchased the bottle earlier from a sketchy roadside liquor store behind iron bars surrounded by a gaggle of men.

"Maybe," he says thoughtfully. "But maybe because we're not from here, it's not as ingrained, we know a different way."

Paul lights another Coronation Rocket that takes off improbably high and then explodes in a shower of green stars.

***

The official night of Diwali arrives. Joanie and Ruma wear gorgeous, colorful gowns, and Hasan and Noora are summoned upstairs to help prepare the house for the celebration. Joanie looks especially radiant in a cheerful canary yellow salwar suit which is a striking contrast against her dark raven hair. Ruma fills dozens of small clay pots, diyas, with oil, places a thick, waxy wick into each pot, and arranges them strategically around the apartment, particularly around doorways and the puja[20] table that she and Joanie have set up. As we light each diya, one by one, the room takes on an increasingly soft, yellow glow. I help Ruma arrange marigolds and purple aster petals in beautiful designs around the puja alter and front entrance. Sweets and fruit are offered to Ganesh and Lakshmi in a solemn ceremony while traditional

---

19 Many buildings in India have a designated "watchman," who is charged with monitoring the comings and goings of individuals, deliveries, building maintenance, trash collection and recycling, and helping tenants with various tasks. In this case, Hasan and Noora's father was the watchman and he lived with his family in a grim small concrete structure in the basement/garage of the apartment building.

20 Puja (or pooja): offerings and prayers as part of ritual worship of Hindu deities.

Indian music plays on the computer. A red bindi is marked on each of our foreheads, pressed with a grain of rice.

We then proceed to light an incredible amount of fireworks from the roof-top, as do all the households around us. Fireworks, one after the other, mushroom into a kaleidoscope of color overhead and snap and snake ferociously and erratically along the ground. I've never seen such a protracted, loud, and potentially hazardous display of fireworks. It seems part celebratory, part war zone, with the smoke and deafening noise.

Later that night as the festivities finally draw to a close, I am reprimanded when I begin to pick up the paper garbage strewn about the terrace, remnants from the exploded fireworks. "They'll clean it up, Virginia," Joanie and Ruma admonish, gesturing toward Hasan and Noora. "You mustn't spoil them," Joanie whispers to me. I swallow, stare at her. I don't even know how to respond. But Paul, who has overhead Joanie's comment, does: "Don't listen to her, Virginia. You spoil those kids like crazy. Like *crazy.*"

Tinnāvā?

The higher authorities need to know what nursing care really is, and what is a nurse.

Sister Meena, general ward nurse

You wouldn't believe it, I struggled a lot. I see these patients here, and if I feel any pain, if my child gets a fever, I feel frightened—I think, 'is this cancer?' When I started working here, I thought—'what is this cancer? It comes at any age, old, young or children of 2 or 3 months of age, in the pediatric ward. Why is this happening to so many patients?' I was shocked to see so many patients. And they would tell us—'he was okay till just yesterday; he returned from school just the day before; he was okay. He said he had leg pain, then he got fever, and we brought him to the hospital and now he has leukemia.' I thought—'Just in two days, does it go to that stage? Even now, I still have that fear...But still, I feel sad all the time here when I see the patients...They have pain mostly. They cannot breathe properly. Also, when they are given chemo, they have vomiting, vomiting, vomiting. If it is lung cancer, they have cough, breathlessness, and they are dyspneic [short of breath]. They cannot sleep. They make sounds all night. If they have stomach cancer, they have stomach pain. Because they have cancer, even if we give pain killers, it is relieved only for some time.

Sister Chaaya, general ward nurse

After delays due to festivals, room scheduling conflicts, and bureaucratic hurdles, it is finally time to formally introduce myself to the entire hospital nursing staff. Up to now, I've mostly been spending time with the palliative care clinic staff and Sisters Asha and Agnes.

A few minutes before I am scheduled to start speaking, a senior nurse approaches me and asks bluntly, "I am a diabetic patient, also with high blood pressure. Can I take herbal therapy?" I am caught off guard by her question, but I want to be helpful—and credible. She is unable to tell me exactly what herbal therapy she has been taking but says she has been feeling better the past few months. I hedge my bets and tell her that diabetes and high blood pressure are important conditions to be monitored, but without more information, it is hard for me to advise her about what is the best therapy. I tell her that herbal therapy isn't my area of specialty, and that the herbal therapies they have available in India are different than what are available in the U.S.

"Oh, I thought you would know this information," she replies, clearly dissatisfied with my answer, and doing little to hide her disappointment with my underwhelming response. She takes her seat and begins whispering to her colleague. I imagine what she is saying: *Nurse from the U.S. who knows nothing! What a waste of our time!* This does not seem like an auspicious beginning.

A total of 25 nurses attend, with some trickling in at the very end. Having Mayank by my side—the calm, articulate law student Dr. Madhu recommended as a translator—is invaluable; the nurses do not know him and he is neutral and objective and I feel confident he is delivering my message accurately and thoughtfully. The nurses laugh when I smile and emphasize that no one is required to talk with me; it is completely voluntary. But, suddenly, with this one statement, the nurses want to talk: hands fly up and mouths open: *"Will you share the knowledge with the Director so change may arrive?"* *"Do you know we are mixing chemotherapy in so much of a dangerous way?"* *"When will you come visit our ward, Madam?"*

Reassured and optimistic, I hand out study information and consent forms, along with my business card and mobile phone information, and then we relocate to a small conference room next door for samosas and chai, which savvy Jasmine, the SICH administrative coordinator, suggested I offer after the meeting. The nurses devour the spicy vegetable samosas and drink the tea. Some paper cups have fallen from the table to the floor, and as we are preparing to leave the conference room Jasmine calls to someone down the hall to dispatch someone else to clean this up. Once I realize what is happening, I say, quickly, "Oh, I'll get it, it's no problem," and bend down to pick up the crushed paper cups. But Jasmine grabs my forearm, pulls me upwards before I can pick up all of the cups. "Ma'am, no, no!" She slaps her open palm against her forehead and shakes her head. She and Mayank break into laughter. "We have people to do that!" Mayank says.

I shrug, smile uneasily, and toss the cups I have managed to collect into the garbage can a few feet away.

***

"Veerginniaaa!" Joanie sings in her lilting Hindi as she walks into the apartment later that afternoon. "Have you eaten yet?" When I tell her no, she says, "Let's have some of this fruit!" She hands me a piece of mysterious produce. I turn it over in my palm.

"What is this? It looks like an artichoke."

"No, no! It's a custard apple. The most delicious fruit you will ever taste!"

I admit that I've neither seen, heard of, nor eaten one.

"Here, you do like this," Joanie instructs, gently pushing up against the bottom of the fruit until its segments split open at the top. We pick out the soft, pale, yellow flesh, eating around the black dewdrop-shaped pits.

"This is *amazing*! I've never tasted a fruit like this," I gush. "It's delicious…it tastes…," I pause, working the delicate flavors in my mouth, "well, sort of like a pineapple."

Joanie wrinkles her nose, disapproving of my comparison. "Umm…I don't think you have had pineapple in a while. You're just saying that because it rhymes, custard *apple*, pine*apple*."

I shrug. "Maybe." (When I later introduce custard apples to Paul, he makes a much better assessment: "This is no fruit, Virginia. This is a *pastry*!")

"You must eat the seasonal fruit here. You *must*. It will keep you from falling ill," Joanie advises. We finish the custard apples and Joanie retreats for a nap. "Don't drink any water right away," she cautions. "Why not?" I ask. "You'll catch a cold." As I try to make sense of this unusual advice, Joanie pauses and turns back to face me. "Oh, and we *must* wax your arms," she says randomly. "It is the first thing Ruma and I noticed about you."

"What? Really? The first thing?" I ask, more incredulous than embarrassed. No one has ever accused me of being particularly hirsute.

"Oh, Veerginia…," she says, visibly repulsed as she inspects my arm. "We *must* do something about this! We *must*. Only the *most* deprived in India, *villagers*, do not remove this hair…everyone is noticing. You cannot have that here in India. We will take care of it tomorrow." And then she disappears into her bedroom.

As promised, Joanie takes me to the Chinese Women's Beauty Parlor down the street and I pay the equivalent of 2 U.S. dollars to have my arms waxed, much to Joanie's relief and my amazement. My virgin arms are rapidly and simultaneously assessed by a young Indian girl and an elderly Chinese woman, who mutter to each other in words I cannot understand.

The extent of my problem established ("not good"), a blue bowl on a rolling metal tray—the kind one sees in an operating room—is produced from the back room, and they descend upon my arms with concerning zeal, one focusing on the left, the other the right. Spreading hot wax with small spatulas up and down my arms, they press white pads to my flesh, and then vigorously tear them off. *Rip, rip, rip.* Joanie looks on approvingly, examining their progress and occasionally directing the shop owner to redo an area: "Auntie, here, this needs more." *Rip, rip, rip.* On the walk home, I can't stop rubbing my hands over my arms, marveling at their new silky smoothness.

"You must do this when you get home, back in the U.S.," Joanie instructs.

"Well, it's pretty expensive in the U.S. and not as convenient."

"Yeah, yeah I know. Here, there is a Chinese Beauty Parlor in every lane. It's not like that in the States."

"You've been to the U.S.?" I ask, curious.

Joanie hesitates. "Umm, yes. Actually, Virginia, I lived there. For one month, outside Boston."

"Really? I didn't know that."

"Yeah. I don't talk about it much." I nod and do not press, but Joanie continues. She lived in Massachusetts for a month while she was married—a fact I also did not know, assuming she was single and never married, like Ruma. "I got divorced 4 years ago." Joanie relates this fact casually, but her voice, which wavers and hesitates, belies the trauma of the experience.

"It was an arranged marriage. I met him once before we got married, he seemed like a nice guy, and I married him. Five days after the marriage, he left for the States, for a job, and the plan was for me to join him there," she explains. He stalled for a painful year. "And when I finally went there, after 1 month, he sent me back to India." Joanie links her elbow with mine as we cross Road Number 14 and turn left on to our unnamed street. We fall silent, listening not to each other's voices, but now to the fringed palm fronds and banana leaves rustling high above in the evening breeze, the close-by staccato barking of dogs that punctuates the dusk that falls gracefully, like the draping of a chiffon sari. "Twenty-eight days later he sent me back," she repeats sadly. I don't have the heart to ask why, and I suspect that even she is unsure.

"Is getting divorced in India difficult?" I ask.

"No," Joanie says, quickly. "Not if you don't ask for anything."

Safely ensconced back in our apartment, I share my own demoralizing tale of divorce and she listens intensely. "Getting divorced, it is not looked well upon here. People will judge you," Joanie warns, looking directly at me with her flashing silver eyes. "Yes," I say, feeling the burden of her story, heavy and cumbersome like the loads of wood men heave onto their thin backs or the jugs of water women balance improbably on their heads and carry through the streets of Dandaka.

"I was so humiliated. I felt like such a complete failure," I say to Joanie who lingers in the doorway of my bedroom. My voice chokes with more emotion than I intended.

"I guess some things are universal," Joanie says, and I see her eyes soften and swell, pregnant with her own tears about to fall.

***

I show up at 8 am to meet with Sister Asha to finish our interview, as she requested. We started yesterday, but finding a quiet and private place to talk had been impossible, and the impressive amount of ambient noise and constant interruptions forced us to stop. When she asked me to come early the following day, she said, "No one will be here then."

And she is right. As I wait for her, I realize there are no nurses on the ward. The ayahs are there, cleaning, and I am in their way. In an effort to not be underfoot, I squeeze myself behind the break room door, but still manage to get inadvertently splashed with antiseptic flung vigorously from a plastic mug on to the floor, which is then later swept with a short-handled straw broom toward small holes in the corridor wall which serve as ad-hoc drain spouts. The smell of the antiseptic cleaner is overpowering. I hear a patient moaning toward the back of the ward. Most of the family attendants are not on the ward; they are out in the front parking lot of the hospital by the adjacent temple getting food. I saw them this morning, standing grim faced in a long snaking line, tin plates and tiffins in hand, waiting to be filled with heaps of free rice.

After the nurses arrive, the day starts with a familiar question: "Tinnāvā?" (Have you eaten?)[21]

While still unsure as to the culturally appropriate answer to this question, I am beginning to sense that the correct answer may be "no," because if I say "yes," the nurses seem skeptical and disappointed, and when I say "no," they gleefully ask me to join them, which I do. I am generously fed rice and roti and a variety of spicy curries. They are completely intrigued by what I eat, who cooks for me, that I like spicy food, and that I am vegetarian. I, in turn, am amazed by their generosity, culinary skills, and pleasure they seem to take in feeding me. Before eating, I go to wash my hands. The one sink for the 50-plus bed ward does not have running water today, so next to it is stationed a blue jumbo-sized plastic trash can filled with water and a small plastic mug floating on its surface. I lather my hands with a pink bar of soap carefully squirreled away in one of the cabinets and then use the mug to rinse with water from the trash can.

---

21 A local phrase translated as "have you eaten?" or "did you eat?" In the beginning of my fieldwork, I misinterpreted this common greeting as a literal question. As my fieldwork progressed, I came to understand it was often asked in a way more akin to the generic American greeting of "how are you?" to which one does not necessarily expect, or even desire, a factual response. However, there were times when I was asked this question and sensed the nurses wanted me to say "no" so we could share a meal together, or when I answered "yes," and they probed with additional follow-up questions to more fully understand what I had actually eaten, as if they *did* actually want and expect a detailed response. A colleague conducting fieldwork in North India during the same time period related to me a similar experience, where residents would greet her with the phrase, "where are you going?" to which she initially replied with a literal answer until she also discovered that this was intended as a generic greeting to which a detailed and honest reply was not expected.

The nurses eat first, before the ayahs. I am slow and finish last, so while I am still eating the ayah creeps into the small break room and squats on the floor, her sari gathered in folds around her knees. I gesture to one of the multiple empty plastic chairs at the table, but she ignores me and continues to eat her meal on the hospital floor.

After breakfast, chaos ensues when the doctors arrive on the ward to make their rounds. Patients and family members crowd around the table where physicians sit sifting through charts that are thrust at them haphazardly by the undulating mass. The ward is packed.

I follow Sister Pooja as she is dispatched to administer the medications and insert IVs. We stop at each bed that has a visible pile of syringes and IV bags at the patient's feet, where she inserts an IV if the patient doesn't already have one and gives the medication to the patient lying in the bed. We do not consult any charts, and there is minimal, if any, conversation with the patient or family member, who is typically hovering close by. Pooja's aseptic technique is erratic or absent. She wears the same pair of gloves as she moves from bed to bed down the impressively long row of patients, the one nonworking sink further and further away. Bloody, used needles are left on the edge of patient beds, their sharp ends exposed like miniature bayonets. Family members sometimes clean this up and dispose of the needles (where I am not certain) or hoard them by the bedside. Without the benefit of curtains or hospital gowns, female patients must pull up their saris, loosen their blouses, and expose their buttocks for injections in the presence of men they do not know.

I see an ayah adjust the flow of a chemotherapy infusion for a patient, and a family member disconnect a bottle of Adriamycin from the intravenous tubing full of red fluid and spike the saline flush bottle. Sister Asha sits at the documentation table close by and observes what is happening; she nods, and gestures for the family member to proceed.

***

Across the hall, on Female Ward II, I am again greeted by the now-expected, *Have you eaten?* and the familiar follow-up questions: *How old are you? Are you married? What is your salary in the U.S? When do you go to church? Where do you stay? Can you take me to America?* I do my best to answer succinctly and honestly and change the subject.

Female Ward II has 40 beds, the census is 63. Dr. Rama, a professor of radiation oncology, sits down at the physician's table with two of her residents and invites me to join them. Her long, dark, thick hair is tied back in a low ponytail, and she emits a calm, stately, healing energy that contrasts with the chaos swirling around us. The perspective from the table is positively claustrophobic: above us, and on all sides, we are surrounded by patients and family members thrusting charts and papers toward us, pressing closer. Dr. Rama and her residents talk quietly and calmly to each patient and family member, flipping through charts and making notations, making eye contact, smiling, and occasionally even laughing.

As a radiation oncologist, Dr. Rama not only administers radiotherapy to patients with cancer, but is also trained to give and manage chemotherapy for certain tumors, like breast, ovarian, and head and neck.

There are so many patients I ask Dr. Rama how she possibly attends to everyone. "I separate out who is really sick, who needs the most attention," she says, referring to the rapid triage process many of the doctors have told me they follow, a survival skill quickly honed to cope with the massive influx of patients. But there are dilemmas in identifying those that are really sick, especially when patients need services they cannot afford, or are simply unavailable: the patient with chest pain who may be having a heart attack—but there is no cardiologist in the hospital after 2 pm[22]—or the patient who is bleeding from her rectum and urgently needs a transfusion of platelets. When the latter happened, Dr. Rama mobilized family members, and even donated herself, to keep the patient's platelet count at a safe level for ten days. "Suppose if we had a full-fledged blood bank with all the blood components…," she says, wistfully. Accepting a patient's death from incurable cancer, that's one thing. But when a patient dies due to a complication or treatable condition? Well, that's a different level of frustration. In the end, the staff make do with what resources are available—and compromises are made. "In that compromise, sometimes we will lose," Dr. Rama concedes. "Losing the patient without proper treatment is really very painful for us sometimes."

* * *

I'm grateful Sister Meena is one of the medication nurses, as it is getting tedious watching nurses copy information into ledgers all day. Meena has been a nurse for 30 years and worked in Kuwait at one point in her career. She was also a senior supervisor at one of the most prestigious corporate hospitals in Dandaka. Like many, she pursued a government position at SICH for the job security, superior salary, and excellent benefits, and became a nurse due to family pressure. "I wanted to do higher studies," Meena says, 'but, my father told me to do nursing. So, I joined as per my father's wish, at an age when I did not know anything!"

Meena moves around the ward in her white uniform and slightly tattered white cap pinned to her curly hair, which is swept into a bun at the nape of her neck. She has a round face and kind eyes that crinkle at the edges when she smiles. White stockings peek beneath the open toes of her white sandals. She doesn't seem content to be bored and I see her taking initiative when she is finished one task, seeking out another, or helping others.

---

22 It is common for many government-employed physicians to run clinics in the afternoon at private hospitals/clinics.

Sisters Gowri and Meena mix pre-medications and chemotherapy at a furious pace; at one point, I try to visually follow the path of one syringe—from the opening of its package to ultimate disposal—but it proves impossible with the flurry of activity. Glass ampules are snapped open with a well-practiced, forceful downward *whack, whack, whack* with scissors or Kelly clamps, the jagged pointed tips scatter on to the floor, some near the trash bin, some not. Dozens of IV bottles are lined up on the cluttered table in assembly line fashion, jabbed with a needle to provide a vent, and frantically injected with a combination of Decadron (steroid), Kytril (antinausea), and Rantac (antacid). It's unclear to me how Meena and Gowri keep track of which bottles they have injected and which still need medication. The process seems simultaneously haphazard and rushed, and yet formulaic and mechanized. Gowri and Meena pause only occasionally to verify the medications they are mixing against the patient's case sheet (doctor's orders form) in the chart. Family members crowd around the table and Meena admonishes them to move back, *give us space to work*. Earlier in the morning, Meena called hospital Security because family members were "bunching up around the doctors," which apparently they don't like. Security showed up 45 minutes after Meena's call and did little except walk authoritatively around the unit.

Both Gowri and Meena wear gloves, but the same pair the whole time, and they are plain latex gloves, not the thick rubber hand-to-elbow ones I remember being required to wear when handling chemotherapy. Adriamycin squirts on the table as the chemotherapy is rapidly drawn up from vials in to syringes and I notice Meena's gloves are covered in red stains. At one point, another nurse steps in to help; she has been doing documentation because Meena tells me she is pregnant and cannot stand for long periods of time. The pregnant nurse does not wear gloves or a mask and begins mixing Taxol.

Both Gowri and Meena mix drugs as a team for an hour, then they split up. Gowri continues to mix drugs, while Meena starts medication administration. Meena moves from bed-to-bed, patient-to-patient, inserting IVs, hanging premedication, giving chemotherapy. She works steadily from 11 am to 2 pm with only a short five-minute break for tea.

Over thimblefuls of milky, sweet chai, Meena confides to me. "Ma'am," she leans toward me, conspiratorially, "Sisters, we know the right way, proper way. Keeping things clean, safe needles, we know. In training, in books, we know this. But it is not done here." She shakes her head, makes a soft, clucking noise: *tsk, tsk, tsk*. Meena chalks this up to lack of supervision and protocols, and the strong sentiment among government nurses that they cannot be fired. "Government employees think, 'No one can do anything to me. They cannot expel me even if I do something wrong.' But in private jobs, it is not like that—if you make a mistake, they will fire you, dismiss you."

Perhaps because I am observing or perhaps simply because this is how she works, Meena diligently and carefully administers medication. She carries one square-shaped metal bin for clean supplies and another in which she places all used needles, syringes, and cotton. Meena is the most careful nurse I have seen with sharps: she doesn't leave them on the patient bed; she carefully collects them all in the metal tray and disposes them in a red trashcan at the front of the ward.

Meena is working hard. Her forehead and upper lip bead with perspiration as she starts IV after IV for chemotherapy. I look over to see Head Nurse Hema positioned at the front of the ward, slouched in a wooden wicker-backed chair with her eyes closed, chin propped in her cupped palm, her right arm and elbow extended like a triangular wing on the front table. I resist the urge to go over, shake her out of her stupor, and demand that she help.

Meena starts about 25 IVs for chemotherapy. As we examine arm after arm, hand after hand, she encounters the same challenges oncology nurses everywhere face—fragile, damaged veins, infiltrated lines, edematous limbs. She inserts either a butterfly needle, securely taped down, or an IV cannula, "if the patient is receiving a vesicant," she says astutely.

Meena is unfailingly patient as she moves from bed to bed, caring for the sick individuals curled in the cots and the family members who hover over them, pointing out possible IV sites. If she is annoyed or frustrated that she is working solo while her colleagues leisurely eat lunch, she does not show it. We encounter one patient whose veins are so delicate that Meena does not have a small enough sized IV cannula. Meena writes down what is needed and the patient's young daughter, who looks about 12, is dispatched to buy it at a local medicine shop. When the daughter returns with the appropriately sized IV catheter, Meena deftly inserts it. One patient in her 50s is deaf, mute, severely developmentally delayed, and cannot walk. She has terrible veins, and after three failed attempts Meena tells the family attendant that the patient must go to the OT (operating theater) for an anesthesiologist to put in a line.

Meena has to give two injections—one IV (intravenous, into the vein) push and one IM (intramuscular, into the muscle) injection—to a nine-year-old girl, Priya, who I am surprised is not on the pediatric ward. Priya howls in pain when Meena pushes the medication in to her vein, while her mother strokes her forearm tenderly. Meena makes no attempt to comfort or distract the child, she simply tells her to turn over, injects the second medication into her buttocks, and quickly walks away. When we are in the middle of the ward, a family member approaches Meena and tells her the patient's first IV bottle is empty. Meena tells him to get an ayah who will change the bottle.

Finally, at 2 pm we have finished. I am exhausted. And all I've done is shadow Meena. Meena tells me that tomorrow will be easier because the IVs are already in place.

* * *

The following morning, Sister Meena and Head Nurse Hema sit at the front table, documenting: Sister Meena diligently transcribes information from the patient case sheets to the chemotherapy indent book; Head Nurse Hema idly flips through one of the ledgers and then stares off blankly into space.

Patients and attendants approach the table and are intermittently ignored, swatted away, or addressed briefly with minimal eye contact as charts and ledgers are tossed around and plopped down on the table. One young woman approaches the table and asks when her sister's medication will be administered; no one responds. The nurses stare straight ahead as if no one has spoken. They are frustrated that family attendants relentlessly ask the same questions, over and over—*when will they get their medications? When will they be cured? Why did their medication not come yet?* "The patients and attendants know the situation, we have already told them!" the nurses tell me. "But they still go from one sister to the next and again they will ask the same question to a different person. They keep asking, over and over."

Meena is kind enough to let me follow her again as she administers medication to the far row of beds in the ward; Gowri takes the other row. Meena isn't as careful today in handling sharps. She can't be because today she only has one tray, Gowri is using the other. Meena partially or completely recaps used IV needles, but they are left on the patient's bed and attendants are told to throw them away. The attendants seem a bit confused about what to do with the used needles; most take them to the communal bathroom in the hallway and dump them in a blue trash bin.

Meena is called over by one of the ayah's to check a patient's foley catheter. Apparently, the ayah inserted it earlier that morning, but is concerned about its placement since no urine is draining from the tube. This is the one time on the ward I see a small green curtain partition around a patient's bed, but it isn't adequate to provide full privacy and the ayah yells at a male attendant who is standing too close. The patient with the problematic catheter is lethargic and does not seem particularly concerned about what is happening between her legs. Meena beckons me over. "I think it is in the vagina. The urethra is deeper," she says. She removes the errant catheter, adds more lubricant and reinserts it—this time into the correct orifice. Urine immediately fills the tubing and drains into the bag. I try not to think of the urinary tract infection this woman may get due to the lack of sterile technique, but I am nonetheless impressed with Meena's ability to correct the catheter and the initiative she took to remedy the problem. It occurs to me that this is really the first proactive nursing task I have seen so far on the general wards.

As the shift wraps up, it is again Meena who remains behind to wait for the evening shift nurse to arrive. While she and I talk, another day shift ward nurse, her uniform removed and transformed back to her saried-self, emerges from the break room and begins talking harshly with Meena. It is clear Meena is being reprimanded. Meena hangs her head and mumbles, "Sorry, sorry." After the other nurse leaves, I ask, awkwardly, "Is everything okay?"

"Yes, ma'am. She was just saying that I do too much, helping there, helping here. I need to learn to share the work with others."

"She was saying you are doing too much, doing more than your fair share?"

"Yes, ma'am."

Meena folds her hands in her lap and looks down, embarrassed.

Privacy at a Price

Nothing happens physically, but mentally, I feel something like depression. Now, the patient will be there. When I come the next day, the patient will not be there and he died, I feel sorry.

Sister Nalini, general ward nurse

My first uncensored thought as I enter Female Ward III is that this must be where the stray cats roaming the hospital urinate. The acrid smell of ammonia is pungent and overwhelming as I make my way to the nurses' documentation table where the now-familiar line of questioning begins:

How old are you? (*They guess 29, I let it stand.*)
Are you married? (*'Not yet.' They are incredulous.*)
Is your ring platinum? (*'No.'*)
Had your breakfast? (*'Yes, thank you.'*)
What did you eat? (*'Cereal, coffee, a banana.'*)
When do you go to church? (*'Well, um, it depends…'*)
Can you take me to America? (*'You'd be really far from your family, that would be difficult, no?'*)
What is your salary in the U.S.? (*'Enough to be comfortable.'*)

These frequent, persistent, rapid-fire sessions always peter out with the distinct and uneasy feeling that I have fueled further disappointment and frustration by so inadequately providing the personal information the nurses seek.[23]

---

23 This pattern of persistent questioning resonates with a passage from a memoir about an Australian woman who falls in love with an Indian man and begins a new life in Mumbai:

> *In Indian culture there exists an overwhelming compulsion to classify and rank people based on certain qualities. The way a person is treated in India is very much based on their position in society and the power it affords. Upon meeting someone, the first thing an Indian will do is determine that position, and act accordingly. This is one of the reasons why they ask so many intrusive questions. 'What does your father do?' 'where do you live?' 'are you married?' 'do you have children?' 'what's your qualification?' and even 'how much do you earn?' are all questions aimed at uncovering a person's social standing. Caste, which is usually revealed by a person's surname, has, in the past, been the overarching factor. These days, it's not enough to make an accurate assessment. Other factors also taken into consideration include occupation, relationship status, skin colour, ability to speak English, and whether the person has any important connections. Ultimately, it's money and looks that count the most.*
>
> (Sharell Cook, *Henna for the Broken-Hearted*, 2011, pp. 255–256)

Female Ward III is purely a surgical unit with 55 beds in three different wings. It is a unique unit because no chemotherapy is given. Four sisters are posted on Female Ward III: three government nurses—Sister Eliza, Head Nurse Badari, and Sister Indira, and one contract nurse, Anjana. It becomes clear that good-natured and hard-working Anjana is getting the short end of the stick—she provides almost all of the patient care (which essentially involves giving out medications), while the other nurses sit at the nurses' table, occasionally writing in the ledger books. Anjana mixes and administers medications, and she seems to make a concerted effort to keep herself busy. Her interactions with the patients are kind and gentle. In contrast, Sister Indira scolds a family member for not standing up when the doctors walk by during rounds, while I watch the ward ayah remove a child's IV.

At one point, a 12-year-old girl with a renal mass admitted for surgery stumbles into the nursing station with her parents. She looks petrified. Her father tentatively asks Sister Eliza a question. Eliza makes fleeting eye contact, does not get up from her chair, but says something quickly, gesturing to them to go next door to the preoperative area. Sister Eliza, who does 20 minutes of actual work during the six-hour shift, looks so incredibly bored I actually feel sorry for her. She is clearly smart, but her face and demeanor radiate disinterest. Again, I see nurses wearing the ubiquitous face mask, even though they are sitting in the nurses' station, writing in ledgers, far removed from any direct patient contact. Curious, I ask Eliza, "Why do you wear the masks?" She looks at me condescendingly.

"Chemotherapy, to protect ourselves."

"Yes, I know. But here—on the surgical ward, when you are not giving chemotherapy, why do you wear the masks?" She looks at me as though she has serious concerns about my intelligence.

"This is a surgical ward. Open wounds here."

I nod, even though this doesn't make sense from an infection control standpoint.

These interactions are further contextualized within Isabel Wilkerson's compelling non-fiction work, "Caste: The Origins of Our Discontents" (2023, Random House), which discusses parallels between the caste system in India, the rise of the Third Reich in Nazi Germany, and the Civil Rights movement in the U.S.:

> Indians will ask one's surname, the occupation of one's father, the village one is from, the section of the village that one is from, to suss out the caste of whoever is in front of them. They will not rest until they have uncovered the person's rank in the social order.

(p. 175)

My interpretation of the repeated line of questioning I experienced at SICH—and it happened almost every day, sometimes multiple times a day, up until the very last day of my fieldwork—is that the nurses were attempting to evaluate where I stood in the social order. As a white, female, middle-aged unmarried American without children or a clear family lineage, in a low-status profession but with advanced education, I likely presented quite a puzzle.

"And smell. Bad odors," she adds as an afterthought.[24]

* * *

"Your parents? They are responsible for you?" asks Eliza, as I look through a medication ledger.

"I'm not sure what you mean."

"Your education, your marriage?"

The other nurses at the table listen to our conversation intently. "No, no, they are not," I say. "Well, they helped pay for school when I got my Bachelor's degree, but otherwise, no."

She arches her eyebrows. "And marriage?"

"No. They are not responsible for that either."

They are incredulous. "No dowry?"[25]

"No, no dowry."

"Free? Free to marry?" Eliza asks again, disbelieving.

"Yes. Where I am from there are no arranged marriages."

"Just love matches?" Indira giggles.

"Yes, love matches." I pause. "Although, some have more love than others!" I say playfully. This elicits a round of hearty laughter.

They ask me to draw a map of the U.S. and point out where I live, where my sister lives, where my Mother and her husband live. I try to explain that my Mom remarried after my father died, but they seem confused by this. They are appalled at how far I live (Arizona) from my sister (Pennsylvania) and my Mom (Virginia), and equally shocked when I tell them I left home after college and have been living independently since.

Promptly at 2 pm, Sisters Badari, Eliza, and Indira leave Female Ward III. Anjana is left to wait for the evening shift nurse, and I have a feeling this is the norm. She is a willowy girl with a homely, elongated, oval face, and eyes set a bit too close together to be pleasing. She takes out her phone and shows me a series of pictures of her family and friends, and then asks to take my photo. After she snaps my picture she giggles, and confides, "I call you 'The

---

24 Again, it is important to contextualize the wearing of masks pre-COVID-19 pandemic. During my fieldwork, many nurses and staff members wore face masks in the hospital when there was no clear clinical indication to do so and did not wear masks when it may have helped (e.g., while mixing and administering chemotherapy). Oftentimes, the masks seemed more of a way to create additional distance between patients and nurses and served as a visual reminder that patients were unclean and smelled badly.

25 The payment of property or money a bride's family gives to the groom's family upon their marriage. Traditionally, a dowry was intended to provide the bride with their own financial assets and security within the new family. In my experience, however, dowry was viewed as an incentive for a groom's family to assume the "burden" of the bride and to ensure a high-quality groom. Dowries have been technically illegal in India since 1961, but the practice persists. See Families are at war over a wedding tradition India banned decades ago, CNN, 2021.

Laughing Doll.'" Her joy and laughter is contagious and, fittingly, I cannot help but burst out laughing too. She waits until 2:30 pm and when the evening shift nurse still hasn't arrived, she stands up abruptly and announces, "Time to leave now."

And so we do.

* * *

Needing a break from the drudgery of Female Ward III, I walk up one floor to the Elysian Fields of the hospital: Paying Wards. Here sits the pleasant faced and plump Sister Nalini. Her seniority has earned her the plum position of a permanent posting on the Paying Wards while she waits to be promoted to Head Nurse. There are ten beds, two rooms are private, the rest semiprivate, and the cost is 500 to 300 rupees per day, respectively. The rooms are dingy, poorly ventilated, and isolated. The only obvious advantage is that it is quieter with more privacy than the general wards below.

But this privacy comes at a cost: Dr. Rashi told me that Paying Wards is the most dangerous place in the entire hospital, isolated on the third floor and frequently left unattended. "Sometimes in the evenings and nights there is one nurse for all of Female Ward III, Male Ward III, and Paying Wards," she said. Patients on the paying wards have to pay for everything out of pocket. "So, if you're septic with a blood pressure of 40, but don't have the money on you for the saline, well, you're in trouble."

There are two patients now on Paying Wards, but one is still in the Intensive Care Unit (ICU). The other patient is a male palliative care patient. I talk with the granddaughter of the patient who is in the ICU. She is a lawyer in Dandaka and it is her 83-year-old grandmother who had surgery for uterine cancer. They are paying 500 rupees (approximately $10 U.S. dollars) per day for a private room. She tells me that they were referred to SICH for the expertise of a particular surgeon, and she has found the physicians "very nice" and feels her grandmother has received good care at the hospital. It wasn't difficult for them to secure a private room—they simply asked the DMO (duty medical officer) for a private paying room. "We are grateful to have it because the general wards have major sanitation problems with only one shared bathroom," she says in her soft and gentle voice.

Sister Nalini seems kind, but tremendously bored. Even though the much more favorable nurse-to-patient ratio (right now, one nurse for one patient) would certainly allow it, it doesn't appear that patients in the Paying Rooms receive specialized nursing attention. I spend two slow hours on Paying Wards without seeing any interaction between Sister Nalini and the one patient or the patient's attendant. Instead, Nalini helps the ayah clean out and organize some of the metal storage cabinets in the break room, her ample behind situated on a cot, peeling an orange in an impressive, continuous curl of rind, while she instructs the ayah who squats on the floor what to keep and what to throw away. Afterwards, Nalini then sets to work repairing one of the ledger books by re-gluing and re-taping the cardboard spine that has split apart.

Nalini admits that her job can be depressing. It's upsetting to give chemotherapy to a patient one day, and then come back the next day and find out the patient has died. But it doesn't help to dwell on the inevitable: "In 1 or 2 hours, it will become routine again," Nalini says pragmatically. Before leaving Paying Wards, Nalini pinches me—hard—on my right cheek, and tells me, not to worry, she will find me a good Indian husband.

***

The next day at lunch, in the palliative care clinic, the nurses are transfixed by the food I pull out of my bag. I know from past experience at this midday communal meal that the group will generously feed me, but I am having a hard time eating rich Indian food three times a day, and more importantly, I am feeling guilty consuming so much of their own food. So today I produce a sandwich, a container of apricot yogurt, and an apple from my bag. They all watch, fascinated. Hindi flies around the small room. They insist I peel apart the two pieces of wheat bread and they each dubiously inspect the peanut butter inside.

"You know about the nursing strike?" Dr. Rashi asks me, after the group has finished their thorough investigation of my lunch. Laughter erupts. I can't tell if they are making a joke or if they are serious. They are serious. Apparently, as I have been sequestered on Female Ward III, where no chemotherapy is administered, the government nurses throughout the rest of the hospital have been refusing to give chemotherapy for the past four days.

"Really?" I ask incredulous, thinking about the flyers I recently distributed around the hospital advertising the chemotherapy class I am scheduled to teach next week. Since arriving, I'd been peppered by the nurses with questions about cancer—*What causes it? Is it ever curable? How is it treated? How does it kill people?* After realizing how little oncology training and education the nurses receive, I asked the Nursing Superintendent for approval to teach some classes—a lengthy, bureaucratic process, but one that finally resulted in permission granted and a room reserved. Almost all of the nurses expressed concern about administering chemotherapy, so teaching an "Introduction to Cancer and Chemotherapy Administration" class seemed like the logical place to start. The nurses happily took the flyers, smiled, nodded, told me they would come. No one mentioned they were not giving chemotherapy. I panic, fearing a connection will somehow be made between my class and the nurses' refusal to give chemotherapy, especially since I clearly stated on the flyer that part of the class will be about chemotherapy safety.

"What about the patients?" I ask, the distress in my voice obvious. Everyone is still laughing, but I don't get it. Why is this funny?

"I told them, 'That is good. No one should get chemo here. The quality of life will be better for the patients,'" Dr. Rashi says sarcastically. "Pediatrics too?" I ask, confused.

"No! Not my lovely Sisters," Dr. Rashi says, smiling at the pediatric nurse seated next to her and patting her on the shoulder.

"The doctors are giving the chemotherapy," she explains. I look over at Dr. Madhu. "At least they didn't strike AFTER the class," I say, seriously. Dr. Madhu giggles.

"Virginia is going to give out hand sanitizers to the nurses who attend her class and … " Madhu says. Rashi interrupts and says cynically, "Don't waste your money on the government nurses. Give them to me!" Again, the group roars with laughter.

I leave the room a little traumatized. Clearly, the rift between the government nurses and the rest of the hospital is even deeper than I realized. I stop by Female Ward I and see Sister Asha. She is in the middle of adjusting a bottle of chemotherapy. Maybe the palliative care team was mistaken, maybe there is no strike after all? Asha approaches me and we clasp hands, she smiles at me warmly.

"I've been on Female Ward III," I start. She nods, she knows. "I just heard there is a strike and nurses are not giving chemotherapy. Is this right?"

"Yes, yes, that is right."

"For how long now?"

She pauses, considers. "Umm, 4 days."

"Who is giving the chemotherapy?"

"The unit doctors. The nurses want more money from MHS to give chemotherapy."

"But," I point to the infusion I just saw her adjusting. "That is Adriamycin. You are giving that?"

"No, duty doctors are giving," she clarifies.

"I hope it gets resolved quickly." It's all I can think to say. She smiles at me as I leave the unit, confused and strangely discouraged.

* * *

Female Ward II is abuzz with activity. I see two nurses making a bed—the first time I have witnessed this. Head Nurse Hema is actually out of her chair circulating around the unit, doing what I am not exactly sure, but she is moving. I sense that all of the nurses are making a concerted effort to look busy. They have identified so much of their role with the administration of chemotherapy I wonder what they are left with without that task.

I spot Meena and Agnes and hope they can shed some light on the situation. Agnes looks very stressed and barely says hello to me; she snaps at patient attendants who crowd around the table. I ask Meena about the strike. She tells me it is because the doctors are not giving the required 10% from the MHS to the nurses for administering chemotherapy. I try to find out who ordered the nurses to strike—the Superintendent? A Union? Meena shakes her head vaguely. I'm also unclear with whom, exactly, the nurses are upset—the physicians? The government? MHS? The Director? And what exactly are they seeking? Meena isn't sure either.

The PGs (medical residents) are administering the chemotherapy since the nurses are not. Meena and Agnes stand at the medication table, assisting. I feel badly for the residents—have they ever been taught how to do this? All the residents I have ever met in a U.S. hospital would have no idea how to mix or administer chemotherapy. There is an unexpected tenderness and sweet camaraderie in watching the nurses help the physicians. The strike seems like an odd formality as I watch Agnes hold up the IV tubing, tell the resident how to prime the line, and basically do everything except draw up the chemotherapy into the syringe. The nurses seem to want to help the doctors; they are not simply sitting idle and watching the doctors do the work. The PGs work calmly and slowly; they wear masks and gloves. I stop one of the PG-3s and ask her how it is going. She doesn't understand why the nurses are striking either. "Really, they just said, 'the nurses aren't giving the chemo, so now you have to do it.'" She sighs. "It is hard, because I have so much other work to do and this takes a lot of time," she laments.

I see one nurse lead a physician to the bedside and help him insert an IV for chemotherapy. I even see Dr. Rama pitch in and step up to the chemotherapy mixing table. She doesn't seem bitter or upset as she starts proficiently cracking off the end of ampules with a Kelly clamp.

I observe this strange non-strike strike for a while. On my way out of the hospital, I peer back into Female Ward I. I see three nurses crowded around the chemotherapy mixing table. They are laughing and smiling, helping one of the PGs mix chemotherapy. I recognize the PG—it's Dr. Raja, my ill-fated suitor whom I attempted to interview—and he is laughing and smiling too. It's contagious: I smile as I walk down the hall. This has to be the happiest strike ever.

***

The strike continues, and I remain somewhat fuzzy as to the details. The next morning, I find Pradeep in the palliative care clinic and I ask him what is really going on. He explains—as I suspected—that it is all about money. Apparently, the government gives a percentage of reimbursement to physicians for providing cancer care and a smaller cut of that goes to the nurses within the hospital. Pradeep adds a slightly different spin, telling me that the government nurses do not want any of their "cut" to go to any nongovernment nurses, that is, contract nurses, palliative care nurses, or pediatric nurses. He leans against the doorframe of the clinic and tells me this is the first strike like this, where nurses are refusing to give chemotherapy.

"We are being careful to stay out of this," he says. "Once this is done, we will go and request a special incremental, the contract nurses. See, they don't understand the work we do," Pradeep continues. "They think because we are not giving chemotherapy, we are not working. They don't understand the maggots, and wounds, and pain control, and procedures. They say because we are not giving chemotherapy we don't deserve any of the government funds."

I head over to Female Ward I to see how things are going. The PGs are mixing the chemotherapy, again assisted by the nurses. I see Sister Asha and ask her take on the situation. Her story is similar to Pradeep's. "See," she says writing on a piece of paper, "The physicians, they get 100%." She writes "100%" out slowly in clear, blue penmanship.

"We are only asking for *10%*." She writes 10% in slanted blue script below the 100%.

Another nurse, Praveena, whom I don't know well, joins our conversation and starts aggressively asking me questions. She is persistent and criticizes the Hindi I mangle.

"Enough," Asha finally shushes. Praveena asks me if I am married. I say no. She says something quickly to Sister Asha.

Asha says, "Oh, I thought you were married." I shake my head no.

"Any children?"

"No. Maybe when I get back from India," I say with what I hope is a convincing and optimistic smile.

Praveena isn't finished: She asks if I can take her to the U.S. for a job, how much salary I make, if I drive my own car, what I ate for breakfast. And she wants details— where I live now, what type of house I live in in the U.S., who cooks my dinner. She is surprised when I tell her I drive my own car in the U.S. "No driver?" she asks, disappointed. I tell her that having a cook, a maid, and a driver is uncommon in the U.S. except for the very rich.

Finally, Asha rescues me. "You are being interviewed, no?"

"I feel like I am at a police station!" I say, laughing, trying to keep a sense of humor about the interrogation.

Just when I think I've completely ruined any chance for rapport, Praveena compliments me on my salwar suit, maroon satiny pants with a dupatta of the same color, and a black and white kurta. She looks me over, critically, then peels the red bindi off her own forehead and affixes it firmly to mine with a press of her thumb.

"There!" she says proudly, taking a step back, looking me over approvingly.

I leave Female Ward I, happy, until I pass Head Nurse Hema in the corridor. Glancing at me, she zeroes right in on my forehead. "Why are you wearing that? Christians should not wear bindis," she admonishes me sharply.

I smile, shrug, and leave it.

A few days later the nurse strike ends. I am told the nurses will now get 20% of the MHS money for giving chemotherapy, even more than they asked for.

* * *

The chemotherapy class is scheduled to start at 1 pm. No one shows up until 1:30 pm and I know they won't stay much, if at all, past 2 pm. I focus on the basics, and try to talk quickly, but clearly, and still allow time for translation. Esha, my new translator, a retired woman who is friends with one of the palliative care department volunteers, seems to be doing a good job, but I suspect by her lengthy responses, and the smattering of English words I catch, she is adding her own interpretation.[26] Esha has the loving face of a kindly grandmother, and her hands flap endearingly by her sides as she speaks. When she puts on her glasses, her already owllike eyes get even bigger. I asked her to come because I know that many of the nurses do not understand English well, and even the ones who do sometimes have difficulty deciphering my accent.

At the end, a nurse stands up and says, "What can happen to us if we are giving chemotherapy?"

I try to answer her question as honestly as I can, acutely aware that personal protective supplies at the hospital are limited or simply unavailable. I tell her that these are serious drugs and they need to be handled carefully to reduce the risk of unnecessary exposure.

"Remember," I say, "the chemotherapy is for the patient, not you!"

Adishree, from the ICU, stands up and announces her throat is sore, her hair has fallen out, and she is always tired: is this from giving chemotherapy?

Another nurse pipes up. "The doctors told me there is no problem giving chemotherapy and it doesn't matter if we are exposed. Is this true?"

Before I can respond, Agnes says that *all* the nurses who give chemotherapy at the hospital have problems with their hair thinning.

I struggle to respond to their rapid-fire questions, stumbling over my responses, and talking in circles. I feel like I am failing. I want to protect these nurses, but OSHA[27] guidelines (specific regulations that dictate how chemotherapy and hazardous drugs are handled in the U.S.) are completely unrealistic here. Somewhere there must be middle ground?[28] And while it

---

26 This is a good example of the influence of gender. My first translator, Mayank, was a superior translator but culturally problematic as an unmarried male interacting with me as an unmarried female. Esha, although not quite as good of a translator, was much more culturally acceptable as a married woman spending time with me and the other female employees I interviewed.

27 Occupational Safety and Health Administration; a governmental agency in the U.S. that sets standards for workplace safety.

28 Chemotherapy guidelines for low-resourced settings do exist; see https://www.paho.org/hq/dmdocuments/2014/safe-handling-chemotherapy-drugs.pdf. However, even they are often unrealistic based on available resources and cultural norms (e.g., the expectation family members assist with chemotherapy administration). See von Grunigen et al. (2022 March). The safe handling of chemotherapy drugs in low- and middle-income countries: An overview of practices. *Journal of Oncology Pharmacy Practice*, 28(2), 410–420. https://doi.org/10.1177/1078155221995539 for a discussion of the persistence of unsafe chemotherapy handling practices.

is true they don't have the right masks, gowns, gloves, or ventilation hood, I can't confirm any definitive links between their symptoms of sore throats and hair thinning and potential chemotherapy exposure. I flounder, trying to explain this. I wait for the Nursing Superintendent to interject, but she remains silent.

I finally stop talking and a nurse asks, bluntly, "Can we leave now?"

"Yes, of course," I say. "I hope this was helpful."

The nurses smile and laugh and seem satisfied with the small bottles of hand sanitizer and the candies I distribute. At least they came.

* * *

That evening I meet Paul for dinner. I tell him about the chemotherapy class, about my fear that I botched an opportunity. "It feels so complicated. Like I said not to re-cap needles,[29] put them directly in the designated trash bin. And now I'm wondering if that even makes sense. It makes sense at home, but does it make sense here? I don't know."

"Because they don't have proper sharps bins, do they?" Paul asks, referring to the sturdy plastic boxes in U.S. hospitals designed to safely discard used needles and syringes.

"Exactly. No, they don't."

"So," he says, "who empties those trash cans? That poor person could get stuck with uncapped needles. I guess it depends on who you want to protect. The nurses or the people who empty the trash or the general public who will sift through the trash after it leaves the hospital?"

I think of the young children Paul and I saw squatting in a large trash heap in Chennai sorting through the garbage, syringes glinting in the sun by their small, bare feet.

"Maybe it's actually better that nurses *do* recap needles here, you know? If kids or other people are going to be in the trash, then we don't want them to get stuck either." I sigh. "I don't know, Paul. Everything is turned around here. It's like every suggestion that seems logical back home doesn't work here, doesn't translate. Solving one problem seems to create another, bigger one. It's like a domino effect of problems."

We both sit in silence, turning this complexity and its implications over in our minds. As I consider my next planned set of observations in the intensive care unit, I feel anxiety rising, along with an equal measure of hope that perhaps it will be different.

---

29 Recapping needles is generally considered an unsafe practice as it increases the risk of the nurse being stuck (punctured) by a used needle which can expose them to blood-borne pathogens.

References

Brand, N. R., Qu, L. G., Chao, A., & Ilbawi, A. M. (2019). Delays and barriers to cancer care in low- and middle- income countries: A systematic review. *The Oncologist*, 24(12), e1371–e1380.

Cook, S. (2011). *Henna for the broken-hearted: When the search for meaning takes you all the way to India*. Sydney, Australia: Pan Macmillan.

Mayra, K., Matthews, Z., & Padmadas, S. S. (2022). Why do some health care providers disrespect and abuse women during childbirth in India? *Women and Birth*, 35(1), e49–e59.

Pan American Health Organization (PAHO) and the World Health Organization. (2013). Safe handling of hazardous chemotherapy drugs in limited resource settings. Washington, DC. Available at: https://iris.paho.org/handle/10665.2/28554

Sood, A. (July 31, 2021). Families are at war over a wedding tradition India banned decades ago. Available at: https://www.cnn.com/2021/07/31/india/india-kerala-dowry-deaths-intl-hnk-dst/index.html

von Grünigen, S., Geissbühler, A., & Bonnabry, P. (2022). The safe handling of chemotherapy drugs in low-and middle-income countries: An overview of practices. *Journal of Oncology Pharmacy Practice*, 28(2), 410–420.

Wilkerson, I. (2020). *Caste: The origins of our discontents*. New York: Random House.

3 If We Don't Shout, They Won't Listen

If we don't shout, they [family attendants, patients] won't listen. They push and shove and want their patient to be seen, 'We want that, we want this.' I say—'you first must sit. The doctor will call you. Why are you behaving like this?' If we shout at them, then they will be okay; but sometimes they will come back and shout at us. I say—'Why? The sister is seeing patients; the doctor is seeing patients. Why are you getting upset? Sit there.' Then they sit. If we shout at them with anger, then they listen. If we shout normally, they won't listen. If I make an angry face and shout at them, then they will sit. I tell them, 'I have told the doctor, I have given your file and told that you have pain. We gave you a tablet. What more do you want?' I scare them by saying—'the doctor will scold you. He won't see you.' Then they will sit.

Radha, ayah

As a nurse...one thing we find is that we should give full comforts ... it's not only medications. Even like, psychological, and social and spiritual, we would like to give complete freedom to the patient. We would like to satisfy them, do what they are expecting...so, would like to give them, it is my desire...But now I am praying, that, "Lord, [help] me treat [them, patients]. Give full strength. Because You gave me good job, so I would like to fulfill what You are expecting." Daily, I'm praying. Because sometimes I failed in ICU. Yeah, that makes me a little bit sad in my heart nowadays. We should be completely perfect...that time, I'll pray to God, "Lord, I failed in this matter. It makes me hurt." So. [Crying] That means, what God expects from me, as a nurse, so I should fulfill 100% [Crying].

Adishree, ICU nurse

I descend into the darker, more cramped, and markedly less well-ventilated part of the hospital to shadow Adishree in the Intensive Care Unit (ICU). Adishree greets me warmly and enthusiastically. She is an experienced ICU nurse; before coming to South Indian Cancer Hospital (SICH) she worked in the ICU of a large corporate hospital. "Everybody always asks me, 'why are you working here? You could go to another hospital!' No, no, no, no. I decided to work here only, because I want to help others in need," Adishree says, definitively. The

DOI: 10.4324/9781003413158-6

green epaulettes stitched with bright yellow lettering S.S.N.S. (Southern State Nursing Service) provide a vivid contrast against her white uniform. She is petite and her quick, dark eyes shine like onyx. Adishree is very curious about my project, what information I am seeking, my clinical background and training. The head nurse of the ICU is much more interested to know if I am Christian, where I am staying, and what I am eating.

The ICU is an austere, narrow, ten-bed unit, with small, high windows that are sealed shut. The air feels stagnant, and the lack of cross-ventilation felt in the open-air wards upstairs is conspicuously absent. Almost all patients after surgery pass through the ICU and stay for an average of two to three days before being transferred to the general wards. It is exclusively a Surgical Intensive Care Unit (SICU). I ask what happens to medical, nonsurgical patients who become critically ill. "There's not many options for them," Adishree explains. "The prognosis is very bad, so they are managed on the ward." The ICU has two ventilators and Adishree tells me that patients on the ventilator stay longer, sometimes for weeks.

The three shifts are the same as the general wards (8 am–2 pm, 2 pm–8 pm, 8 pm–8 am), but the staffing is better: three to four nurses on days, two on evenings, and two on nights. And the ICU nursing staff, a total of nine nurses, do not rotate to the general wards—they remain in the ICU. Patients are attached to basic vital sign machines, but there are no IV pumps or complicated cardiac monitors. There is one sad looking sink at the very back of the ICU in the utility and supply room, but the faucet isn't working, so similar to the set-up on other wards, water is scooped from a large bucket with a smaller mug to wash hands. A communal towel is kept at the front of the ward.

A group of surgical doctors begin rounds, moving from bed to bed to assess patients, and Adishree joins them. "Come observe!" she says, gesturing me to follow. She is assisting a doctor who is trying to insert a nasogastric (nose to stomach) tube in to a patient with head and neck cancer as a way to provide supplemental nutrition. The patient lies flat on his back as the doctor inserts the tube roughly into the man's right nostril and tries to push the tube down the esophagus and into the man's stomach. The man reaches out, and Adishree does her best to comfort him. Adishree places a stethoscope over the patient's stomach to verify placement: she shakes her head "no." After two tortuous, yet unsuccessful, attempts, the tube is yanked out of the man's nostril and the physician announces that the patient must go to the operating room to have it placed. A basin of fresh blood lies under the patient's gurney and the attending surgeon wearing a lovely sari brushes against it with the tip of her open-toed sandals. After the team moves on, the ward boy[1] reattaches a portable metal crank to the end of the bed and elevates the patient's head.

---

1 A ward boy is roughly equivalent to what is termed an orderly in the U.S. health care system. A ward boy does not have any formal medical training and assists the nurse with certain tasks. Similar to ayahs, the scope of practice is highly variable, depending on the nurse, patient needs, and the specific situation.

A lanky, animated man with slicked back brown hair wearing crisp white pants, a white shirt, and a blue and white sweater vest has been holding a large flashlight during the procedure. His efficient, bright demeanor and nautical-style outfit reminds me of a cruise director. This is Rajeeb, the Dresser, who prepares the bandages and sterile packs for the operating room and assists physicians with dressing changes. Surveying the number of patients with saturated and visibly soiled bandages it seems this task is overdue.

The last bed, at the back of the ward, is occupied by a depressed looking woman who stares up at the ceiling. A cardboard tag hung with string on the siderail of her bed reads "HBSAg+ve" handwritten in black ink. Adishree catches me looking at the sign. "Oh," she says, "yes, that means the patient is positive for hepatitis B."[2]

Family members crowd outside the entrance to the ICU, congregate in huddled clumps along the staircase that leads up to the third floor. Some are allowed in, and others are harshly admonished if they try. Family members who are allowed into the ICU do an extraordinary amount of physical care: they empty catheters, feed patients, assist patients to the small bathroom at the back of the ward, give baths, help patients up into wheelchairs.

At one point, the woman in the last bed, the hepatitis B positive patient, motions to Adishree and asks to be repositioned. Adishree promptly pushes open the glass door that separates the ICU from the hallway, walks around the corner to the mass of waiting family members, finds the patient's family attendant, and asks them to enter the ICU: their family member needs assistance. The family member hurries in and dutifully helps the woman turn and sit up; Adishree does not.

I am intrigued at the amount of care delegated to family members, and then confused and disturbed by how they are treated. Despite the much more favorable nurse-to-patient ratio, I observe similar exchanges in the ICU as I do on the general wards. One woman tentatively enters the ICU with a young child on her hip. The head nurse seated at the desk barks at her to exit the unit immediately: "*Doesn't she know children are full of infection?*" All family members are required to remove their chappals (sandals) before entering the ICU. They walk barefoot on the tile floor smeared with blood.

Of the three nurses on duty, Adishree engages in the most amount of patient care; the head nurse works on documentation for the entire shift, slowly writing in registers similar to the ones I have seen on the general wards: Indent Book, Diet Book, MHS Register Book, Maintenance Inventory Book, Night Instruction Book. The other nurse, Sonia, stocks supplies, organizes cupboards, and assists Adishree in taking vital signs.

I ask Adishree about pain control in the ICU.

---

2 It was not uncommon for patients with blood-borne and stigmatized illnesses, such as HIV or hepatitis, to be visibly identified. In my experience, preserving patient privacy was not seen as a general concern or priority.

"Is morphine ever given here to patients?"

"Oh no," she says. "Only in palliative care, they give the tablets and the IV morphine. But not on the general wards, and not here." Adishree leads me to a medication cart at the back of the ward where ampules lay like larvae in dozens of small cardboard boxes. "Pentazocine, you know this?" she asks, holding up an ampule of what I know as Talwin, an older opioid no longer used in the U.S.

"And this one, for pain," she says, handing me Promethazine, a common anti-nausea medication.

"You mean for nausea, not pain?" I say, thinking she has grabbed the wrong vial.

"No, for pain," she says definitively. "It's a sedative." She also shows me ampules of Tramadol, a weaker opioid, and Diclofenac, a Motrin-like anti-inflammatory medication.

The woman in the first bed who had a neck biopsy and is in the ICU for short-term observation indicates that she is in pain. Adishree and Sonia check her chart. "Hmmm…they've only written for oral pain meds," says Adishree. "That won't work. We'll give something else," she says and Sonia walks to the ampule cart to prepare something IV.

There is no need to call the physician for a different order, they assure me, it is fine to give this in the ICU. This level of autonomy surprises me, although I have seen more proactive nursing tasks in the ICU than on the general wards. Earlier, Adishree examined an X-ray film before contacting the physician, holding it up to the light, scrutinizing the shadowy images of the patient's lungs; the ICU nurses routinely check bloodwork results and notify the physicians if abnormal results are reported, they perform finger sticks to monitor a patient's blood glucose levels, and do hourly vital sign monitoring.

A fresh postoperative patient is wheeled into the last bed of the ICU, recently vacated by the patient with hepatitis B who returned to the general ward, and is left unchecked while Sister Sonia continues to talk on her cell phone. I realize that patients who have not been visited by family members have also not been turned or moved in hours. Finally, an alarm sounds on the monitor for the patient next to the recent admission. Sonia rises to check the persistent beeping.

Hoping to prompt Sonia to assess the new postoperative patient, I state the obvious: "So, this patient just returned from the operating room?" "Yes," she says and, almost as an afterthought, begins to attach a pulse oximeter to the patient's finger to monitor his oxygen levels. She doesn't say anything to the patient who looks up at her, glassy-eyed. I notice the cardboard "HBSAg+ve" handmade sign still dangles from the bed. "Should we remove this?" I ask holding up the cardboard sign slightly. "No, no! Him too," she says.

* * *

The ICU is busy—nine out of the ten beds are occupied and a few of the patients look gravely ill. I am particularly worried about the 60-year-old man with metastatic parotid cancer who wears a non-rebreather oxygen mask, and the young, exceedingly frail 30-year-old with ovarian and colon cancer who has had a fever since surgery. As we make rounds, Adishree intermittently assists patients to an upright position and roughly slaps their fragile backs with her open palms in a crude adaptation of chest physiotherapy. Patients' throats are pressed and they are encouraged to produce sputum, and while they all valiantly try, few are able to meet the expectations of the team. The young 30-year-old looks at me with wild, frightened eyes as she inhales quickly, and ineffectively, on a plastic, incentive spirometer machine, a handheld device designed to expand the tiny air sacs of the lungs and prevent pneumonia. I notice a pale greenish liquid that has puddled underneath her stretcher and is slowly oozing across the floor. Adishree says something to the patient's elderly mother who waddles away to get a towel and then stoops over to mop up the liquid.

After rounds, one of the surgical oncologists approaches me. He asks where I am from, what I am doing in the hospital. He seems genuinely interested.

"You will see," the surgeon says, "civilization is moving forward, but India is moving backwards here. This is all very substandard. Very substandard." His eyes dart around the ICU. "Somehow, there is not much mortality." He says this like he cannot believe it. He lists off the cases, bed by bed, ticking them off on his fingers: head and neck, head and neck, ovarian, lung, parotid, head and neck, breast, cervical, gastric. As he is leaving he turns to me and warns, "Put a mask on. You will get infected here." Adishree promptly opens a cabinet and hands me a thin light-blue paper mask. The mask is not adequate to protect against tuberculosis—the main thing I am worried about contracting here—but I tie it around my head dutifully anyway. Not for the first time I wish the nurses were as diligent about handwashing, a critical infection control measure, as they are about wearing the flimsy masks, whose purpose seems dubious.[3]

The three sons of the 60-year-old with parotid cancer struggle mightily to help their extremely ill father back to bed after they have taken him for a short walk. Adishree hollers instructions to them from the back of the ward, while the other two nurses remain at the desk talking to each other and documenting. It takes every bit of self-restraint I have not to run over and help; the man looks like he is about to fall and the three sons are doing the best they can, but really have no idea how to mobilize their critically ill father, a man who, in my opinion, looks like he is actively dying. A patient in the

---

3 Another important reminder to the reader to contextualize this observation pre-COVID-19 pandemic, when wearing masks became an essential strategy to mitigate transmission of the coronavirus.

bed closest to the nurses' desk, whom I saw earlier happily eating some food wrapped in newspaper, sits up and begins to retch and vomit. The nurses at the desk, sitting less than three feet away, do not intervene. A family member holds a basin under his head. The patient finishes and falls back to bed, spent.

* * *

The ICU is particularly busy today because the Dresser is absent, so the ward boy and the nurses fill in to assist the physicians with the many bandage changes. The young 30-year-old and the elderly man with the parotid tumor are still there, looking extremely ill. New patients have appeared and I am particularly struck by a man with a bulging cheek mass and tracheostomy. He stares blankly ahead and does not say a word nor make eye contact with anyone. I watch him get suctioned by one of the physicians, the tracheal catheter touching the bed, the patient, the doctor's shirt, before it is inserted into the hole in the patient's throat to pull mucus from his lungs. The ward boy, changing a bed, jettisons the pillow and red blanket on to the floor, then picks them up and puts them back on the bed after he has changed the bottom sheet.

Adishree begins performing vigorous chest physiotherapy on patients as they are roused to sit up in bed, one by one. The physicians do it too, roughly and haphazardly slapping backs and encouraging patients to cough and spit. The young 30-year-old with metastatic ovarian cancer is whacked by Adishree with such force that she begins to moan and cry. I can tell Adishree thinks she is doing the right thing, doing what has to be done, but the patient looks miserable and terribly frightened. Her thin face is creased into a grimace, and she leans forward, eyes closed, supporting her forehead with one small, bird-thin hand. She looks utterly and completely despondent.

A patient's wife shuffles into the ICU and the head nurse suddenly looks up, her face contorting in to a fierce and unattractive expression of disgust and disdain. There is an ominous pause and then the head nurse begins to scream, shrill and strident, at the young woman who tries to interject, but is cut off by the head nurse who continues to yell. Watching the nurse berate the woman is unbearable, and I become anxious, wondering if I should say something.[4] Finally, Adishree intervenes, says something quietly to the patient's wife who then walks away.

"What happened?" I ask Adishree a few minutes later.

---

4 This was one of the most difficult interactions I observed during my fieldwork and one I have reflected upon many times since returning from India. It was terribly painful to see a vulnerable patient's family member berated and publicly shamed by a fellow nurse. While I cannot fully understand all of the complex dynamics at hand, especially given the language barrier, I interpret this as a manifestation of caste and a nurse asserting their power and control over a patient's family member of lesser rank/status. This is further discussed in Chapter 10.

"She put a bag of blood in the deep freezer, and now it is ruined. It cannot be used."

"But was she told to do that?" I ask.

"Yes."

"Hmmm," I say slowly. "I guess it really wasn't her fault. She didn't know."

"Yes, she didn't know," Adishree echoes.

Adishree opens the door of the small red refrigerator in the corner of the ICU. It is overflowing with bags and tubes and boxes of medication. No wonder the patient's wife squeezed the bag of blood wherever it would fit.

One of the surgeons walks into the ICU and now the head nurse begins yelling at him. Adishree, again the peacemaker, talks with him, again something about the refrigerator.

"He," she nods her head to where the physician was standing, "he tells people to put their blood products in our refrigerator, it's the only one here, in the ICU. But we can't have all of this here," she explains. "So, we told him not to say that anymore."

* * *

Adishree is on leave, so I shadow Sonia, the tall ICU nurse with an odd sense of humor. As soon as I walk into the ICU, she and Rajeeb, the cruise ship-appearing Dresser, ask me with a sense of urgency, "Had your breakfast?"

I smile. "Yes, thank you, I have eaten."

But they want to know *specifically* what I have eaten, and they both wait as if the recounting of my simple breakfast is occasion for true suspense. I try to explain a bagel to them, but am not particularly successful.

I watch Sonia and another nurse pound and slap on patients' backs again in their rough rendition of chest physiotherapy. Labs are drawn, medications are given. Asepsis is arbitrary. Needles are recapped using a technique that guarantees an eventual fingerstick. But I can say this: Sonia stays busy; she seems to want to interact and care for patients, not be stuck behind a desk doing paperwork. There is a patient on one of the ventilators today in the ICU. He is a 43-year-old man, conscious and alert. Sonia tells me that he is very sick and recently had his leg amputated.

"From a sarcoma?" I ask, referring to an aggressive soft tissue cancer whose initial treatment typically involves amputation of the affected limb.

"Yes, sarcoma," she says from behind her paper mask. The bunched up red blankets at the bottom of the patient's bed make it impossible for me to tell if the man has two legs or not.

Later that day, the surgeon comes to check on the ventilated patient; Sonia and I stand next to him at the patient's bedside.

"This patient had a Whipple," the doctor tells me. "It's a specialized surgery to remove pancreatic tumors," he instructs patiently. I nod, familiar with the complicated surgery and the often difficult postoperative course, but am confused: isn't this the sarcoma patient with the leg amputation? I wait for Sonia to say something, to correct the diagnosis and surgery, but she doesn't appear bothered by this significant change in information.

After rounds are finished, Sonia and I stand at the end of the ventilated patient's bed. "So, this patient, did *not* have an amputation, right?" I clarify.

"Yes, amputation," she says again.

"No, I don't think so," the nursing instructor in me feels compelled to correct her. "This patient had a Whipple for a pancreatic tumor, a totally different type of surgery. That's what the doctor was saying in rounds. Here," I say pulling out the surgical report form and pointing to the description of the surgery.

She reaches over and pats the red blanket bunched over the patient's lower body. "Oh! Two legs!," she exclaims. "No amputation!" She giggles and returns to the nurses' desk.

***

"You know how to insert IV cannula?," Sonia asks me later in the afternoon.

"Yes," I say.

"Oh, please, please do this patient." She gestures to the 60-year-old with parotid cancer.

"I'm so sorry, but I cannot do that."

She looks upset. "There are rules about what I can do here and what I cannot do here as a nurse. But I will help you look for a good vein," I suggest as a compromise.

She lifts up the patient's incredibly edematous (swollen) arm, which has a slight bluish hue and is concerningly cool. I don't see any promising veins at all. Sonia presses and presses the patient's forearm and hand, denting the skin with her touch. Neither of us find anything. While I examine the patient's other arm, Sonia notices my very simple earrings, a present from a good friend back home.

"I like those," she says.

"Thank you."

"Can I have them?" she asks brazenly. I am taken aback by her request and can't tell if she is serious or not.

"You want my earrings?"

"Yes," she says matter-of-factly. I'm not sure if this is some sort of test I seem likely to fail.

"These are a gift from a dear friend, I'm afraid I can't part with them," I say. She looks crestfallen.

A research coordinator enters the ICU and tells Sonia that a patient participating in a clinical trial needs to be admitted to the ICU for an infusion of Taxotere (a type of chemotherapy) that will require additional monitoring. Sonia says they have only given chemotherapy once before in the ICU as she examines the benign-appearing white and green box. I give her a crash course in chemotherapy administration. "This is a very toxic drug," I say bluntly. "You need to wear gloves and a mask when you mix it, and you must be very careful with it."

I hear Sonia say "Saturday" quickly to the study coordinator who promptly hands her a 100-rupee note before he exits the unit. She stuffs it in the pocket of her uniform. She sees my quizzical look and tells me vaguely that patients on clinical trials must pay to come to the ICU.[5]

* * *

Somehow, Adishree seems to have escaped the quagmire of documentation, as she busies herself helping with dressing changes, changing bed lines, and doing chest physiotherapy. At one break in the action, I ask her about patient deaths in the ICU. I tell her that in the U.S. many patients die in the ICU. I ask her if it is the same here.

"Oh no," she says. "Very rarely. They are here, two, three days, they get better and go to the ward. Maybe some do not improve and they expire here. But it is not common."

I also ask Adishree what happens if a patient's heart or lungs stop, if the nurses are required to initiate CPR (cardiopulmonary resuscitation).

---

5 I did not ask Sonia why she received the 100 rupee note, and so I cannot be certain of the reason. However, it seems possible this could have been payment from a patient's family. One SICH nurse explicitly told me, unprompted, during her interview that hospital staff routinely accepted payments by patients and family members, which were given to increase the odds staff would respond to the patient's needs: *"Here, many people take money from the patients: nurses, ayahs, but in secret. They take bribes. If a nurse is going to do their job, they take bribes, they harass the patients for money. Even in radiation, an ayah gets 15,000 to 20,000 in salary, but will take a minimum of 50 rupees from each patient. Why are they doing this? Why aren't they being held accountable? Everybody knows they are taking money, but nobody is holding them accountable."* This is not unique to SICH, or India, and is a normative practice in many countries. It is also not isolated to the hospital setting. One Dandaka native told me: *"You cannot believe the level of corruption here. It's everywhere. Say you don't pay your taxes. You make 15% profit you are supposed to pay taxes on, but you don't. And I also make 15% profit and I pay all my taxes. You pay off someone for 1%; that person is happy, you are happy, and you have retained 14% of your profit. How am I supposed to compete with you?"* This individual considered anti-corruption initiatives in India completely ineffective: *"a joke."* During my fieldwork, I was personally asked for a bribe—or told I would be taken to the police station for questioning—when I attempted to legitimately extend my residency permit but there was an issue with my stated address on the form; I paid the money. I was also advised that if I wanted to successfully reserve the hospital auditorium for nursing education classes, I needed to pay the room scheduler additional money, which I very reluctantly did. Of note, a placard posted within SICH from the Director stated:

The treatment at this hospital is free of cost. Patients are requested not to pay anything to any staff while taking treatment or staying in wards. Patients and their relatives are requested not to hesitate to consult their doctor for any problem. Please help us to maintain the hospital discipline.

"Oh, I would like that training!" she says, excitedly, when I explain that nurses in the U.S. are required to be certified in basic CPR. "Can you teach me? How long is the course?" I immediately regret even bringing the subject up. Clearly, Adishree is a bright, motivated, caring nurse who wants to learn and do right by her patients. I would love to teach her CPR. But how do I explain to Adishree that I am not certified to teach CPR? That it is a team effort and all staff would need to learn it for it to really be effective. And what would be accomplished by teaching everyone CPR if there is no way to support the patient after they are successfully resuscitated, which is extremely unlikely in itself for someone this ill, even given the best of resources?

As I contemplate this, the small ICU is suddenly deluged with a group of nursing students from Desai General Hospital. A group of eight students, bright-eyed and eager, crowd into the unit, short, smiling, and nervous. They are like a troupe of freshly starched miniature nurses. At 5'2" I tower over all of them. Adishree tells me they come for one week a year, and I feel lucky to be here when they arrive. They are in the second year of their three-and-a-half-year General Nurse and Midwifery (GNM) program.

As a former clinical instructor, I am curious as to how this educational experience will work, as the number of students is four times that of the nursing staff. I watch as the head nurse removes a large roll of gauze from one of the cabinets and abrasively instructs the students to cut up the material into folded squares. The students move in the way nursing students around the world move—cautiously, slowly, diligently. The head nurse then unearths a large plastic jug of "surgical spirit"—a ubiquitous antiseptic, largely composed of ethyl alcohol. The students hold their gauze squares over the jug's opening, and tilt the bottle, saturating the gauze.

The head nurse barks a command and the students disperse like tiny ants throughout the unit with their saturated gauze squares in hand. And then I see them all begin to reach up and start: cleaning.

They stand on chairs and stretchers to reach the monitors, wiping the screens furiously with their gauze pads. They scrub the side rails of stretchers and the raised backs of gurneys. Every now and then, Adishree and the head nurse correct the students, redirect them to clean something again, better. I want to cry. These young, energetic, impressionable students are *cleaning*? What kind of message does this send? What kind of socialization is this? What a missed opportunity! One of the surgeons walks into the ICU, glances with a bemused expression at the students cleaning, climbing around, up, under and on top of beds. One student finishes early and Adishree puts her to work cleaning out the disastrous overflowing red refrigerator. Bags and bags of expired blood products are thrown in a pile to be discarded.

After about an hour, the students are restless and unanimously decide they have had enough of cleaning. They crowd around me at the front of the unit.

"Teach them something!" the head nurse says to me spontaneously. The students look at me expectantly. I hesitate and then launch into an impromptu oral quiz. They all know that handwashing is the primary way to prevent infection. Most of them know the signs and symptoms of infection. Few of them know much about cancer or side effects of chemotherapy or postoperative care of the patient. I want to do more, and am thinking of what to do next when one of the smallest students abruptly announces, "We have to leave now!" Before they leave, they each hand me their individual notebooks and ask for my address and autograph. Afterwards, they link arms with me, walk me through the hospital, back to their waiting bus.

4 Behind the Wall

Night Shift

[Before we had morphine] they used to roll on the ground in pain. I used to think these patients are seeing hell on earth. It is not somewhere else, somewhere they go if they are bad. Hell is right here in front of our eyes. The pain, and the agony, the bad feelings. Sometimes I used to cry, I used to become so emotional. I used to feel so bad seeing those patients.

Sister Agnes, general ward nurse

Sister Agnes apologizes for being late; she has to take two different buses to reach the hospital, over an hour-long journey, and tonight a bus was labeled incorrectly, causing her to travel way out of her way before she realized the mistake. I am happy to see her warm, smiling face. The first question she asks me is about my transport; she wants to be assured that I am safe getting back and forth this late at night. Then she whips in to action, gathering supplies from the metal cabinet at the back of the ward. There is a ward boy working with Agnes tonight. He seems very competent, and Agnes tells me he is one of the good ones, and subsequently is allowed to do more. Apparently, some assistants briefly show their face and then disappear for the rest of the night. I watch the ward boy administer some IV medications; Agnes says they can only do this in the presence of the nurse. This seems loosely interpreted, however, because the ward is massive and standing with Agnes at the front of the ward, I can barely see what the ward boy is doing. There are 36 patients on the ward currently, and Agnes is the nurse for all of them.

Unbelievably, more ledgers have appeared. Agnes opens the "Night Instruction Register" book to find the list of patients that need medications during her shift. Fifteen patients are listed; most of the medications are steroids, anti-nausea medications, antacids, and antibiotics. I don't see any pain medications ordered. There is one chemotherapy to give—Cytarabine.

Agnes stands behind the front desk and loudly calls out patient names. Patients or family members shuffle forward and silently hand Agnes the ampules and vials they have been issued earlier that morning. Agnes consults the night register and draws up the medications into syringes. She tells me she learned in

DOI: 10.4324/9781003413158-7

her Bachelor's courses about safe handling of chemotherapy—wear an apron, use special gloves, wear a mask. "We should have an isolated area, much better ventilation. That is not possible here. But the nurses do wear the gloves and mask." She pauses. "Well, some do, and some don't," she concedes.

Family members stand around the table and help agitate powdered medications that need to be reconstituted in sterile water or saline. Agnes tells me that sometimes there is a shortage of needles so they try to combine the medications that they can in to one syringe for injection. I notice a small, tattered poster hanging by the table that lists the qualities and rewards of being a nurse—it mentions "incredible responsibility, but limited authority."[1]

Agnes does not mix the Cytarabine, the chemotherapy, at the front table—instead she returns the small box to the patient's mother to take back to her son's bedside. She does this to remind herself this medication is to be given subcutaneously (under the skin) and not intravenously (into the vein)—which could be a fatal mistake. Agnes works fast, snapping the ends of glass ampules with a sharp downward slap of the narrow end of a Kelly clamp. Some of the broken glass bits fall into a trash can, a lot lands on the floor. I get splattered on my arm and face with a blast of the antibiotic ampicillin. I make a mental note to stand further back when the nurses are preparing chemotherapy.

After all the syringes have been prepared and distributed to family attendants, we start down the row of patients to administer the medications. The ward boy is ahead of us and has already started some. Patients do not wear name wristbands and there does not appear to be any consistent method to verify a patient's identity. Agnes does not take any vital signs, nor conduct any physical assessments of the patients. Family attendants sleep on the concrete floor, row after row, blankets pulled up over their heads. We step over and around them.

Going from bed to bed, Agnes injects the contents of each syringe that the family attendant hands to her or that we find lying at the foot of the patient's bed. There is no double-checking with the register before medications are given and no syringes are labeled. As we move further and further away from the front desk and the security of the documentation table and ledgers, I feel

---

1 This poster especially caught my attention as it alludes to the concept of "moral distress," the idea that nurses experience an ethical bind when they believe they know the right thing to do to help a patient but are somehow blocked in this effort. Nurses are generally believed to be a profession at high risk for moral distress, as they are often charged with significant responsibility but have limited autonomy. See Jameton, A. (1984). *Nursing practice: The ethical issues*. Englewood, NJ: Prentice Hall, for a seminal work on the topic. My fieldwork in India suggests that nurses practicing within a different ethical and sociocultural framework, and with a different perception of the moral obligations of nursing practice, are less likely to experience moral distress as it has traditionally been conceptualized. For a fuller discussion of this, see LeBaron et al., (2014). Nurse moral distress and cancer pain management: An ethnography of oncology nurses in India. *Cancer Nursing*, 37(5), 331–344.

myself becoming strangely uneasy and anxious. On our medication rounds, I see a man whom I'm afraid may be dead, he is lying so still and looks so frail. We pass another man who has an orange-sized oozing wound emerging from the side of his mouth and another man who weakly lifts up his soiled tracheostomy dressing as Agnes walks by to reveal a gooey, bloody mess. Agnes gives a cursory glance, but we do not stop.

Agnes administers the Cytarabine to a young patient who looks to be in his 20s. This is the one medication she will mix at the bedside. Agnes draws up the chemotherapy in a syringe and then squirts some out as she expels the air from the syringe. Droplets of chemotherapy fall on the bed and possibly on Agnes and possibly on the patient and the patient's mother. The patient grimaces as Agnes gives the injection, but there is minimal discussion or eye contact between Agnes and the patient or his mother. I find this interaction particularly sad since Agnes told me last week how she wished she had more time to spend with patients and families: "*Usually in the evenings or nights it's okay, we can spend some time with patients.*"

After we give all the medications, which takes about an hour, it is time to document. We sit at the front table and Agnes begins by copying all of the medications in the Night Instruction Register to a different page in the same register, indicating that they have been administered. As I watch Agnes engage in this laborious task, I sense there is security in hiding behind all of the documentation amidst the grit and chaos; it's safe, it's clean, it is controllable, and it is predictable. It is manageable. In a sea of un-meetable needs, you control what you can.

* * *

Agnes seems particularly eager to show me another register on the Female Ward. We head upstairs, leaving Male Ward I without a nurse, and I am introduced to friendly and lively Sister Ruth who is full of questions—about nursing in the U.S., how the national licensing exam works, what the shifts are like, what documentation is required, and then the most critical question of all: what is the salary of a nurse in the U.S.? They tell me that nursing in India used to be seen as a "cheap" profession, but they feel it is changing. Ruth decided to become a nurse after watching a nurse in her village, impressed with the quality of her work, but her parents were initially resistant. "In my family, ladies do not go outside and work. Women are working in the home only. Cooking, housework." She eventually either convinced her parents—or ignored them, I am not sure which—and secured a job at South Indian Cancer Hospital (SICH). "With my own interest, I am the first to 'come out,'" she says proudly, using the common expression for women who leave their natal home to seek out a more independent, professional lifestyle.

Ruth has no shortage of stories, and she offers them up freely. Her face is small and delicate, and her voice high-pitched, with a singsong cadence.

She tells me about the time she inadvertently caught a medication mix-up between two patients with similar sounding names; luckily, she realized it right before the patient received the wrong infusion of chemotherapy, but it was a close call.[2]

She also tells me the harrowing account of a patient who committed suicide during her shift.

"Once a patient slit his throat with a surgical blade," Ruth says abruptly, catching me off guard. "He was a postoperative patient, in the ICU. Maybe he was not able to bear the pain, I am not sure." Ruth was on night duty in Male Ward III and went across the hall to relieve the ICU nurse. For two hours, Ruth watched the ICU patient—he finished his IV fluids, he slept; all seemed okay. Ruth remembers the patient was in the last row of beds, by the cart where supplies and medications are kept. And because family attendants are not allowed to stay in the ICU, he was alone. "I called the other sister as I was sleepy, so I handed over the sister's duty back to her and I went up and slept,"[3] Ruth recalls. "About 15 minutes later, the patient got up. There was a surgical blade on the dressing trolley beside his bed. He took that and slit his throat. He died."

Ruth's face is calm. I wonder if Ruth has ever told this story before; I get the sense from her animated and rapid speech, perhaps not, and she seems almost relieved to confess what happened. "There was blood all

2 When I asked Agnes how the nurses at SICH confirm the identity of patients, as patients don't wear identification or name bands, she explained: *Many of the patients are here for many months; they are like family, we know them well. Also, the documentation nurses alert the medication nurses if there is someone with a similar name and then they verify more than just the patient's name, they will ask the husband's name and address to be sure it is the right person.* However, this wasn't always failsafe, as evidenced from my conversation with Sister Ruth: *But I had an experience once, when there was a mix-up, and I felt very bad. Two patients were there, Ashwina Kumar and Ashwina Kumari, on the same ward. We called 'Ashwina Kumar,' but Ashwina Kumari came forward. I asked, 'Is this your name?' She said, 'yes,' and I gave the medicine to her, but it was not for her. The first bottle will be common for all: Zofran, Rantac, and Decadron [a standardized combination of anti-nausea, antacid, and steroid medicines given before chemotherapy]. But the second bottle is chemotherapy—and that is different, based on diagnosis, age, weight, everything. The first bottle finished, and when the second bottle started, I told Ashwina Kumari, 'you won't get your medicine today.' Sometimes it gets too late for the order to be signed, but the patients will still wait for their medicine to come. I didn't want her to have to wait, so I said, 'you did not get your medicine today, I will give it to you tomorrow.' She said, 'I am already getting it!' I said, 'How?! How can you be getting your medicine?' Then I checked the two patients, the two names, case sheets, their addresses, and she said, 'That is not my name.' I realized that the medicine that belongs to one patient was being taken by another patient! Immediately, I stopped the medication and gave it to the correct patient. But if I had not told the patient that her medicine was not coming—and we don't usually do that—then the wrong medicine would have gone to the other patient and would have resulted in something. That is the main reason there should not be crowds in the wards.*
3 It was not uncommon and generally expected that nurses on night shift would sleep during part of their shifts.

over. The ICU sister came running out. She was waking up another sister—'Come, come!' The sister wouldn't come. I said—'What happened, what happened?' and came down. I was not able to look at the patient. The ward boys held him and tried to put clamps; but the patient died as he lost a lot of blood."

There are other patients, too, that Ruth cannot forget. Like the patient six years ago who accidentally pulled out his abdominal drains and bled to death. Ruth remembers waking up to the patient's wife crying, hitting herself on her chest and yelling, "I don't know, I don't know, I didn't do anything!", afraid she would be accused of pulling out the drains and killing her husband. Ruth called the duty doctor, but the patient had already died.

"Those are very sad stories," I say, thinking of the ward full of patients Agnes and I have left unattended.

"I was not able to forget it for a long time," Ruth says quietly.

When Ruth first started at SICH she used to ask all of the patients, "How did you get cancer?" Some people answered, "I was hit by a cricket ball, a wound formed, and the wound became cancer." Some said, "My leg broke; then it became cancer." Or "I was running a fever for many days, it did not come down; we did many tests and then I was diagnosed with blood cancer." When they told me about their experiences, I thought "Oh! Do people get cancer like this?!" "If anything happened to me, I felt sure it was cancer, after seeing all these patients." Ruth still feels like this, even now, worried that a headache means she has a brain tumor. Ruth smiles when I tell her I have had the same experience as a cancer nurse—being hypervigilant about any slightly unusual symptom and worried everything is cancer.

Agnes and Ruth, like other nurses, find the incessant crowds of family attendants irritating and stressful, especially when they have to repeat information over and over to patients and family members—specifically that receiving chemotherapy the same day of admission is not possible. "But, still they'll come and give the case sheet like this,"—Agnes demonstrates by shoving a piece of paper aggressively toward me— "and they'll ask, 'You'll give medications today?' Some patients come from far away, from remote districts for chemotherapy. They say to us—'We have to go today, the train will leave.' They plead with us that they have some festival or marriage at home. 'Give the chemotherapy today, sister,' they repeat over and over; over and over we repeat the same answer: 'no, we'll give your chemotherapy tomorrow.' It's exhausting. Sometimes we have to even shout at them a little bit, only then will they understand."

Ruth attributes the problem to family members being illiterate and uneducated and essentially incapable of understanding. But sometimes, it is not about education. Sometimes, even educated family members do not listen, and that creates confusion. Recently, a man came to SICH with a patient admitted to the ward, believed to be his mother-in-law. Unbeknownst to any of the nurses, the man was a high-ranking official in the Indian government. When Ruth asked the man to vacate the ward, he initially agreed—"I will go, I will go, I will go." But he didn't leave. "The doctors don't like it when there are too many attendants on the wards. Dr. Suresh, the Orange Unit attending, he is *very* strict. He says only patients should be inside, no attendants on the ward. 'I don't want any attendants,' he tells us. 'If the attendant is here, I won't see the patient,'" Ruth explains. So, Ruth told the man over and over he had to leave. "When someone looks like an educated person, we don't want to tell him repeatedly. If he were illiterate—'Why are you not going even after telling you so many times? Why are you making us shout? We are losing our voice.' We can say like that. But this man did not listen," Ruth recalls. The man kept requesting that the patient receive her chemotherapy that day, and even sat down in front of the doctor, which was highly unusual. This got Ruth wondering: who actually *is* this man? Is he a doctor? The mystery family member even tracked down the Resident Medical Officer (RMO, the second highest physician position in the hospital, under the Director) and brought up all the patient files. Now, Ruth was really curious and she asked him directly, "What do you do?" But the man was vague, saying only that he worked in the city of Pondicherry and that no, he was not a doctor. By this time, the other staff had had enough and another nurse shouted at him, "Why are you standing here, how many times do I have to tell you, go!" The man eventually left the ward. Later, he returned when Ruth was mixing medications, and she asked him one more time, "What do you do?" Finally, the man coughed up the truth—"I am an IAS."[4] The nurses were shocked. "We didn't know! So many times we are telling and he did not listen!" Ruth laughs, remembering the story. "If he had introduced himself that way first—'I am an IAS officer; just give the chemotherapy early,' then we would not have shouted at him so many times, and we would have given the medication. But, when he does not say anything to us, how are we supposed to know?"

* * *

Back on Male Ward I it is quiet. The ward boy has dimmed the lights and absent the daytime cacophony, the rhythmic whine of the ceiling fans and the buzz of the fluorescent lights overhead are pronounced. Agnes tells me she will spend the rest of the night reading the Bible or sleeping in the side room. Cots for this purpose are set up in the break rooms. I ask Agnes what happens if a patient has a problem or needs help and the nurse is asleep. I can't

---

4 IAS: Indian Administrative Services officer; the highest ranked employee of the Indian government.

stop thinking about the stories Ruth just told us. Agnes tells me not to worry, an attendant will knock on the door and let her know.

* * *

The following night, Agnes and I walk by a patient with a huge facial tumor partially obscured by multiple bandages held in place by a mask tied on sideways; his visible left eye is swollen and weepy. He stops Agnes as she is moving quickly to the next patient who needs an injection and shows her a small bottle which is empty. The man has a prescription for morphine but he took his last tablet tonight, so he will not have any for his 6 am dose.

"What do you do in this situation?" I ask.

"I told him he will need to wait for the doctors to arrive around 9 am, and then they will give the prescription and his wife can go to the pharmacy and get the tablets." She doesn't say this unkindly, just matter-of-factly. I look at the man with his grotesquely bulging face and his wife standing close by in a teal sari, her hair pulled back in a single barrette. I think about how long it will actually take for him to get his next dose of morphine; even an optimistic 10 am means he will go 12 hours without pain medicine. We move along to the next patient, the young man who gets the subcutaneous injection of Cytarabine.

When we get back to the nurses' desk to document the medications given, I cannot help myself and ask about the morphine patient again. "Is this a situation when you could consider calling the DMO?" I ask gently, referring to the Duty Medical Officer, or doctor on call. The thought of this patient going all night and waiting until tomorrow morning for morphine makes me feel sick. "Is that an appropriate reason to call them?"

"No," Agnes shakes her head. "The DMO is for emergencies only, and they won't want to take responsibility. Better to wait for the patient's regular doctors."

I acknowledge it is a difficult situation and don't say anything further, but I can see Agnes thinking. After a few minutes she says, "Well, there is one other option. Maybe we can call the pediatric oncology unit. They may have some extra tablets." Agnes calls; they have 10mg morphine tablets. Agnes beckons the patient's wife over to the desk to let her know what is happening and also to reiterate the importance of not running out of the morphine. "I told her they cannot wait until they are all out of tablets to let us know. When he has 1 or 2 days left, then they need to tell us. Or else he will suffer very much from the pain. I told her she cannot know how much he is suffering." Agnes writes something on a slip of paper and sends the ward boy upstairs. He returns 20 minutes later; he doesn't come to Agnes. Instead, he goes straight to the patient's bed and ostensibly gives them the tablets. "This way he will have one overnight if he needs it and then his dose for 6 am," Agnes says. "That's good," I say, relieved.

The nurse who is posted on Male Ward II comes over to Male Ward I and tells Agnes she has to leave an hour early, can Agnes keep an eye on her patients? Agnes, already responsible for 37 patients, calmly agrees to watch the additional 40 patients in a ward opposite the courtyard, and not within eyesight. When it is time for me to leave, Agnes walks me out to the cab and talks to the driver to be sure he is clear about the directions to drive me home. She smiles her beatific smile, clasps both my hands in hers, and says if there is anything I need, anything at all, to call her, anytime.

* * *

The patient from the previous night—the man with the huge facial tumor who ran out of morphine tablets—shows up the next morning at the palliative care clinic. He has been referred to have maggots removed from his wound. The patient's sister, whom I mistook for his wife, recognizes me from the ward, and smiles. We each press our palms together in front of our chest, "Namaste."[5]

The patient lies down on the cot, covered with an old sheet. Daya removes the tattered bandage—I wonder when it was last changed. The wound is not quite as bad as I anticipated, but still horrible. Red and pink cauliflower-like eruptions extend along the patient's left cheek, up to a ragged half-dollar sized hole. I don't see any immediate evidence of maggots. Daya is handed a large bottle of Terpint, a turpentine solution, by the patient's sister. Using a syringe with a purposely bent needle for a better angle, Daya expertly irrigates and saturates the wound with the solution whose pungent smell quickly overpowers the small room and makes me feel rather lightheaded. And then she waits. The Terpint will help bring the maggots, if there are any, to the surface for extraction. Daya has the man open his mouth: no maggots. She shines a flashlight directly into the hole in his cheek: no maggots. Pradeep is called over to confirm her finding. Pradeep is upset the patient's sister had to buy the big bottle of Terpint for no reason. "They didn't even look, before sending this patient here." He shakes his head in disgust. "They didn't even look."

After Daya has finished cleaning and redressing the man's facial wound, she grabs my arm and pulls me in to the back room of the clinic. Daya has been at SICH working in the palliative are department for the past four years. She came here from a corporate hospital in search of the security and salary of a government job. "Palliative Care is *entirely* different," says Daya. In her previous job, she took care of patients with diabetes and simple surgeries and tuberculosis. "I had never seen cases like this," Daya tells me. "I had no idea cancer could be like this."

---

5 A traditional Indian greeting that involves placing the palms together in front of the chest and offering a slight bow; a way to formally and respectfully honor and acknowledge another person. It has been translated as "the divine within me bows to the divine within you."

Daya later learned, however, that the palliative care department nurses are actually contract nurses—and therefore do not qualify for the same benefits as government employees. Despite this disappointment and her initial fears and misconceptions about working with cancer patients, Daya stayed—and found that she actually enjoyed working in the palliative care department: doing procedures, dressing changes, managing colostomies and difficult wounds—things general ward nurses don't, or won't, do. Like many nurses I spoke with in India, it was not Daya's choice to become a nurse, but a result of familial—largely paternal—pressure. "I have done my master's degree," she tells me, "but the reason I came into this profession is due to my father forcing. He forced me to do nursing because we get jobs quickly."

A breast cancer patient who completed therapy a year ago arrives for a lymphedema treatment, and Daya has received specialized training in a type of massage that can help promote lymph drainage and reduce swelling in women who have had mastectomies. This patient does not look like the typical SICH patient; she is well-dressed, educated, mobile. She is back at the hospital today to tie up some loose ends before finalizing a move to Chennai. While in the clinic, she and her husband make a 5,000 rupee ($100 USD) donation to the palliative care department.

Sequestered in the privacy of the clinic's back room, the woman unwraps the top of her olive green sari and unhooks the matching blouse to reveal a normal left breast and a lumpy, scarred line where the right used to be. I watch Daya as she gently rubs paraffin oil onto the women's arms and upper torso. Daya talks to her softly in her hypnotic blend of Hindi and English, occasionally turning to me with explanations: "First, we start above the clavicle," she says, deftly moving the pads of her three middle fingers in a gentle circular motion. For the next hour, I watch transfixed as Daya gives the woman a thorough lymphedema massage, instructs her in self-care techniques and range of motion exercises, and demonstrates diaphragmatic breathing. Daya even lovingly massages the woman's ample, intact left breast. Daya's eyes are soft and kind and her presence conveys she has all the time in the world. It is nursing at its finest: *I care about you, I can help you, I want to teach you.*

This act stands in such stark contrast to other interactions I have witnessed, I find myself formulating uncharitable questions: is this patient receiving better treatment because she has money and made a donation to the clinic? And then: don't we *all* do this to some extent, sometimes overtly, sometimes subconsciously—in India, the U.S., everywhere? Is a patient's economic status really a—maybe sometimes *the*—primary driver of the kind of care nurses provide, even if we don't want to admit it? As Radha continues the lymphedema massage, I am humbled to think how I have done the same thing as a nurse; the times I have been pressured, or expected, to make an extra effort with influential patients, patients who have made sizable donations, patients with connections to senior administrators, all the while telling myself I treat all patients equally.

You Have to Manage

What you see here, it may be very different from what you are used to, you will wonder about the way things are done. But you have to remember: it works here. It works for the volume of patients, it works for the facility. It works here.

SICH Surgical Resident

Male Ward III is located directly across the hall from the Intensive Care Unit (ICU) and is a mixed medical and surgical ward with two distinct wings—one side houses radiation and medical oncology patients, the other, postoperative surgical patients discharged from the ICU. Situated between the two wings is a large nursing station, which has an attached small break room where the sole sink is located. Two communal patient bathrooms flank the end of each wing.

What is immediately disconcerting about the layout of Male Ward III is that while the medical wing is connected to the nursing station by a fairly large window cut in to the concrete wall, there is no such "window" to the surgical side. For nurses to see patients on the surgical wing, they must exit the nurses' station, turn right in to the hallway, walk a few feet, and then turn right again to enter the surgical wing.

"It may be a little hard to see what is going on with the surgical patients the way the ward is set-up?" I suggest to Preeti, a nurse who has worked at SICH for two years, thinking about the myriad of complications that can befall postsurgical patients—bleeding, breathing problems, stitches bursting open, severe pain, drains falling out.

"Oh, nothing will happen. The attendants will come and get us if they need something," Preeti reassures me.

Preeti seems bright, but is clearly bored. "It's routine," she says, yawning and taking a break from making notations in the Diet Book. "We come, we give medications, we go. We have children and families, this is just routine." She asks me to help with some of the documentation by noting what medications have been given in the expenditure log book. I gently tell her I don't think it would be appropriate for me to document in their records. "Oh, it's okay," the head nurse confirms. "We'll check and make sure it is correct." I hesitate long enough that they eventually give up, assuming perhaps I am too dense for the task.

* * *

Only two chemotherapies are scheduled today, a light day. Calm and gentle, there is a soothing quality to Preeti's relaxed speech, languid movements, and serene face. With practiced competence, she snaps open vials and draws up the various medications in to syringes, squirts them in to IV bottles. At 11 am everything stops for tea, but the nurses are angry because the tea doesn't taste right and the ayah is sent back out for a new batch.

Preeti wants to know if I am married. I tell her I am not; I don't dare mention that at one point in time I was.

"How are marriages arranged in your place?" she asks.

Preeti is shocked when I tell her people generally date for months, sometimes years, before they decide to get married, generally without any real input or formal approval from their parents.

"I talked to my husband once before I got married," she says. "It is very difficult." Preeti acknowledges that there is a three-month engagement period where one could *technically* extricate themselves from an arranged marriage, "but it is very difficult. Very difficult," she repeats. "You cannot say no, for the parents' sake. And then," she pauses, and exhales deeply, "it is over for the woman." She says this not with melodrama, but with such a visceral sense of resignation and finality that I am startled. She seems entirely too young to be so defeated.

A patient attendant enters the nurses' station from the surgical side of the ward. He seems to be indicating that a patient is having trouble swallowing? Breathing? Eating? I cannot quite tell. My immediate instinct is to run next door and make sure the patient is okay. Instead, another nurse, Mary, opens a cabinet, pulls out some tubing and hands it to the man.

"The patient needs to be suctioned. Family members do that here," she explains.

"Oh," I say disappointed that a nurse is not going to at least check on the patient. "Really, that is the job of the ward boy, to suction," Preeti adds. I am beginning to wonder what nurses are supposed to do on the general wards, since every traditional nursing task seems to be delegated to others—family members, ayahs, ward boys, physicians. So, I simply ask.

Preeti hesitates a long time before she answers. "Well, the senior nurses, they have to document, the diet book, the nominal register, indent all the medications." In my observations thus far, this takes at most, an hour to do. "And the juniors, we give medications, do rounds with the doctors." Then she is silent.

* * *

The next morning the Male Ward III hallway is still dark. The power is out again. A few of the ward boys are there and so are the ayahs, splashing water on the cement floor with mugs and pushing it with a long-handled squeegee type broom. Ayahs give themselves modified sponge baths using the ward's one sink, rubbing handfuls of water over their faces and arms; hiking up billowing clothes above wrinkly knees, washing legs and bending to scrub feet, their navy blue saris serving as both cover and towel. Skittish, stray cats with skinny frames and skin lesions that have taken up residence in the hospital weave strategically between the beds searching for food until they are chased out of the ward by shouting ayahs who stamp their feet and wave their brooms menacingly at the desperate animals. Some of the patients and attendants on the medical oncology wing peer through the cement window and stare at me. We all seem confused: where are the nurses? While I wait, a young man wanders in to the nurse's station. His name is Sunil and his father had surgery for stomach cancer. He tells me his father is recovering well, but they had to travel very far to SICH—their village is over 150 kilometers away.

Sunil wears worn black slacks and an impressively crisp blue dress shirt too big for his thin torso. His father—the patient—is clearly not feeling well with a nasogastric tube hanging from his nostril and a concerning pallor. I wonder what exactly the family has been told about the patient's prognosis, as the son seems incredibly confident and hopeful about his father's recovery. I tell him I am a cancer nurse researcher, studying pain management.

"I am the eldest of three brothers," he tells me. "My family is a poor family," he says. "My parents are farmers, but I have my Bachelor's degree," he says with pride.

Sunil's father trajectory fits with what I've been told about how patients arrive at SICH—his father was seen by a village doctor who referred them to a private hospital where 30 treatments of radiation were given. "But the mass didn't shrink," Sunil says, "and the doctors recommended chemotherapy and surgery. But then that hospital stopped taking MHS (the government subsidized health payment plan), and so my father was referred here."

Sunil tells me his father has had pain, but he feels the staff is attentive and the pain has been managed well. "My father takes all his medications without argument. He complies fully!" Sunil doesn't know the name of the medication his father takes for pain, but his face lights up in recognition when I suggest Tramadol. I ask him how things have been going in general and how he helps his father in the hospital.

"I am satisfied with the care provided to my father," he says quickly, almost too quickly. "I monitor for all symptoms and report them to the nurse—nausea, if a medication has run out, pain. I have experience in government hospitals," Sunil says, "so I know what to report to the nurse. I can find the nurse in the duty room. I help with all the daily care, bathing, helping with toileting, emptying drains, feeding."

"At first," he admits, "I had trouble adjusting to the smell in the ward that was coming from the Operating Theater," he says. "And it is difficult because only 1 attendant is allowed to stay on the ward, and they prefer it to be a male attendant. But I sleep under the veranda outside, so my mother can sleep on the floor by my father's bed. I also feel very bad seeing other patients suffer... with pain, vomiting, passing motions. I want to help them, but I feel helpless."

And with that he smiles, and leaves—this temporary distraction complete— and returns to his primary purpose: caring for his father.

***

Preeti arrives, and in her unflappable manner announces, "no one else is coming today." It seems there was a miscommunication about leave requests, and both Mary and the head nurse will not be at work today. A series of phone calls are made, and relief staggers in throughout the day—first a nurse from Male Ward I comes and administers the medications on the surgical wing. Then, Sujatha pops in from the Paying Ward to help start IVs. She is a waif of a thing, with tiny spectacles and elfin-sized feet in white stockings. And then another nurse arrives from Female Ward III to help Preeti with documentation.

Preeti's posture uncharacteristically stiffens when the Orange Unit attending physician arrives on the ward for rounds. She whispers, "we are all scared of him. For the tiniest thing wrong, we will get scolded. *Scolded*," she emphasizes. The physician swaggers intimidatingly among the beds, wearing a white and blue checkered dress shirt, thick black-framed glasses, and sporting the ubiquitous male Indian moustache. He grills the resident as they move from patient to patient, quizzing her about detailed aspects of cancer biology and treatment. Patients push their palms together in a "Namaste" gesture when he stops at their bed, but the attending physician only talks to the resident in English; he does not address the patient. Nothing is translated into the local language. At one point, he pokes at a patient's clavicle after a long, one-sided conversation with the resident about locally and nodular recurrent cancer, and announces, "this treatment is not sufficient," and then abruptly proceeds to the next bed.

The next bed is a man with a white blanket wrapped completely around his neck and face, as if he is protecting himself from a violent dust storm. Only his brown, blinking eyes peer out.

"You, where are you from?" the attending physician suddenly barks at me. I didn't think he'd even noticed me.

"From the U.S.," I say, trying to sound confident. "I'm a nurse researcher."

He accepts this easily. "You won't see this in the U.S., only in a picture that you can take and show people at home," he says, and he motions vigorously for me to come forward, which I reluctantly do. Clearly, this patient is hiding a horrific wound; I don't want to make him feel more stigmatized and like a spectacle than he must already. In a culture that puts a high value on personal appearance, I cannot imagine the challenge of navigating daily life with the burden of deformity.

The patient is instructed to unwrap his covering, which he does, slowly and deliberately. His arms circle around his head in a well-practiced maneuver, uncoiling the cloth, loop by careful loop, apologizing with his eyes for what he is about to reveal. He draws his hand away, finished, and we are confronted with a man with only half a face. Below his eyes, there is no cheek, no chin, no nose, a partial mouth. The entire right side of his face has been eaten away by cancer and resected by surgery. All that remains is a pulpy, dark hole. I swallow hard and feel my throat tighten. *Please God, don't let me throw up.*

Early afternoon sun slants through the open windows, illuminates a panel of dust particles that hover, suspended, by the man's bed. They shift and dance in the warm, still air and pellucid light. There is a sacredness in this man's open offering of pain, the acceptance that there is simply nothing left. Except, of course, everything.

"Take a picture," the physician encourages me.

"No, no, it's okay," I quietly decline. The doctor looks disappointed by my refusal.

"Tobacco chewing, it causes much cancer here," the doctor lectures, clearly viewing this as a teachable moment. "Buccal malignancies are very common." He lists the challenges: the patients are very poor, they come from so far away, they present with late-stage disease, they continue to use tobacco. "There are no counselors, the doctors are expected to do it here," he says. "But how can the doctors do it? I see 80 patients a day in clinic."

The man is receiving palliative chemotherapy. "There is no point," says the attending physician bluntly. "Try to stop it," he tells the resident as they move along to the next patient. I glance back as the man stares straight ahead, slowly twisting and rewrapping the blanket around his head.

After the doctors leave, I notice attendants streaming back on to the ward, barred from being there with the physicians, but now returning to their job at the bedside of fathers, brothers, sons, and uncles.

*   *   *

Preeti is preparing medications for the surgical side of Male Ward III with a ward boy whom I don't recognize. I start to follow her as she gives medication, but she stops me.

"Wait outside, I don't have a mask for you," she says simply and then proceeds down the narrow, cramped aisle of cots. I watch as she becomes swallowed by the crowd.

While I wait for Preeti to finish, a middle-aged man approaches me. He introduces himself as Akil, and he is wearing a red t-shirt which says in block white lettering: *The four stages of life: (1) believing in Santa, (2) knowing Santa is fake, (3) playing Santa, and (4) looking like Santa.*

"My father, he is 68 years old," Akil points to one of the first beds on the ward that I can see from the corridor; it is occupied by a depressed looking elderly gentleman with a large bandage covering his face. "Two days ago, he had surgery to remove some cancer, basal cell." Basal cell cancers, a common form of skin cancer, are generally not aggressive and easily curable with a straightforward outpatient procedure. From the extent of the surgical incision and flap on his father's nose, I judge this is not the case, and I wonder if he, in fact, has a more extensive head and neck cancer. "He was in the operating room for five hours," Akil tells me, further raising my suspicion.

"Do you have anyone here to help you?" I ask. Akil looks completely depleted. He tells me he is an only child and his mother died when he was young, so he is the primary caregiver for his father. "I do have an uncle, he'll come shortly so I can rest. I didn't get much sleep last night."

"Where do you sleep?" Akil points again to his father's bed. "There, by his bed, on the floor." The concrete floor.

"That is not easy," I say, inadequately.

"It's life," he says, half-smiling. "You have to manage."

While I observe Preeti mixing more medications, I glance behind me and see Akil and his uncle, who has arrived, talking with one of the surgery residents. Akil shows the doctor some tablets and asks him a question about one of the creams he is to apply to his father's face.

When they are finished talking, I sit at the table in the nurses' station with the surgical resident. His shirt pocket is stuffed with folded bits of paper and his shaggy jet-black hair curls around the collar of his wrinkled lab coat.

"Can I ask you a question about the patient you were just talking about?"

"Sure," he says, looking up at me from the chart he is writing in.

"What is his diagnosis? He has head and neck cancer?"

"No, no. He had surgery for a basal cell carcinoma and then as an incidental finding we found an enlarged lymph node, so we dissected that, all at level 1, very difficult surgery to remove while preserving all structures, and it looks like he has lymphoma too. He's very fortunate we caught that."

I wonder how fortunate the man thinks he is, but I don't say anything.

"You know, I psyched out when I first got here," the surgical resident admits. "All these bald patients from chemotherapy, all these emaciated people, tubes coming out of their bodies. I couldn't handle it. I left. I thought about another specialty. I tried it, taking care of kidney stones that aren't really a big deal, you know that sort of stuff. But then I came back. I said to myself, 'if I don't do this, who will?'

"You will find that the nurses here do not have much responsibility at all, it's trivial," he continues, affirming what I have observed. "The nurses do not take much personal interest in the patients. Adishree is different, the ICU nurse, she is the exception. And Preeti, this sister here today, she is very cooperative. On a scale of 0–10, she is a 12 for cooperation. You tell her to do something, and she will do it. But there are others, who are a 2 or 3 on a 10 scale, and it is much more difficult."

"Why do you think that is, that the nurses do not take much personal interest in the patients?" I ask.

He stops writing and looks up at me like I am an idiot. "Do you know how much money they make?"

He scrawls a quick calculation on a pad of paper. "It's about $100 dollars a month, that's all. What do you expect for that amount of money?" he asks rhetorically. "And they can lose their jobs, like that,"[6] he says, snapping his finger.

The resident asks me about differences between SICH and U.S. hospitals. "Well, some things are very similar, and some things are very different. The sheer volume of patients is different, and some of the social challenges are different," I say. "And family members are expected to provide a lot more of the care here than what I'm used to."

---

6 The surgical resident is referring here to contract nurses, who made significantly less money and had less job security than government nurses. During the time of my fieldwork, on average, SICH government nurses made 35–40,000 rupees per month (approximately $500–600 USD); SICH contract nurses made about 10–12,000 rupees ($150–200 USD) per month.

This surprises him. He tells me that a male attendant is required before a patient can go to surgery.

"Why a male attendant?"

"Well, sometimes there is a way around it. Someone may have two female attendants who are very aggressive and can get things done. But we need someone strong, someone who can go out and get blood or get supplies or medications, and we can't expect females to do that."

This is first time I have heard anyone mention a gender requirement for attendants. I'm about to ask him more, when Preeti gestures that it is time to eat.

In the break room, Preeti is eating chapattis and curry. She insists on sharing her meal and generously offers me the most prized part of her lunch—a hard-boiled egg mixed in with her rice and curry, which I try to refuse, but as a compromise, we split. I go over to the sink to wash my hands and find the pink bar of soap missing.

"Is there any soap?" I ask.

"Maybe in the cabinet?" she suggests. I open the metal cabinet and Preeti points to a packet of powder that says, optimistically, "*Clean Anything!*" on its side.

"Is this okay to use on your hands?" I ask, dubiously examining the package. It looks like the kind of powder that needs to be diluted for institutional type cleaning.

She shrugs. "I used it," she says. I put a small amount of the mysterious white powder on my hands and then go to the sink, scrubbing with as much friction as I can.

After lunch, Preeti wants to go to the hospital nurses' lounge, a significant distance away in the older section of the hospital. I'm concerned about leaving the ward unattended, Preeti is not. The nurses' lounge is empty. It is a surprisingly bright room, with lockers, a table, an old wooden vanity with a cloudy mirror, a cot, a large table with chairs, and a tall rack where saris are hung after nurses change in to their uniforms. We sit for a while. "Come," she says, rising from her chair, "we will go to Male Ward II, there are some Sisters who will talk with you."

On Male Ward II I meet Lavanya and Naveena. Lavanya looks suspicious and unhappy, but Naveena is full of questions: How many siblings do I have? Am I married? Where do I stay? How much is my rent? What do I eat? How am I finding the food? What is my salary in the U.S.? How do I get back and forth to the hospital?

Naveena grabs my hand and says urgently, "I must ask you one important question! In America, why is everyone so, supersti...," she cuts herself off, "so, with black magic, and ghosts?"

I laugh. "What do you mean?"

Naveena consults Preeti for linguistic support. "You know, in the movies, always ghosts and aliens and evil forces."

"What movie did you see, can you give me an example?" I ask.

"Harry Potter!" she shrieks.

I burst out laughing. "That's just entertainment, fantasy. People in America don't really believe in that." She seems disappointed, so I tell them about Halloween and that seems to cheer them up.

***

Today, the hospital medicine store (pharmacy) has made a large delivery, so Preeti and the head nurse are busy organizing ampules and vials into small cardboard boxes spread out on a table in the nurses' station and on a rolling metal cart. I notice a young man is helping Preeti; he wears a wool cap and pants and a shirt that are too large for him. I ask if this is the ward boy I haven't met yet.

"Oh no," Preeti says, "he's a patient here, and he helps us." Suresh is a 15-year-old with acute leukemia who spends long periods of time on Male Ward III receiving his treatment. To help alleviate his boredom, the nurses allow Suresh to assist with certain tasks, similar to Hameeda—the young female patient with osteosarcoma—who occasionally prepares bandages in the palliative care clinic.

Suresh draws up syringes of fluid from the vials, assisting Preeti and the ayah in preparing the medications. He does this as any typical male teenager would—somewhat sloppily and carelessly, playing a little ad-hoc hacky sack with an empty vial box that falls toward the floor. From my vantage point, I cannot tell if he mixes any chemotherapy, but I do see him handle it: he gives an IV bottle that has been injected with ifosfamide to a patient's attendant who accidently turns the IV bottle upside down, causing fluid to rush out the bottom, spilling chemotherapy on to the medication preparation table and the floor. Suresh grabs the IV bottle, rights it, and then hands it back to the attendant, telling her how to carry the bottle and to be more careful. Preeti calmly continues what she is doing.

I don't say anything at first, but eventually feel compelled. So many people are barefoot. I approach her and say quietly, "Preeti, some of the chemotherapy from that bottle spilled on to the floor..." I wait for a response; there is none. I think back to my days as a chemotherapy nurse and the intensive protocol we had to follow if chemotherapy spilled. I try again.

"Should I call the ayah and ask her to come clean it up?" I ask trying to be helpful. "It's chemotherapy..."

Preeti remains unconcerned, and even as I ask the question I realize that asking the ayah to clean it up will put her at risk of exposure to the toxic drug. There doesn't seem like any good solution.

"I'll call her later," Preeti tells me. I sit back down.

On the surgical wing of the ward, Preeti and Suresh work together dispensing tablets to patient attendants, who then are responsible for administering the pills to the patient. I see Akil standing patiently, waiting to collect medications for his father, the patient with basal cell carcinoma and lymphoma. Preeti stands behind the medication cart; I count 18 attendants crowded around her diminutive frame. Even watching from a distance it feels claustrophobic.

I return from medication rounds on the surgical side of Male Ward III in time for the nurses' mid-morning tea break. The head nurse sits at the documentation table drinking her small Dixie cup of chai. When she's finished, she casually pushes the used paper cup out the hospital window onto the street below, seemingly unaware of the blue trash can a few feet away.

* * *

I am enthusiastically invited to the nurses' Christmas party. In preparation for the party, I have worn one of my better salwar kameez suits and the nurses are delighted that my turquoise colored sparkly hairpin and bangles match my dupatta and trim of my kurta. It is different than any other hospital holiday party I have ever attended, as it is less a party and more a church service, complete with hymns and a bombastic sermon. All of the nurses have changed out of their uniforms and into bright, dazzling saris. They are perfectly and beautifully pleated, draped, and folded, like vibrant, walking origami.

The Director of the hospital, along with a few other high-level guests I do not know, are seated at a dais and given flowers to officially begin the party. A small Charlie-brown-esque artificial Christmas tree is laden with shiny ornaments. It is an odd mix of church and work and party. A blanket is draped over the projector stand and a large cardboard box placed on top. After the sermon, the lid of the box is removed to reveal a large birthday cake with "Happy Birthday Jesus!" written in pink icing. The Director makes the first cut, and then the Nursing Superintendent, a no-nonsense woman, picks up the piece of cake and places it in to the Director's mouth. It's a funny and intimate picture to my Western eyes, and now I feel like I am at a wedding.

More pieces of cake are cut and fed to the other special guests, neatly or messily depending on the server. Everyone wants in on the action and head nurses leap up to feed cake to each other. I am called forward and a chunk of cake is stuffed in to my mouth, complete with the requisite mess of pink icing. After all the guests and senior administrators have received their cake, mayhem ensues as the audience rushes forward to get their slice, and also pick up cookies and small snack bags that are being frantically distributed. I feel like I am caught in a cake mosh pit, with a baked good being sacrificed on the altar of a Christmas party. I am jostled and pushed and ultimately squeezed out the auditorium door in to the hallway by the laughing and jubilant crowd.

Namaste

Because this is a government referral hospital, 99% of our patients are poor—below the poverty line—and they don't have any education, they don't have the money to go for early detection. For women, most of them they will be in the house, doing household things; only when their disease is incapacitating them to the point where they cannot do their daily work, then male family members will bring them to the hospital. Especially some of the young girls with cancer; their husbands leave them and the parents do not want to look after them either. Particularly HIV patients. So, our patients are very poor, they come in a late stage and they have many problems. That is the scenario.

Dr. Rama, oncologist

Naveena, the nurse who asked me about Harry Potter, grabs my arm as I walk onto the ward. Sister Lavanya approaches, her voice barely audible, which she attributes to a bad cold and a sore throat. Her lacey Bachelor's cap looks much too small for her large head.

"Had your breakfast?" she rasps, followed by, "What did you have?"

Three nurses listen intently as I recount the specifics of my morning meal: Special K with milk and a banana cut up on top, coffee with milk and sugar. They seem positively baffled by this bizarre combination of foods, and collectively decide it is horribly inadequate and insist that I eat their dosas, rice, and okra curry. I try to request small portions, but this proves impossible. While eating, we are interrupted by one of the Green Unit attending physicians who bursts into the nurses' break room; the nurses scramble to hastily stand up. The physician launches in on Naveena for allowing the ayahs to be mopping the unit at this time.

"You need to be sure they are finished with this business before I come to do rounds!" he demands. Naveena's head bobbles so vigorously I fear it may detach from her neck. "We need to be able to fully concentrate, not deal with *this*," he extends his arms in exasperation, gesturing toward the ayah mopping in fast, furious sideways strokes at the end of the ward.

I watch as Naveena mixes medication; it is similar to what I have observed on the other wards, so I turn my attention to the documentation books. I count 18 scattered on the table. I am intrigued by the last one—the Doctors Call Book—as I have not seen any like it on the other wards. The book is blank except for one lone entry from over a year ago. I study the Night Instruction Book for a while, then look up and realize both Naveena and Lavanya are gone. They disappear for over an hour, leaving one nurse—Lakshmi, a gaunt-faced contract nurse with a pronounced overbite—to administer medications to 56 patients. Sitting at the front table, I quickly lose sight of Lakshmi's white uniform as she disappears among the rows of beds. Patients and their attendants, looking confused, approach me and try to hand me medical files and charts. Embarrassed, I try to explain in broken Hindi that I cannot help them. One attendant hands me a green folder, repeating "new admission, new admission." She looks desperate and on the brink of tears. I nod and clutch the folder to my chest, pantomiming its importance. As the minutes tick by with still no sign of Naveena or Lavanya, I become increasingly agitated.

When they finally return, Lavanya grabs a stack of charts and slams them down on the documentation table, visibly annoyed. Her face is pinched and tight. She pulls folders off the top of the stack, one by one, opens to the Case Sheet and copies the doctor's orders in to the Night Instruction Book. Attendants tentatively approach the table; Lavanya keeps her back toward them, she does not turn to speak to them or make eye contact, but shoos them away with a disinterested flick of her wrist. The rebuffed attendants shuffle backwards, barefoot and silent.

I observe what I have before: patient family members yelled at, dismissed with snarls and brushed away, a general disinterest in what is happening on the ward, the delegation of traditional nursing tasks to ward boys, ayahs, and family members. Chemotherapy is mixed haphazardly and dangerously and splatters everywhere. Naveena's uniform looks like it has a case of the chicken pox.

The only bright spot is when Dr. Rama arrives with her students and sets up shop at the front table. Her calm and gentle energy pervades the entire unit, and suddenly, unbelievably, Male Ward II feels relaxing. After observing so many negative interactions, it is a relief to watch her make eye contact, smile, and attempt to make a genuine human connection with the dozens of men who crowd around the table, holding their files, awaiting their opportunity to speak with her.

"Hello, Virginia," she says to me, holding up a CT scan and patiently talking with her residents about the images. "You must join us in clinic one day," she offers. "You'll get a better sense for how things operate."

* * *

Lavanya wants to know what jewelry women in the U.S. wear—ankle bracelets? *No, not really.* Nose piercings? *Well, sometimes, but I wouldn't say it is common.* Bangles? *Hmmm, not generally.*

"Really, I think the difference is that the jewelry women wear here is more ritualized, more structured. It's not quite like that in the U.S.," I say. I purposely don't say "the jewelry *married* women wear," because I don't feel like having another conversation about my marital status.

But I am unsuccessful.

"You're married?" Lavanya asks me.

"No, not yet. Hopefully soon," I respond, providing the answer I know I am expected to give.

"Will you marry family or outside?"

"Do you mean will I marry a blood relative?"

"Yes," she says.

"No, I won't. Is that common here?" I ask.

"Yes, yes," Lavanya says quickly.

"How close is not okay?"

"A sister's sister and a brother's brother is okay," she tells me. I'm not entirely clear what she means but we move on.

"Are marriages arranged in your place?" Lavanya asks.

"No."

"What will your parents say?"

"Well, I don't have to get their permission." Lavanya seems amazed by this revelation.

"The family structure is stronger here," she asserts.

I find myself strangely eager to defend my culture. "Well, I think it is a different strength," I say. "In the U.S., most people when they reach 18 or a little older leave the home and set up their own independent house."

"They live with their parents?"

"Not usually. They live separately."

"Do they have to take care of their in-laws?"

"Sometimes, but that is not generally an expectation," I explain.

"Is there a dowry?" she asks, referring to the Indian tradition of the bride's family providing the groom's family with lavish gifts as additional incentive to marry their daughter, a practice that is technically outlawed, but remains commonplace.

"No," I say.

"The divorce rate is much higher in the U.S.," Lavanya says smugly, as if that settles everything.

"I think in part that's because it's very difficult to get divorced here," I challenge. "Maybe impossible." There is silent acknowledgment of this reality.

"Do men beat their wives in the U.S.?"

In the familiar litany of questions, this one stops me: it is the first time I have been asked this. Lavanya's face is as unreadable as an outdated map. My heart softens.

"Yes, sometimes that does happen. But it is considered very, *very* wrong."

Lavanya looks at me blankly and does not say anything. If she is surprised by my answer she does not show it. Her mobile phone rings, and she excuses herself.

***

On my way to the outpatient department to spend time with Dr. Rama and her team, I stop by Female Ward II to visit Hameeda, the 19-year-old palliative care patient with osteosarcoma. She has been getting progressively weaker and she looks terrible today—worn out and utterly exhausted. She tells me she has horrible pain and hasn't slept. I ask her if she has told the nurses. She shakes her head no.

"Nothing is working," she says dejectedly.

"Would you like me to talk to the nurses? See if we can change your medication?" I ask optimistically, although as soon as the words leave my mouth I dread that nothing will happen. Thankfully, Agnes is working on Female Ward II today, so I find her and tell her about Hameeda's pain.

Agnes looks at me with her kind eyes. "I'm worried about Hameeda, Agnes. She doesn't look good today and she is telling me she has horrible pain. Could you assess her and see if there is anything else to be done?" Agnes nods thoughtfully and I leave Female Ward II, hoping Agnes will follow-up.

* * *

The outpatient clinic hallway is packed with people: men limping, women pulling their dupattas over their faces to avoid breathing in the unpleasant odors permeating the tight space, people lined up outside of clinic rooms, crowding around doorways. I have to literally push my way through the throngs of people, through the green OT (operating theater) drape that hangs as a makeshift divider between the hallway and the clinic room. Dr. Rama and her colleagues sit at a table, encircled by people holding colored folders; I count 16 people. I can barely see her, let alone get close enough to ask her a question. I wait, wedged in the corner. A small, electric fan rhythmically billows the edge of her lab coat. Once again, she is the epitome of calm in a sea of chaos. Finally, there is a small break in the crowd and we make eye contact.

"Hello, Virginia!" she says pleasantly. "Welcome! I told you not to expect a chair!" she says, smiling.

Behind the front room is a smaller exam room with a sink, metal table, and a rack of rewashed latex gloves hung up to dry. Patients are assigned to different medical teams—Orange, Red, Green, Purple, Blue, or White—not based on disease, but on the day of the week they register at the hospital, and they are seen by whichever clinic practitioner grabs their folder off the pile first.

The clinic room swells with patients and attendants, until the ward boy or ayah, standing sentry at the door, decides a critical mass has been reached, and then barks commands as people are pushed back in to the hallway. From the corridor, anxious and curious faces peek around the green drape. The ayah's voice is strident and shrill, and I find her immediately distasteful. She sits on a wooden stool by the clinic entrance like a toad, waiting to strike at the next fly, wearing an olive-colored blouse and a white sari that reveals rolls of flesh that ripple like waves when she moves.

The ward boy and ayah behave unpredictably. Sometimes they let the crowd grow to almost 20 people huddled around the doctors at the table; other times they chase out a few stragglers. Their words are harsh, their body language abrupt, and they are at times physical: the ward boy roughly grabs a woman's arm and pushes her out of the clinic; the ayah takes hold of a ten-year-old boy, bald from chemotherapy treatments and wearing a gray cap, who has been standing—waiting—over an hour for a 15-second interaction with Dr. Rama, by the arm and pushes him out the door, scolding and scowling. The doctors let the ayah and ward boy do their thing; only at one point when the ward boy continues to yell loudly at a man does Dr. Rama say something and he quiets down. The patients who come to clinic are very, very sick; women's scapulae push out from too thin torsos like plates.

I am told the simulator (the machine which marks the areas of the body to be targeted with radiotherapy beams) is being repaired and is only available one day a week, so patients are marked for radiation by hand using anatomical landmarks with a black marker. The marks are then outlined with a thin tape that contains a material that can be confirmed by X-ray. Patients return weekly to get remarked. "PG-1s (first-year residents) are allowed to do the abdominal markings, because it's much easier," Dr. Sita explains, herself a first-year resident. "The head and neck patients are harder, so the PG-3s (third-year residents) and attending physicians mark those patients."

Dr. Rama beckons me to the exam room to see a woman with breast cancer. The woman sits on the high metal table, her flat and scarred chest exposed.

"This patient was initially treated, but then had a recurrence," Dr. Rama explains to me, as she runs her fingers expertly along the woman's dark, ridged scar. "She did not follow-up with her chemotherapy and radiation and now has a paralyzed left arm from nerve damage related to the growing tumor." The woman supports her flaccid and swollen left arm with her right, like a bird protecting a broken wing. Her round face and crinkly eyes radiate kindness. She bobbles her head and smiles at me.

"Do you know why the patient wasn't able to follow-up with treatment?" I ask Dr. Rama.

"Ignorance," she says simply. "Many of these patients are illiterate. We tell them things over and over and they do not understand."

I press. "Why don't they understand?"

She pauses to consider this. "Because of ignorance," she says again, matter-of-factly but not unkindly.[7] She exits the small exam room.

I linger. The woman looks down at her shirt and then up at me beseechingly. She makes a feeble attempt, but clearly cannot refasten her shirt with her heavy and limp left arm and the lack of feeling in her fingertips.

"Do you need some help?" I ask, uncertain if she understands my English, but gesturing to her open shirt as I move toward her. She nods and smiles; I button up her blouse, poke the small white plastic circles into their respective slits with a renewed appreciation for the difficulty of the task. Using her strong right hand, she then grasps her swollen, paralyzed left arm, heaves it upwards with tremendous effort, and forces her palms together in front of her disfigured chest in a lopsided gesture: *Namaste*. My throat catches.

***

7 This is an example of a well-intended interaction but one seemingly limited by a lack of awareness of social determinants that can influence health outcomes. It seems noteworthy that Dr. Rama, one of the most compassionate physicians I met at SICH, did not seem able or willing to consider the multitude of reasons (transportation, poverty, stigma, etc.) that may have impacted this patient's ability to come for follow-up treatment. It is also possible that Dr. Rama was using the term "ignorance" in a broader or different context than I understood, one that was meant to encapsulate these other reasons.

Back at the main clinic table, Dr. Sita, the first-year resident, talks with a young man.

"Virginia," she says, looking up from the medical file in front of her, "this is a case of carcinoid, renal involvement, which is very rare. The team is going to discuss it at the case conference this Saturday." She spends quite a bit of time with the man and toward the end of the conversation, asks Dr. Rama for some assistance.

"Even though it's atypical, you need to tell him the prognosis is poor," Dr. Rama instructs Sita from the opposite side of the table over the crowd and noise. The man sits on the hard metal stool, oblivious to this casual exchange about his fate. He has a well-groomed moustache and wears a worn looking white and blue dress shirt. Sita nods in understanding. I wonder how she will break this bad news in the crowded space. She leans in closely, quietly says a few more words to the man, who then calmly leaves the clinic without any outward sign that he has just been told devastating news.

"What did you say about the prognosis?" I ask her.

"I didn't. That's not the patient."

"It's not the patient?" I ask confused.

"No, that's his nephew. So I told the nephew to bring in more films and then we can talk more."

"Is that common, that you don't see the actual patient in the clinic? They send a family member in their place?"

"Sometimes, yes," Sita says. "And when it is the patient I need to ask how much they want to know about the disease, the prognosis. Some don't want to know much," she says wisely.

A woman with vulvar cancer shuffles into the clinic exam room. She wears a black and white sari that hangs loosely on her emaciated frame. Her hair is stringy and oily, tied back in a messy braid, and her sunken eyes are hollow as caves. She carries a urinary collection bag in her right hand and from my brief assessment, looks weeks from death. With difficulty, she gingerly climbs on to the metal exam table and pulls up her sari over her buttocks. There is no sheet underneath her and she sits with her bare perineum pressed against the cold metal surface. Sita instructs the woman to lie down, but she cannot do it by herself. Even though we are standing right there, available to help, Sita calls for the ayah who comes in and assists the patient to a lying position.

As the ayah helps with positioning, Sita whispers to me, "this is sort of a psychiatric patient."

"Is she having pain?" I ask. The woman looks miserable.

"Yes, she is being seen by palliative care. She's already on morphine."

A second-year resident comes in to supervise as Sita re-marks the woman's radiation field with a black pen. The young residents talk with each other, but say nothing to the patient, and then both exit the exam room. I hesitate. Does Dr. Rama come in now to see the patient? Is there another part of the exam? The woman is lying there on the hard metal table, her genitals and abdomen completely exposed, and she cannot sit up. Uncertain, I step back in to the front room. "Sita," I say, gesturing toward the exam room, "should

we, can I…?" Sita cuts me off. "She'll be fine," she says curtly and yells for
the ayah. But the ayah is not nearby, so the woman lies exposed on the exam
table for an interminable ten minutes until the ayah is located and she assists
the patient to sit up and get off the exam table.

The patient walks slowly into the front room. She stops by the door, turns
to face the physicians at the table, and begins to cry—shuddering, heaving
sobs that radiate from the deepest realm of the soul. Everyone stops. The
woman is talking rapidly and loudly in high-pitched Hindi. Dr. Rama holds
up her index finger in front of her mouth—"shhh"—but the woman continues her distressing monologue. I lean toward Sita.

"What is she saying?" I ask.

Sita whispers to me in the staccato of translation: "She wants to go home.
She doesn't want any more radiation treatments. She wants the tube taken out."

Fifteen onlookers witness the emotional discussion that ensues between
the patient and the doctors. Eventually, the patient pushes aside the green
drape and leaves the clinic.

"What happened?" I ask.

"She wants the catheter removed. Her son won't come visit her with it. He
calls it 'her tail,'" explains Dr. Rama.

"That's terrible," I say, thinking how painful it must be to be rejected by
your own son in such a dire time.

"Is she going to get more treatment?" I ask, confused.

"Yes, she is scheduled for another round of treatment. She must complete
her treatment," Dr. Rama says, who goes on to explain in detail about the
types of radiation and grades of fractions that are required to treat this type
of advanced vulvar cancer. "The tube must stay."

Before I can ask any more questions, a young woman with cervical cancer
comes in to be evaluated for brachytherapy and disappears in to the back
exam room with Sita. There is no partition separating the small exam room
from the front room, so I clearly hear the clinking of metal instruments and
the distinct sounds that accompany a pelvic exam. The ayah assists. After the
exam, as the patient is leaving the clinic she leans her back against the wall,
utters a small cry, and slides slowly down to the floor in a crumpled heap.
She is pale and breathing rapidly and appears to be in tremendous pain; she
holds her head in her small hands.

Sita says something short and rapid to her in Hindi, and the woman stands
up and silently exits the clinic.

* * *

"Would you like to come with me to temple this evening?" Joanie asks. "It is
a beautiful temple, a replica of a much larger one in my home state." It has
been a long day and it sounds like a wonderful idea.

A short auto ride to the temple reveals a stunning sandalwood brown
complex with intricate carved spires; Joanie tells me the original temple that

inspired this one has spires so high you cannot see the tops. There is a calm, friendly, orderliness to this temple and I immediately feel relaxed and included, despite the fact that I am clearly an outsider. Joanie purchases yellow flowers and coconuts and orange thread from one of the multiple stands lining the entrance to the temple. We remove our sandals, store them in a small cubby, and wash our feet.

At the first shrine, to Shiva, Joanie proffers a coconut to the priest who stands in front of the idol wearing a bright orange robe. A quick conversation ensues, the priest will not accept the coconut. Joanie shakes her head and we exit the temple to crack the coconut over a metal rail before we can hand it to the priest. "At home," Joanie says, "you hand the whole coconut to the priest and he cracks it open over Shiva's lingam.[8] Quite messy. Now there is more emphasis on making things cleaner." She leads me toward an exit. "In India the contradictions can be so obvious and painful. You will say, 'oh Joanie said all of the temples have to be so clean, and kept this-and-this a way', but then you will see someone put up a god in a little corner, under a tree, right off the road, and then people pay money to come pray at it, and then later the person who is supposed to be watching and protecting the god is snoring in the corner and a dog is coming up and urinating on the god. It's awful."

We stop at a metal railing outside the temple entrance, and Joanie repeatedly whacks the furry brown fruit against it to avail. Seeing our trouble, a kindly security guard walks over and with one fluid motion cracks the coconut, releasing the sweet white milk, and returns the dripping halves to Joanie.

We go back to the shrine and try again. This time, the coconut is accepted, along with the incense, flowers, and orange thread that Joanie gives the priest. The priest turns to the idol, whispering prayers and making small hand gestures. The orange thread is then returned to Joanie who ties it around her neck, kneels, and prostrates herself before Shiva.

We make the rounds: Ganesh, Lakshmi, Hanuman. At each shrine, the blessing routine follows a predictable pattern: a priest ladles a handful of basil-imbued water into a cupped hand which is drunk, the remaining drops are sprinkled on top of the head, while the priest holds a silver cone over the person's head.

I am officially a disaster at the temple. Joanie has to remind me to hold the diya in my right hand only. I accidently touch my shoes removing them at the shoe kiosk, necessitating another hand and foot wash. When the priests ladle the special water into my cupped hands, I'm a little afraid to drink it, so I splash most of it on the top of my head as instructed, but it's much too much and it trickles down my face and washes off the sparkly gold bindi Joanie affixed between my eyebrows earlier. "Your bindi! It's gone!" she tsks-tsks. We both search the temple floor until Joanie grabs my hand and we give up.

---

8 Lingam: A symbol of divine generative energy, specially a phallus worshiped as a symbol of Shiva.

At Hanuman's shrine, the priest hands me a piece of coconut and a yellow flower. "A very sweet gesture, he is saying, thank you, thank you for visiting our temple," Joanie explains. "Hanuman is a very cool god, Virginia, very chilled out. He's hanging out in the forest, then he helped Rama, then he goes back to the forest and has a good time. I like him. And he's low-maintenance, if you don't pray exactly the right way, or do puja exactly right, it's okay, no problem. Not like the goddesses," she shakes her head ominously. "Oh, yes, you simply *must* do it right for the goddesses. Or else you will have big problems in your life. *Lots* of trouble."

Joanie leads me to a quieter corner of the temple, and we sit together in the soft evening air watching people light diyas and offer puja. I ask Joanie about the origins of her name.

"Yes, it was a bit of a crisis."

I look at her, puzzled. "Crisis?"

"Yes, an identity crisis. Everyone thinks I'm a Christian or a Muslim. My father named me, after Joanne Woodward. He was a big fan. I have very light eyes, fair skin. Always, I have to explain this; yes, yes, I am Indian, yes, yes I am Hindu."

"You were named after Joanne Woodward?" I say, laughing.

"Yes, yes," she says and then she starts laughing too. We sit on the cool temple floor, hugging our knees to our chests, giggling, and suddenly everything feels light and possible again.

References

Jameton, A. (1984). *Nursing practice: The ethical issues.* Englewood Cliffs, NJ: Prentice-Hall.

LeBaron, V., Beck, S. L., Black, F., & Palat, G. (2014). Nurse moral distress and cancer pain management: An ethnography of oncology nurses in India. *Cancer Nursing, 37*(5), 331–344.

5   I Cannot Always Trust
My Heart

When I first came here I was working night duty, I was alone, the only nurse. At that time, one boy was there. He would always ask to eat roti. I used to cook it at home and bring it for him. If I give him roti one day, the next day he will ask again: "Sister, I want roti!" We used to eat together. One night, while he was eating the roti I gave him, he sat up and coughed, and suddenly, blood came pouring out. Everywhere. I didn't know what was happening. I didn't know cancer patients can have blood vomiting. I put my hands, like this [cupping her hands in front of her, like a bowl] "Blood….," [she shakes her head side to side, as if still in disbelief]…" He said—"Sister, call [Dr.] Rashi Madam. I want to live! I want to live!" Five minutes later, he died. Right in front of me. I cannot forget it [grasps her head with both hands, shakes her head both and forth]. We cannot bear it! We cannot bear it! After a child dies, we tell to the attendants— 'God gave us, God has taken back, so we should not cry.' But afterwards, I leave the patient and come outside because I can't… I cannot bear to see it; they will cry and I will cry. One day we were playing with them; the next day the patient dies. It is somewhat better now. But I cannot always trust my heart.

Sister Reesha, pediatric nurse

Kate, the American volunteer who spent part of her childhood in Dandaka and is volunteering at SICH, comes with me to the Consulate Office to pick up my diplomatic pouch, which I mailed from the U.S. before leaving for India—a perk of being part of the Fulbright program. The "pouch" is really two cardboard boxes full of nursing textbooks and gifts for the pediatric patients.

The public affairs assistant meets us at the gate with the boxes that look like they've had a rough trip; one is about to split open.

"Are you sure you don't have rocks in here? These are really, really heavy!" she jokes.

"No, no!," I laugh. "No rocks. But books. Lots of books."

Kate helps me lug them back to the hospital and upstairs to the palliative care office. As soon as I tear open the boxes, Pradeep and Dr. Darshan pounce on the pens that I had intended for the pediatric patients. One of the social workers asks if he can have one of the plastic necklaces for his daughter, a yellow one. I don't have yellow, so I give him a white necklace. My plan

DOI: 10.4324/9781003413158-8

was to distribute the nursing texts equally around the hospital, but Pradeep insists they all stay in the palliative care office and they are quickly squirreled away in a cupboard.

Kate and I take the rest of the contents to the pediatric playroom. I begin to panic as a burgeoning crowd of children gathers around us and I realize I haven't brought nearly enough toys for everyone, and even worse: what seemed logical and appropriate back home, now seems ridiculous. Some of the items, like the purple butterfly barrettes, are an absolutely inappropriate choice for a cancer ward full of bald children—what on earth was I thinking?

Wide-eyed children push toward us; one paralyzed boy is dragged into the playroom by his mother and deposited on the floor in front of me. His mother stands by, staring at me, expectantly. The small blind girl I remember seeing at the Diwali ceremony is there too, in her sparkly sequin yellow and brown dress, her head down, wearing the oversized sunglasses. I give her a small stuffed animal pig to hold because it is soft. She strokes its fluffy pink fur with her tiny hands. Predictably, now others want a stuffed animal too and I don't have enough. The pack of waiting children grows increasingly restless and I nervously look toward the door as still more and more children stream into the playroom. Word that the White Girl Brought Toys has apparently spread rapidly.

Vivek, the volunteer who staffs the pediatric playroom in the afternoons, arrives. He quickly surveys the chaos, says something sharp in Hindi to the children and parents and tells me to place the toys on three plastic chairs. This feels awkward and odd, but I do as he instructs and set up the toys on the plastic chairs in some sort of bizarre version of an auction or yard sale. The children sit quietly around the chairs, carefully eyeing up the goods, which Vivek will not let them touch.

"This is horrible," I whisper to Kate. "I can't believe how badly I screwed this up. What should I do?"

"You have some paper and pens, right? Enough for everyone? Let's give out those," she suggests.

"Good idea," I say, quickly handing out paper and magic markers. But the children aren't sure how to use the markers and pens I've brought, and they have no idea what to do with the stickers of dinosaurs. They look more confused than happy.

After another painful half hour, Vivek starts to lock away the toys I brought—most of them untouched—into the large floor-to-ceiling metal cabinet in the playroom. When he opens the cabinet I see it is crammed full of toys; as he works to wedge in this latest contribution, I cannot help but wonder if they will ever be found or used again.[1]

---

1 This was an extremely humbling example of when "trying to help" actually made things worse. Not having enough of the same toy for every child was a disaster and unfair. Later, during my fieldwork, I tried to rectify this with the help of Paul and we distributed small, identical treats to all the pediatric patients.

After the debacle on the pediatric ward, I am thoroughly discouraged, and Kate kindly suggests lunch at a nearby restaurant.

"I never realized how American I was until I came to live in India! I don't know how it is genetically possible that I am Indian!" she says in her charming self-deprecating manner, referring to her multiple food allergies and intolerance to spicy food. Kate is staying with her elderly aunt and uncle and confides that the toughest adjustment has been going from a single, independent, professional woman living in New York City to an unmarried, chaperoned, sheltered woman in Dandaka. She grew up in a well-to-do Dandaka suburb, across the street from a large slum.

"No one will tell you that you can't be something in the U.S.," Kate tells me, "but here, you are born into your lot in life." Even though caste is technically illegal, we both know it is alive and well. Last week, I opened the *Hindu Times* to the extensive matrimony section and saw dozens of grooms-seeking-brides and brides-seeking-grooms, all organized by caste.

Kate tells me how she witnessed her uncles sitting on the sofa, directing a seven-year-old child servant to carry bags of their heavy luggage up the stairs to the bedrooms.

"They just sat there, watching. And these are educated, sophisticated people. I just couldn't believe it," she says, slowly tearing a piece of naan from its oval shape.

Kate tells me about the families she's met at the hospital who come from faraway villages to Dandaka so that their children can get treatment and live in makeshift huts by the hospital—often for months at a time. She tells me about Anup, a 15-year-old boy with leukemia who has been abandoned by his family because they cannot cope with his disease, nor afford the cost of treatment. Kate is particularly worried about him because he has no one really looking out for him. "I brought in a change of clothes and some towels and other stuff for him, but the hospital staff kept saying, 'don't give it to Anup, here, give it the others.'" Kate isn't sure why, but thinks it is because they see a troublemaker teenager, not an impoverished adolescent with cancer who has been abandoned by his family.

I am impressed by Kate for many reasons, in no small part because she has taken the time to really get to know the families and children on the pediatric ward.

"One woman I became close to had a 1-year-old son, named Faruk. Everyday she'd come and smile and we'd talk for a little while," Kate says. "And one day she came and she was on the floor of the ward crying. She came up to me and was showing me an X-ray and crying. I thought maybe she had been confused and thought I was a nurse, because that happens a lot, so I said, 'I'm not a nurse, I'm not a sister,' and she said, 'I know, I just wanted to tell you as a friend, look at what's happening,' and then my heart broke, and she ran back in to the room sobbing, she was in one of those isolation rooms for the kids who are extra sick. I went there and she was lying on the floor sobbing with her son. She was just holding the X-ray in the air and she showed me his tumor. I think he had rectal cancer and the tumor was *so* infected, it was huge. And he could barely breathe. I sat on the floor with her, and she said, 'Don't sit on the floor!'

"Why did she say that?" I ask.

"Because I am technically of a higher caste, higher class," Kate explains. "Despite everything, she felt she should still be suffering, sitting on the ground. She didn't feel comfortable sitting on a chair, or on the bed. So, I sat on the floor and said, 'no, I'm sitting here with you.' And she started telling me *everything* about her life. A lot of people tell me things with an agenda, they are asking for something. But she wasn't asking for anything. She just needed an outlet. She had no husband, no money at all. Absolutely no money. And no other children. She spent all of her money on treatments for her son and they didn't work. I sat there with her for a very, very long time and the whole rest of the evening I was thinking that even if he recovers, she's just a small step above homelessness. Just thinking, even if he recovers, how many other struggles she has in life. The next day I came and looked for them, but he had died in the night. And it was just, very…that was the most difficult thing. It was so tragic this small child died, but mainly tragic for his Mom. Now she has lost her only son, her husband abandoned her when the boy got sick, she doesn't have any money or anywhere to go. I was so worried, like what is going to happen to this woman?"

Kate tried to find the woman the next day, but she was gone, and no one had her contact information.

* * *

Dr. Rashi is busy at the front desk, seeing a long line of children that stretches out through the ward door into the hallway. I take a seat on a metal stool behind her and try to stay out of the way. One by one, small, bald children with captivating smiles step forward. Some are weighed and measured to calculate their chemotherapy dosage. A chubby-cheeked three-year-old girl wearing a bright pink jacket and a black stocking cap with "Puma" stitched in white lettering shyly sidles past me to the scale. "Many children come alone for treatment," Dr. Rashi tells me later. "We had a 12-year-old who took an auto and a bus alone to come here for treatment, and a 10-year-old whose father had to drop him off, return to work and pick him up after treatment." Out of necessity, the requirement of having a family attendant present is more flexible on the pediatric ward.

After the last patient has been seen, Dr. Rashi slides her chair backwards, parallel to mine. "I'm exhausted," she sighs. "Every day is like this."

Built and designed with private philanthropic funds, the pediatric ward is bright and colorful and as busy as an airport terminal. Beds are arranged in rows, close together, and like the general wards, without any partitions. There are three isolation rooms—private rooms—used primarily for imminently dying patients. "And in a luxurious time," says Dr. Rashi, "if patients are neutropenic they can go in those rooms." I notice that two of the three isolation rooms for the most critically ill children are located outside the main door of the ward, in the corridor.

Unlike the general wards, pediatrics is better staffed during the day—with five nurses—and it is the only ward in the hospital where each nurse assumes responsibility for her own individual patient assignment, usually 10–15 patients. These are not government nurses, they are third-party contract nurses hired to work solely in pediatrics and they answer directly to Dr. Rashi, although they still must abide by hospital regulations—like the multitude of documentation ledgers.

I notice immediately that the pediatric nurses are more engaged with their patients, and I sense a different level of accountability: temperatures are taken, body surface areas are calculated and double-checked, and assessment questions are asked and recorded. The nurses follow better aseptic technique, better handwashing, better universal precautions, and safer chemotherapy administration practices. They carry orange, pink, and yellow plastic bins to the bedside to start IVs. Each nurse is responsible for the medications for their assigned patients, so the administration of chemotherapy feels less like an assembly line. Sister Bharati, one of the more experienced pediatric nurses, proudly shows me the "needle destroyer machine," a device which snaps off the ends of used syringes into a secure box, albeit with a loud grinding noise and concerning sparks.

Trying to control infection on the ward is stressful. "It is not possible to do," Bharati says. "Government hospitals in India involve a lot of risk. Here, there are a lot of patients and they don't listen to what we say. Village people don't understand even when they are told multiple times. We tell them that the kids might develop fever, not to leave their slippers there, not to eat here, maintain neatness, take baths; they do not listen to us even if they are told daily. Some understand, but still won't follow our instructions. Even after we tell them repeatedly, they keep doing the same things. The child gets a fever, yet they do not bathe. When I say, 'how many times do I have to tell you?' they just smile back at me. They might have their own problems, I don't deny that, but it's important that they do these things. They smile to prevent me from shouting at them."

I don't contradict Bharati, but I wonder where these parents would bathe, even if they wanted to. "The way I talk is a bit rude," she admits, "but I have a good heart. I'm very strict in the ward, but it's important to help the patients get better."

Bharati remembers caring for a little boy, four and a half years old, with acute lymphocytic leukemia, who waited for her at the hospital gate every morning. Even though he knew Sister Bharati could be stern, this little patient jumped for joy when she arrived at the hospital. Even when Bharati took a week of leave from work, the little boy continued to wait for her at the gate each morning. Sadly, a follow up bone marrow biopsy showed the boy's cancer had returned, and aggressively.[2] Soon afterwards, his body swelled and his eyes became puffy, so puffy he could not see. Bharati was off duty the day the boy died, but somebody said to him—in a well intended but perhaps misguided attempt at comfort—"Look! Sister Bharati has come!" Bharati was told that even though the dying little boy could not open his eyes, he was still trying to find her, desperately searching despite his swollen shut eyes. "I cried a lot that day, the most I have cried before in life," Bharati says quietly.

"I cried and shouted at Dr. Rashi also," Bharati says, her voice becoming higher and more animated. "She was also on leave that day. I said—'Why weren't you there? Why did this happen, can't we do anything?' I cried for two hours, Madam Rashi tried to console me. I don't usually cry. When I have a lot of communication—when I talk with a patient a lot and get to know them—I cannot take it when they die. I know in my heart that I am doing good, but you have to feel it for yourself to experience what I am saying.[3]"

* * *

The children on the pediatric ward are small and adorable and many of the girls wear bright sparkly outfits. Some of the younger male patients run

---

2 Of all the cancer disparities that exist, disparities related to global mortality rates from childhood cancers are among the most shocking and shameful. In the U.S., survival rates for pediatric cancers are as high as 85%–90%, whereas in LMICs, where 90% of childhood cancers occur, survival rates can be as low as 20% due to late diagnosis, lack of access to treatment and follow-up care, and abandonment of treatment. See Graetz (2023), The most vulnerable cancer patients, *The Lancet*, Regional Health. According to Graetz:
  Although an increasing number of publications have established these disparities in paediatric cancer care, the mechanisms contributing to inequities are less well defined. This is likely because the explanation is complicated and multifactorial. It is also because the disparities are due, at least in part, to entrenched racism, an intentionally unjust healthcare system, and an underappreciation or lack of acknowledgement of the impact of poverty on child health—topics that have been avoided in the scientific literature for too long.
  For more information, see also World Health Organization, Childhood Cancer, Key Facts, 2021 and World Health Organization Global Initiative for Childhood Cancer: Increasing access, advancing quality, saving lives, 2021.
3 This experience and others discussed in this chapter (and elsewhere in the book) corroborate findings from research about the work of pediatric oncology nurses in other low and middle-income countries where participants discussed challenges related to the emotional intensity of the work; feelings of helplessness; knowledge deficit; staffing shortages; and safety concerns related to chemotherapy administration. One Ghanian nurse (Nukpezah et al. 2021) compared the work of caring for children with cancer to "pushing a truck." One nurse from Iran (Borhani et al. 2013) related an experience of a patient loss eerily similar to that of Sister Bharati:
  … He had two big front teeth and he was tall…I took some days off, when I came back, they said he passed away; I couldn't be convinced at all. He was the first patient I really liked. Then suddenly, he was absent at the time of my arrival to the work. Oh my God, I was really sad. I said I wouldn't even cry for this, it might impact my emotion but I wouldn't cry. But I really got sad then. I do not cry in front of others, but I got really sad for him. No! I did not cry, I rarely cry… (p. 351).

around the ward without undergarments, one holds a urinary catheter in his small, pudgy hand. Most look very, very sick. A three-year-old girl with Burkitt's lymphoma, Kamala, wearing a pink jumper and with a swollen face indicative of steroid treatment, needs a new IV catheter. Inserting IV lines into children is always tricky business—they have small, delicate veins and often don't understand what is being done and why, so are reluctant to sit still for a painful procedure. Kamala turns out to be an incredibly difficult stick and I lose count after ten attempts by the nursing staff. Each time a nurse tries to put the needle into Kamala's hand or arm she screams and howls and struggles to get away.

Establishing an IV for Kamala becomes an all-day event: multiple unsuccessful attempts, followed by a short break, then another series of attempts. Kamala's face becomes red and blotchy as she screams and screams. Her young mother, who looks no more than 20, in a green and black flowered sari with a short crop of hair,[4] occasionally wipes tears from her eyes as her daughter is held down by three nurses. Finally, an IV is inserted into the child's left foot; Kamala looks almost catatonic from crying.

The pediatric ward is overflowing. The ward has 46 beds and there are 70 patients, plus attendants. Children double up in beds and parents and children sit and wait on the floor and spill out into the hallway. The ward boy, filling in for the absent security guard, intermittently enforces crowd control, arbitrarily shouting and reprimanding parents and children when he deems a certain area has become too congested. He appears to relish this position of power and I get the distinct feeling he is yelling simply because he can. But there's also a practical goal to his actions. "It's important to control the crowd on the unit; only 1 attendant per patient, unless it is very serious. We must control infection; that is the main reason. Also, if there is a large crowd, the ward becomes like a fish market! Everybody shouting and talking loudly and it's difficult to work properly!" Sister Kavita, a plump and pleasant faced pediatric nurse, explains, laughing.

Sister Kavita is a new mother; her one-year-old daughter recently had a bad skin rash. "I was so worried, so stressed," she confides, her eyes welling up with tears, "And now I think about all these parents, and their children have *cancer*." Kavita pauses a moment, sighs. I watch her administer an injection of Vincristine chemotherapy and am impressed with her technique.

There are a total of nine nurses on the pediatric ward and one auxiliary nurse, who can help administer some medications, but not chemotherapy. There are also four social workers, all frantically busy the entire time I am on the ward. I learn more about Hameeda, the 19-year-old with osteosarcoma who sometimes hangs out in the palliative care clinic, from Vasudha,

4 Women in India who have been widowed may have short, cropped hair. Historically, widows in India have been socially marginalized; see Deepa Mehta's haunting 2005 film *Water*, which depicts the lives of widowed women in India in the 1940s.

the pediatric social worker. Vasudha explains that Hameeda is an orphan, her parents died about ten years ago and she was cared for—how well is unclear—by the family who employed her father as the watchman. I immediately think of Hasan and Noora, the watchman's children, who live in the garage below my apartment building. Would our landlord take them in if their parents died? How would he treat them? Would he care for them if they developed cancer?

"Hameeda has a lot of pain, ma'am, and anxiety," Vasudha explains in her crisp English. "She wants to 'be settled.' To have a family, be married, but her disease will not allow for that." I think of her on Female Ward II, alone and scared and hurting.

I see Kamala, the three-year-old with Burkitt's Lymphoma, who underwent the ordeal yesterday to get an IV placed finally in her left foot. This morning I see she has a new IV in her right hand and the one in her foot is gone. I try not to think about how that transpired.

At one point, a young mother comes to the nursing station, wailing. She has lost her cell phone and is absolutely distraught. Sister Kavita, sympathetic, calmly walks back with the woman to the bed where they find it, hidden among the bunched bed linens. Even after it is located the woman continues to cry.

The unit bellows the entire day with the wailing and crying of pain related to IV insertions and chemotherapy administration. I am invited to observe lumbar punctures (spinal taps) to inject methotrexate (a common chemotherapy), and it is difficult to watch. The doctor's sterile technique is terrible, and I don't see him inject any lidocaine to anesthetize the area. He is, however, soft-spoken and calm, making it difficult to reconcile what he is doing with his gentle demeanor. The younger children cry and scream; I am assured it is not because of pain, but due to anxiety. The older ones, restrained by the ward boy in a tight croissant position as the needle is inserted into the space around their spine, do not cry but stumble off the table after the procedure, looking stunned.

A young girl who was given an injection of chemotherapy appears to have had a possible extravasation and her mother thrusts the girl's reddened wrist forward for Sister Bharati to assess. The girl is given a treatment of subcutaneous injections of hydrocortisone—multiple tiny steroid shots under the skin—and her panicked crying is piercingly loud. After the injections have been given, the girl's mother comes to the front desk with a piece of paper in her hand. She presents it to Bharati and asks a question. There is no one else at the desk. Bharati does not look up, she does not make eye contact with the woman, she does not say anything; she continues to slowly draw vertical columns on a blank page in a ledger with a ruler. The woman waits for a minute, looks at me, looks back at Bharati, sighs, and then walks away.

***

"They tell me we are using too much water," Dr. Rashi announces.

"What?" I ask, confused.

"Yes, they sent plumbers to take pictures of the water we are wasting on the pediatric ward. They told them to take pictures of buckets of water overflowing, of the laundry that the patient attendants do here." When I ask who is "they," she is vague; I deduce it is some hospital administration board.

I tell her that the water supply is erratic on the general wards; sometimes there is running water, sometimes there isn't.

"And nobody says anything!" she says. "They just keep quiet. It's terrible. I can't do that. I have made this pediatric unit my *mission* in life. I will stay here, at South Indian Cancer Hospital, I will stay here, and see just how *bad* it can get," she says passionately, simultaneously laughing while her eyes fill with tears. "So, the plumbers came, good guys, and I said, 'here's the situation, these kids are really sick, they are so sick and they are here for weeks, months getting treatment. Am I supposed to tell their families they cannot do any wash, cannot wear clean clothes that entire time?' I don't know, Virginia, I can't even provide them filtered water to drink. I don't even want to know where they are getting their drinking water. I don't ask because I don't want to know, because if I know I will have to do something about it. The plumbers, they feel for me, they understand. They said, 'we'll come back at night, buy us some piping and we'll hook the pediatric unit up to its own water tank, no one will have to know.'"

I look at Dr. Rashi. Given what I have learned about how India works, it sounds like a reasonable solution.

"But I cannot do that!" she says. "I cannot have my own private water supply for this unit, taken from the other parts of the hospital. So, I told the plumbers, 'you go back to your boss and tell him to wear the same pair of underwear for four weeks and if he can do that then I'll talk to you about the water supply we use on this unit,'" she says, leaning back in her chair, laughing. "Here, look," Dr. Rashi says to me, and she pulls out her mobile phone and I see a series of pictures from around the hospital. "See, I am becoming a photojournalist!" She shows me pictures of water overflowing in bathrooms, of leaky faucets. "I am going around the entire hospital, taking pictures of all the water that is being wasted, they can't just pick on pediatrics."

We commiserate about the irony about trying to enforce hygiene practices with neutropenic children while being simultaneously told the unit is using too much water.

"I have been going back and looking at all the data since 2009," Dr. Rashi continues. "It's unbelievable, all the children we have treated, and how many died. I keep thinking, how different it would be now for them. Now I have a team. I know how to get them properly diagnosed, how better to treat their infections. I look back at those notes, my handwriting even looks immature, I didn't know any better, I was doing the best I could."

Her eyes start to well with tears.
She laughs a little, cynically. "Well, now I'm detached."
I am unconvinced.

* * *

When I arrive the next morning to the pediatric ward, I am surprised to see the two night duty nurses still there, each giving report[5] to the oncoming day shift—something I have not seen anywhere else in the hospital. Immediately, I see nurses begin to engage with their patients, seeking out parents to inquire about their child's symptoms. Certain young children clearly have touched the nurses, and they play little games of peekaboo together. The older children lie in bed, bored and unstimulated. Most spend the day sleeping, whether it's because they simply don't feel well or because it is the only way to pass the time, I cannot tell.

A young mother sits down to talk with Dr. Rashi, holding her two-year-old daughter in her lap. Sister Kavita whispers to me, "Madam is about to give bad news. The CT scan shows hepatic (liver) involvement of disease now." Dr. Rashi speaks low and softly, her tone gentle and understanding. The mother looks stunned, and turns around to look at her husband, standing behind her, who looks equally bewildered. The parents are escorted by Vasudha, the social worker, into the playroom for further discussion. Vasudha generously invites me to accompany her, and I do, interested to observe, but equally hesitant to intrude during such a delicate time. I know how fragile these conversations can be, how they can so easily tip and lose their bearings. But Vasudha doesn't seem concerned. She enters the playroom and arranges a few white plastic chairs in a circle and then invites in the mother. The father stays outside with the child. The playroom is quiet and they are not interrupted. I don't understand all that is being said, but I know it is therapeutic and gentle and kind. I can tell by how Vasudha lets the mother talk. How she uses silence judiciously. How she is empathetic, but focused. How she leans toward the mother, making eye contact, touching her knee every now and then. It is real and genuine and raw. Outside, the child starts to cry, and the mother quickly gets up and opens the playroom door, letting the child and father enter. She picks up her daughter and begins breastfeeding. Vasudha continues to talk with them, slowly, carefully, sensitively. The mother is listening, but stares ahead, her face blank and emotionless while her daughter pulls at her nipple. The father leans forward in his chair, the marks of hardship and poverty exposed like an open sore; soiled clothes that hang loosely on his rail-thin frame, mussed and greasy hair, bare, calloused feet.

---

5 "Report" or "hand-off" is when the offgoing nurse gives the oncoming nurse updates regarding what happened to their patients during the shift and what still needs to be done. It is a structured form of communication between nurses to ensure continuity of care for patients.

"They come from very far away, this family," Vasudha explains. "An overnight train ride. The child was treated on the outside, and then came here. She received three rounds of chemotherapy, but now the disease is in her liver."

"And what did you tell them?" I ask, wondering what you possibly tell a family when their two-year-old daughter has progressive cancer, they are desperately poor, and live hundreds of miles away from the medical care their child needs. "Well, Dr. Rashi says she can try three more cycles of chemotherapy and then we will reassess. This is a conversation for preparation. They need to understand that things are not going well, that things are not good. And I need to make sure they do not abandon South Indian Cancer Hospital and go elsewhere for treatment. This happens sometimes, they leave and go somewhere else and then that place starts all over giving the first chemotherapy again, and it won't help."

* * *

I visit Hameeda on Female Ward I, where she is lying in bed, the first time I have seen her without her hijab. She has a thick glossy mass of gorgeous curly black hair. She looks terrified and panicked, like a trapped bird.

"My legs don't work," she whispers to me urgently, clawing at my arm when I approach her bed. I had heard Hameeda was having some numbness and tingling in her left leg, but I didn't know she was experiencing full paralysis. I see a catheter draining urine hanging by the bed, indicating that her bladder is no longer working properly. She must have spinal cord compression; no wonder she was having such horrific back pain. I feel completely helpless. She is lying on a dirty sheet and I smell stool. "I will talk with Dr. Madhu, Hameeda. I will talk with her," I promise.

Madhu finds me first.

"Virginia, about Hameeda. She is paralyzed now," she says. "I had to tell her very quickly what was going on."

"I know, I wanted to talk to you about her. I went to see her on the ward. She looks horrible. What are we going to do?"

"I am sending her to hospice today, this afternoon," Madhu says.

"Can they manage her?"

"I don't know, I think so. I talked to the doctor there, and the home care team will visit her too. We will get her as much support as possible. But here in the hospital it is impossible. No one is doing anything for her. There is no one to feed her or change her. I brought her diapers and when I went to see her she had soiled them and there was no one to change her."

I think of this paralyzed young woman lying in her own defecation, terrified at how her body has betrayed her. I feel heat rising in my chest, and suddenly I am deeply, deeply angry at the nurses on Female Ward I, angry that no one would see it as their responsibility to provide care to this frightened, debilitated young girl who clearly needs help. What depresses me even more is that this is the unit where Agnes is working: one of the strongest, brightest, and most caring nurses in the hospital, a nurse who has had palliative care training. Why isn't she doing anything?

"When she first got here," Madhu explained, "people did everything for Hameeda, they bought her this and that, helped her with everything. Now no one will touch her."[6] Madhu doesn't elaborate as to why and disappears before I have a chance to ask.

* * *

I am haunted by the screaming and crying and wailing I hear on the pediatric unit as children are repeatedly poked and stuck with needles. One nurse tells me that sometimes if a child is a particularly difficult stick, they will call Dr. Madhu and she will give some sedation medicine, like midazolam (a valium like drug). "But that is not frequently, very rarely," she says. "In my three years' experience, only one child."

Young children, less than five years old, are forcibly restrained. One screaming child is pinned down on the exam table by two nurses and his mother, and when he continues to struggle, the security guard presses and leans his entire chest against the child until he is practically lying on top of the terrified small boy. Sometimes the nurses and parents speak harshly to the children: "*Calm down! Don't move! Don't cry!*"

I watch children poked for blood draws and IVs—sometimes 10, 12 times, in their tiny hands and feet while they struggle and wail and howl. Even worse, the other child-patients stand in line and silently watch each ordeal, waiting for their turn and the pain that will soon be theirs to bear. Their faces are blank with the empty-eyed look of complete resignation.

* * *

The security guard has resumed his crowd control responsibilities and stands at the entrance to the pediatric ward. His large, pudgy hand rests authoritatively on the door handle, deciding who can enter and who cannot, an Indian hospital version of St. Peter. I am beckoned ahead of parents and enter freely even though I have the flimsiest reason of all to be on this unit; I am not a parent; these are not my children, some days from death.

6 The specific reasons why the nurses did not provide care to Hameeda in this situation are complex and were not entirely clear to me during my fieldwork. It is possible, however, that a primary reason was due to the nurses' desire to avoid polluting or unclean work associated with the intimate care of the body, especially of someone considered lower status in the traditional hierarchy of the caste system. Hameeda was an orphan, destitute, Muslim, and now dying a difficult and frightening death; all of these factors likely contributed to a reluctance of the nursing staff to care for her. See Chapter 10 for further discussion related to this topic.

Vasudha, the social worker, finds me at the front desk of the pediatric ward and taps me on the shoulder.

"Ma'am," she says, adjusting her tangerine-colored dupatta, "Hameeda was shifted (transferred) to the hospice yesterday."

"Did it go okay? She got there all right?" I ask.

"Yes, Ma'am, she did, without problem."

"That's good. Vasudha—I have a question."

"Of course, Ma'am. Tell me."

"I'm confused as to why the nurses on the wards were not willing to provide the care to Hameeda that she needed, you know with changing her diapers, helping her eat. Do you know why that is? It's been bothering me," I admit.

She looks surprised by my question.

"Here, they do not do," she answers simply.

"But why not?" I press. "I don't understand why the nurses would not do that here?"

"The patient was alone, she did not have family," Vasudha gives as way of explanation.

"Yes, I know, I know she was alone here. But the nurses are here, I don't understand why they would not provide this care to Hameeda?"

She shakes her head. "I don't know, Ma'am. They do not do that here."

* * *

It's early in the morning, and Pradeep, Jasmine, myself, and a young male doctor I don't know from another department within the hospital sit around the table in the palliative care clinic, chatting. While we are talking, an 11-year-old girl in a long brown skirt, a gold sequined top, dark curls, and an angelic smile enters the clinic room. It seems she is here to see the doctor from the other department. She stands in front of him, and he gently pulls down each of her lower eyelids with his thumb to examine her conjunctivae (membranes of the eye). After he is finished with this cursory physical exam, I notice he keeps the girl close, holding her small hand and stroking it slowly against his palm, with an intensity and intimacy that makes me uncomfortable. He does this for a few interminable minutes, looking at her hand with what could be interpreted as desire, or at least intense curiosity. I can't take my eyes off his attention to the young girl, but no one else at the table seems to be paying attention as the doctor turns over her hand and admires her pale purple nail polish. I also can't help but notice that he has a firm grip on the girl's thin left upper arm and at one point pulls her back toward him when she tries to move away. The interaction, and the doctor's uneasy vibe, deeply unsettles me; it doesn't help that I have been reading extensively about sexual abuse in India, which occurs with alarming frequency in joint family (multigenerational) homes.[7] It strikes me how vulnerable children are here, surrounded by unmonitored adults in positions of power.

"There was a death case yesterday," Pradeep says abruptly, interrupting my thoughts. "A 16-year-old boy, with leukemia. His parents brought him here in an ambulance; he was gasping and died right after. But they wouldn't accept it. They wouldn't let us touch him, saying they are going to pray and he will come back to life. Some people are like that here, they refuse to take medicines, they just pray and think that will fix everything."

As if foreshadowed by Pradeep's story, that afternoon a two-year-old girl with acute leukemia dies. The pediatric ward desperately needs the bed, which is in an isolation room, and the staff urge the mother to take the child's body home right away. But because she needs to wait for her husband to arrive—which could take hours—the deceased child is moved to the palliative care clinic. The mother and grandmother weep quietly, hunched over the small body lying on a stretcher under a white blanket. The clinic room is cleared of other patients; Sarah, Abhipsa, Daya, and Jasmine all sit in the room with the child's body and the two sobbing women, making a clear, demarcated circle of space around the patient and family.

Daya sits at the nurses' table and leans her head against the wall and closes her eyes. Is she napping? A minute later, she dramatically rests her head on the table on top of her folded arms, loudly sighs, and covers her head with her dupatta. The message is not subtle and seems indisputable: I am tired, and I am not here. Abhipsa looks equally disengaged. Sarah sits with her chin propped in her hand and hands me a few photos of the child from healthier days. Jasmine texts on her phone as she sits on the exam table swinging her legs back and forth. Everyone looks like they would rather be anywhere else. It occurs to me that they are all mothers, mostly of young children. This could be their child, this could be their pain. Maybe it is just too real, or frightening, or problematic, to be this close to death, especially that of a child. After a few awkward minutes, I silently excuse myself.

* * *

Dr. Rashi has arranged for a special lunch to thank the pediatric staff for all of their hard work. A generous buffet is set up on tables in the playroom.

---

7 Children are particularly vulnerable in India. According to Fernandes et al. (2021), The Indian National Crimes Records Bureau (NCRB) reports a child is sexually abused every 15 minutes, and 53% of children report abuse by a parent, relative, or schoolteacher. For comparison, the prevalence of child sexual abuse in high-income countries is 20% for females and 8% for males. However, it is difficult to know the full extent of the problem in India, as systems to report, investigate, and intervene in cases of suspected child abuse and neglect are limited, especially in rural areas, and generally the privacy and status of the extended family is prioritized over protecting the child. Films such as *Lion, Slumdog Millionaire, Monsoon Wedding, Water*, and books such as *A Fine Balance, The White Tiger*, and *Beyond the Beautiful Forevers* all explicitly discuss or allude to the exploitation and abuse of children in India. Additional related scholarly references to this important topic are included at the end of the chapter.

Jasmine leads a shy five-year-old girl into the room; she is wide-eyed and it is clear she feels special being allowed in this grown-up space. Jasmine pulls over a small blue chair for the girl and makes her a plate of food.

"I had to tell everyone in the hallway that this is my daughter, they kept asking me 'who is it?' and 'why is she allowed to get the lunch?'" I suddenly realize the girl is the sister of the two-year-old who recently died and whose body lays in the palliative care clinic.

"You are the guest of honor!" Jasmine tells her, as Abhipsa and Vasudha attend to her lovingly, giving her drinks, a napkin, talking to her softly. I am struck by how much more comfortable they seem in providing support with the tangibility of sustenance and am touched by their vigilance in attending to this small child, unknowing and trusting, whose little hand moves skillfully around the green paper plate, shaped and grooved to imitate a banana leaf, scooping rice into her mouth. I wonder how this image will coalesce in her developing mind, if it will lodge in the river of her consciousness forever as one of her earliest memories: the day her little sister died, and she was invited to the lunch party in the pediatric playroom.

* * *

The hospice, not easy to find, is a beautiful house—actually two houses—in a secluded residential area off the busy thoroughfare of Road Number 1. There are two large balconies, a garden, and a peaceful room designated for prayer or group activities. The medical director, Dr. Rekha, explains the hospice is the only inpatient hospice in the entire State and it opened just a few months ago. To date, they have admitted 42 patients, 20 of whom have died in the hospice. There are 12 beds, one full-time medical director, and four full-time nurses who live on the premises. The hospice was opened and funded by a well-known international philanthropic organization, and while patients and families are encouraged to give donations and pay what they are able, no one is charged for the services, care, or food that is provided. They do not accept HIV patients, and Dr. Rekha is vague about why not but alludes to the fact it is a stipulation of the funder.[8]

Dr. Rekha makes a special point to show me what she refers to as the "servants' quarters," for the cook, ayahs, and watchman. "It is so difficult to find a reliable ayah!" she randomly laments, the complaint now with a familiar ring, as I have heard it so often from my roommates in reference to the housekeeper and cook they hired.

The average length of stay in the hospice is days to weeks, but some patients have stayed on for months. "We try to reserve beds for those most in need," Dr. Rekha explains, "and if patients are stable and able to be cared

---

8 This was not the first time in my global health work that I encountered hospice or palliative care organizations that refused to accept and care for patients with HIV. Stigma related to HIV is further discussed in Chapter 7.

for at home, we try to discharge them back home." The hospice is currently working on getting a license for morphine, but it has been complicated. I hand over the five fentanyl patches that Dr. Madhu asked me to deliver.

"Oh, thank you. We will use these," she says and gives them to one of the nurses.

"You know, there was some resistance in the neighborhood and with potential donors when they realized that people would be dying in the hospice," Dr. Rekha tells us, walking us back through the main room. "But now I think they have adjusted to us."

She takes me to the room where Hameeda is lying in a bed. I am relieved to see that she is clean and looks comfortable in the pleasant and quiet room. She is without her head scarf and her wild mass of dark curls explodes off her head. She smiles when she sees me. We clasp hands and a couple of tears squeeze from her eyes down her cheeks. I am particularly worried about Hameeda because I know she will not have a quick or easy death. Despite having terrible cancer, she is a healthy 19-year-old, with healthy lungs, a healthy heart, and healthy kidneys. Her body will not give up easily.

She grabs my arm and repeats the last thing she said to me at SICH before being transferred to the hospice.

"My legs still do not work," she says with breathy urgency.

I squeeze her hands and say softly, "I know. That must be so difficult and scary."

She nods. I lower my voice even more. "Are they taking good care of you here?"

"Yes," she says and I believe her. I ask her about pain. She tells me she has some pain in her arms, but she can move them without difficulty. I make a mental note to share this concerning development with Madhu as it's highly possible that as the tumor grows and continues to impinge on her spinal cord Hameeda will gradually become completely paralyzed from the neck down. I think about bed-bound patients I have cared for and how rapidly they can develop horrendous bedsores. Dr. Rekha tells me they tried to put Hameeda on a water mattress to prevent this, but she didn't tolerate it. I can only hope the nurses are turning and rotating her frequently enough to protect her skin, as Dr. Rekha tells us that she already has one bedsore.

"Is there anything you need Hameeda?" I ask before I leave.

"My legs. Make my legs work again."

References

Aravind, A. (2008). *The white tiger*. Simon & Schuster, New York.

Behere, P. B., Sathyanarayana Rao, T. S., Mulmule, A. N. (2013). Sexual abuse in women with special reference to children: Barriers, boundaries and beyond. *Indian Journal of Psychiatry*, 55, 316–319. https://doi.org/10.4103/0019-5545.120535.

Boo, K. (2014). *Beyond the beautiful forevers: Life, death, and hope in a Mumbai undercity*. Random House, New York.

Borhani, F., Abbaszadeh, A., Mohsenpour, M., & Asadi, N. (2013). Lived experiences of pediatric oncology nurses in Iran. *Iranian Journal of Nursing and Midwifery Research*, 18(5), 349.

Boyle, D. (director). (2008). Slumdog Millionaire (film).

Choudhry, V., Dayal, R., Pillai, D., et al. (2018). Child sexual abuse in India: A systematic review. *PLoS One*, *13*, e0205086. https://doi.org/10.1371/journal.pone.0205086.

Davis, G. (director). (2016). Lion (film).

Fernandes, G., Fernandes, M., Vaidya, N., De Souza, P., Plotnikova, E., Geddes, R., ... & Choudhry, V. (2021). Prevalence of child maltreatment in India and its association with gender, urbanisation and policy: A rapid review and meta-analysis protocol. *BMJ open*, *11*(8), e044983.

Graetz, D. E. (2023). The most vulnerable pediatric cancer patients. *The Lancet Regional Health–Americas*, *21:* 100480.

Nukpezah, R. N., Khoshnavay Fomani, F., Hasanpour, M., & Nasrabadi, A. N. (2021). A qualitative study of Ghanaian pediatric oncology nurses' care practice challenges. *BMC Nursing*, 20(1), 1–10.

Mehta, D. (director). (2005). Water (film).

Moirangthem, S., Kumar, N. C., & Math, S. B. (2015). Child sexual abuse: Issues and concerns. *The Indian Journal of Medical Research*, 142(1), 1.

Nair, M. (director). (2001). Monsoon Wedding (film).

Rohinton, M. (1995). *A Fine Balance*. McClelland & Stewart. Toronto, Canada.

Stoltenborgh, M., van Ijzendoorn, M. H., Euser, E. M., et al. (2011). A global perspective on child sexual abuse: Meta-analysis of prevalence around the world. *Child Maltreat*, *16*, 79–101. https://doi.org/10.1177/1077559511403920.

World Health Organization (WHO). (2016). Child maltreatment. Available at: https://www.who.int/news-room/fact-sheets/detail/child-maltreatment (Accessed July 27, 2023).

World Health Organization (WHO). (2021). Childhood cancers: Key facts. Available at: https://www.who.int/news-room/fact-sheets/detail/cancer-in-children

World Health Organization (WHO). (2021). The global initiative for childhood cancer: Increasing access, advancing quality, saving lives. Available at: https://www.who.int/initiatives/the-global-initiative-for-childhood-cancer

6   No Legs, No Life

Actually, to be frank, it's not my job. It's not my job and it's not my responsibility, and if I don't do it, nobody is there to ask me or question me. But our patients are suffering. They come all the way traveling 600, 800 kilometers just to get this morphine. When they come all the way here and we say, "no stock," they are already in pain, and they leave in more pain. Even if we ask them to buy it outside, from a private hospital, they may not be able to afford it, because the same 10 mg tablet which we buy from the manufacturer at the cheapest cost—90 paisa or 1 rupee—is sold at the corporate hospital for 6 rupees per tablet. So if the patient needs to take 6 tablets per day, how many tablets does he have to buy for a 10-day or 1-month supply? They won't be able to afford that much money.

Jasmine, administrative coordinator

The South Indian Cancer Hospital (SICH) pharmacy or "medicine store" is a large, bright room located next to the palliative care clinic. Cabinets and shelves are stocked with a variety of bottles and packages of tablets and an adjacent air-conditioned room contains vials of chemotherapy. A front counter connects the pharmacy with the hospital corridor where patients and attendants approach with prescriptions in hand. There is a wooden desk, visible from the corridor window, where the pharmacists sit to record inventory and the dispensing of tablets into a multitude of large ledgers. An ayah sits at another table slowly stamping the chemotherapy boxes that will soon be ripped open by the nurses with the message "Not for Resale" in smudgy black ink.

I tell Sima, the head pharmacist, about my research, and explain that I am primarily interested in how they stock and dispense morphine. She is more than happy to oblige. "See, here—we have much morphine," Sima says, opening up two metal cabinets. She points to bottle after bottle of 10 mg immediate release morphine tablets. I pick up one and examine the label. Each bottle has 500 tablets. Prerna, another pharmacist, dutifully opens up a ledger and shows me the current balance of all the morphine formulations;

DOI: 10.4324/9781003413158-9

quantities of other strengths are more limited: 10 mg MSIR[1] tablets: 59,218; 20 mg MSIR tablets: 5 tablets; 30 mg MSER[2]: zero; 10 mg injectable morphine: 377 ampules.

Despite the encouraging numbers of the 10 mg tablets, I know from the palliative care team that stockouts and shortages are still a reality. Even now, with improved procedures and monitoring systems in place to better anticipate when the morphine supply will be depleted, Dr. Madhu told me that two months ago, SICH completely ran out of 20 mg and 30 mg morphine tablets. And prior to getting this last consignment, there was a gap of one week when there was absolutely no morphine at all. There are also additional barriers once the morphine is actually in the hospital. The Drug Inspector must be called to certify the shipment before it can be opened—Jasmine told me once that took 15 days—and the pharmacy staff must be willing to issue and process the incoming stock and have the proper paperwork stamped from the drug controller's office. Bureaucratic breakdowns at any of these points result in patients in pain.

Underneath the bottles of morphine, I see boxes and boxes of fentanyl lozenges, a morphine-like drug that is absorbed well through fatty tissue. This large supply of fentanyl surprises me, as this version of fentanyl is expensive and is often difficult to obtain in the U.S. I tell this to Sima.

"Yes, we have such a large supply. But they are for a clinical trial, they will be shifted (moved) to CityStar Hospital next month," she explains.

All medications are dispensed free of charge to patients with MHS certification letters. If the pharmacy doesn't have what has been prescribed in stock, then the patient must go and buy the drug from one of the dozen private pharmacy shops that line the two main roads that intersect at SICH. Today, they are out of Tylenol tablets and Metrogel (Flagyl) tablets.[3]

"But Tylenol is cheap," Sima says. "1 rupee per tablet." About 2 cents.

---

1 MSIR: Morphine Sulfate Immediate Release; short-acting opioid tablets that are typically dosed every three to four hours.
2 MSER: Morphine Sulfate Extended Release; long-acting opioid tablets that are typically dosed every 12 hours.
3 Additional details about morphine procurement from an interview with Dr. Madhu:

> *[I ask Dr. Madhu if the small medicine shops found everywhere throughout the city sell morphine]: "They used to, but back in 1986 there came a strict regulation by the Central Government saying that if you are found in possession of an unauthorized stock of drugs like morphine or found in any way to be misusing the drug, it is a nonbailable offense with 10 years of rigorous imprisonment. The moment that strict regulation was issued, all the pharmacies stopped stocking morphine because it was too much of a hassle to keep track of what is happening to morphine within their pharmacy and whether patients are taking it properly or not. Even today any pharmacist can stock morphine, provided they have all the required licenses, but the licensing process is so complicated they don't want to bother with it. Also, because morphine is really cheap, all of the huge effort to stock it isn't worth*

"And here," she says, opening a series of drawers. "We divide morphine tablets into smaller quantities." I see plastic baggies filled with 50 or 100 tablets of morphine. "This makes it easier for us to dispense," Sima explains.

I ask Sima how patients know how to take their medications, as many cannot read and even if they could, tablets are dispensed without any written instructions. Some prescriptions brought by patients are scrawled with symbols of instruction I am unfamiliar with; others list only the medication name and quantity to be dispensed: *Rantac 10.*

"Yes," she confirms, "many cannot read or write." She pauses. "But they are intelligent in other ways," she says wisely.

I smile at her. It's the first time I've heard anyone acknowledge the patients in such a positive way. When a patient approaches the counter, Sima counts the pills out in her hands.

I am optimistic about my day in the pharmacy but become discouraged when I observe similar interactions as I have witnessed elsewhere in the hospital. The pharmacist Prerna is extremely interested in the details of my breakfast and what Indian foods I like, but blasé about the patients and attendants who approach the counter to fill prescriptions. When she is handed a prescription, Prerna glances at it and simply takes a large pair of scissors and cuts the designated number of prescribed tablets from the prepackaged foil strips and hands it to the patient or attendant, some of whom stand there looking baffled before being pushed aside by the next waiting patient.

Frequently, medications are dispensed without any verbal exchange between the patient or attendant and the pharmacist. A few brave souls ask questions, but they are given instructions very quickly and I'm unclear how they will keep track of the schedule for four or five different medications.

"So, how do patients know how to take their medications?" I ask again, still trying to figure it out.

"They go back to the outpatient department, talk with the doctor," both Prerna and Sima tell me. Prerna cuts strips of tablets with lassitude and foil strips fall to the counter with a soft, tinny clatter.

I picture the very sick patients, or overwhelmed family members, who must fight their way back through the outpatient clinic melee for what is likely to be a five-second explanation by a harried physician. It seems highly probable that many patients, frustrated and exhausted, may simply leave after receiving the tablets from the pharmacy.

A young man comes to the pharmacy desk clutching a palliative care green medication booklet. His eyes fill with tears and the anguish on his face rises up like waves.

---

it because you're not going to make any significant profit. Now, other narcotic drugs, like the fentanyl patch, are more freely available in the market."

"Why?" I ask. "Because it's more expensive?"

"Yes, exactly. Because fentanyl is very expensive, so there is more profit to be made, which makes the effort to stock and dispense it worthwhile. Suppose you prescribe a 3-day supply of 25 microgram fentanyl patches; it's 300 times more expensive than an equivalent dose of morphine."

"My mother, stomach cancer," he chokes. "She will die in a few days." His voice cracks on the last word, and the look of terror and pain on his face makes my own stomach cramp. He starts talking very quickly to Prerna: he is the only son; he is not married. Prerna's face softens slightly, she makes eye contact, and she listens, briefly. She then asks him to sign the back of the prescription. Instead, he uses the inkpad to stamp his thumbprint in lieu of the signature that he cannot provide.

* * *

At 1:45 pm, Jyoti, another pharmacist, and Prerna sit down for a snack at the wooden table, the one clearly visible from the patient counter. The sign by the pharmacy door indicates that the pharmacy is closed for lunch from 2 to 3 pm.

Prerna is the designated dispenser of medications today; Jyoti is responsible for issuing chemotherapies to the wards. Three patients approach the counter, awaiting assistance. Prerna looks up, sees they are waiting, then turns her back and continues her leisurely conversation with Jyoti. The patients look at me, and I look back at them, awkwardly. One of the waiting patients, an indigenous tribal woman, wears the traditional chunky, white plastic bangles—from her wrists to past the elbows—on both arms, and the bright pink, orange, and blue dress decorated with tiny, reflective mirrors. Audibly exhaling, Prerna pushes her chair back from the table, scraping the wooden legs along the cement floor. She dispenses the medications wordlessly, barely looking up. I find this encounter so disheartening that I take it as my cue to leave.

Back at my apartment, I call Paul and share my frustration with him.

"Why don't you yell at them?" he challenges. "You're just like all the rest, letting them pretend that everything is okay, that they're doing a good job when clearly they're not. You're just going to hide everything, aren't you? Write up a neat little report that sugarcoats the truth."

His words cut deep, and I start to cry.

"Oh God, are you crying?" he asks roughly.

"Yes," I say through choked sobs. "I don't want to talk to you anymore." I hang up.

I lay down on my bed and I cry and cry. I cry for the beggars I see on the street twisted and contorted into impossible shapes wheeling themselves around on small wooden platforms; I cry for the old women who bang on the side of my autoricksaw at the intersection of Mirza Talab and Tripura Hills and for the fact that I stare straight ahead and ignore them; I cry for the stray dogs and skeletal cats that wander the streets resigned to their miserable fate; I cry for the ayahs and the family members who squat in squalor instead of feeling like they are worthy of sitting in a chair; I cry for my inability to take a stand and my own selfishness and fear and privilege; I cry for the desperately poor patients who are riddled with cancer and who are ignored, dismissed, and yelled at; I cry for the fact that everyone seems only to care what I have eaten. I cry myself to sleep.

* * *

If medication instructions seem arbitrary, so too do the logistics of dispensing the medication. Some patients who do not provide their own containers for the morphine tablets are abruptly told by Prerna to go buy one at a local medicine shop and come back. To others, she gives small plastic bags to hold their morphine tablets. I watch many patients step away from the counter looking terribly confused. If the pharmacy is out of stock of a medication, Prerna writes the name of the medication on a small scrap of paper and simply says, "Buy this."

Prerna sits down at the table with Sima and Jyoti and strikes up a social conversation. A woman approaches the pharmacy counter. She stands and waits. She waits and she waits. No one acknowledges her presence.

"What does she need?" I blurt out rhetorically in an attempt to prompt someone to action.

"Tablets," Prerna responds simply. She continues to sit and talk, a conversation of the deliberately bored. Nothing in her tone or body language suggests she is going to get up anytime soon. The woman waits patiently, shifting her weight side to side; she and I make eye contact.

Completely exasperated, I finally say, "Should we help her?"

"I will," says Prerna, but she continues to sit for another few minutes, which stretch out like an eternity. She is no longer talking, but sits immobile as a statue, her eyes fluttering shut as if she is about to take a nap. I get up and position myself at the counter. Still, no movement from a pharmacist. Minutes pass, and finally Prerna moves languidly over to the counter and fills the woman's morphine prescription.

Upset and angry, I tell them it's time for me to go, I have to get ready for the hospital fundraising event tonight. They all know it's my first debut in a sari. Prerna grabs my arm and smiles warmly at me, "Best of luck tonight! Be sure to bring us pictures!"

* * *

At home, I proudly display the sari to Joanie that I will be wearing tonight.

"Ohhh…" she says fingering the blue chiffon material and stroking the gold sequin detailing.

"How much did you pay for this Virginia?"

Good grief. What is the right answer? Too much and I'm a stupid American who got ripped off. Too little and I didn't get a good quality product. I whack off 500 rupees.

Joanie smiles approvingly. "You got a good deal."

She pulls out the petticoat. "Why didn't they tailor this?" she asks harshly.

"They did."

"It's too big, Virginia, look at all this," she says critically, bunching up the turquoise cotton material in her hands. It does look like an awful lot of material, but I decide to ignore her as there is nothing I can do about it now.

"Wait—look at the shoes I got in Delhi! They just happen to match!" I show her my gold sequin flats. She looks at them and scoffs.

"Flats? You need to wear heels. What on earth is wrong with you Virginia?"

She offers me a pair of hers, but I can't squeeze my size 7 feet into her size 5 shoes.

"And what sort of function is this for?"

"It's for a fundraising event at …," but I am interrupted.

"And you're wearing *this* Virginia? This is for a wedding! What on *earth* is wrong with you?" Joanie says again. She seems genuinely distressed.

"Someone from work helped me pick it out, they said it wasn't too over the top…" I counter.

"Well, they don't know what they are talking about," she says bluntly. "Everyone is going to stare at you."

"Well, then they will have to stare. This is what I am wearing."

* * *

Sarah and Jasmine help drape me in the blue and gold sparkly sari. It takes them about 20 minutes and an equal number of safety pins, but the final result is amazing. I feel like a princess, a blue mermaid sparkling princess. The fall and twist of the sari fabric is shockingly flattering and I love the bright blue peacock color.

"Thank you so much!" I say, spinning around, checking myself out in the bathroom mirror. I show them the matching blue hair clip I serendipitously bought last month. I start to pull my hair back from my face and clip it on top of my head.

"No, ma'am. Oh no," Jasmine says disapprovingly.

"Not good, huh?" I ask, smiling.

"No."

"Hmmm…how about this?" I move the clip to the side.

"Much better, ma'am, much better." Despite my insistence, Jasmine still won't call me Virginia. Sarah smiles approvingly. She and Jasmine both agree to be my "spotters" for the evening, to be sure I don't trip or reveal skin inappropriately.

When I exit the bathroom, it is immediately clear that I am, as Joanie aptly predicted, extremely overdressed. But I don't care, and everyone seems thrilled that I am trying my hand at wearing a sari. After the event, some of the attendees change venues and go dancing. It is a testament to the draping skills of Jasmine and Sarah that I do not come unraveled. I get home late—Ruma and Joanie are already asleep—and am so tired that when I cannot figure out how to undo the multitude of pins hidden throughout the reams of folded fabric, I eventually give up and fall asleep in the sari. Luckily, the material is tougher than it looks. In the morning, I awaken to find my bed awash in a sea of gold sequins glinting in the early sun.

* * *

An elderly, immaculately groomed gentleman wearing silver-rimmed spectacles meticulously peruses a patient's file at the medical oncology outpatient table. He has a laptop in front of him and I notice the screensaver is from Houston, Texas. He is the only physician at the hospital I have seen using a computer in the care of patients, and I notice that he pulls up National Comprehensive Cancer Network (NCCN) guidelines[4] during the course of patient consultations. I sit down as unobtrusively as possible, not wanting to disturb him, observing the flow of patients oozing in and out of the clinic room.

He turns to me and kindly begins a discussion about the treatment of lymphoma. I ask him about his screensaver. As it turns out, he practiced medicine in the U.S. but recently returned to India to care for his aging parents. His name is Dr. Varun and as a retired oncologist, he helps Dr. Rashi in clinic when he can.

"I'll tell you a story," he says, leaning back in his chair. "A couple of my friends, relatives, knowing I am an oncologist and am back in India—came to me and asked, 'Can you please help us? My son has cancer.' I said—'That isn't a problem; I made a living treating these conditions.' So, they brought me a child with leukemia, and I said—'Wait a minute. Before I start this, I need to get some assurances from various departments at the hospital[5].' First, I went to the nursing staff and told them—'the treatment of leukemia, it is not the doctor who takes care of the patients; it is the nurses who take care of them. Can you do that?' I went to the lab people and said—'I need lab support. By the time I come to make my rounds, I need to have the CBC (complete blood count) results on the patient's chart; can you do that?' I went to the Blood Bank—'I might need platelets; I might need plasma, blood transfusion... Can you keep at least 6 units of random donor platelets on hand?' I got nowhere. The worst answer I got was from the Blood Bank guy. He said, 'You bring the donor; whatever you want, I will give it to you.'

I said, 'if I run around the streets, trying to find donors, then what I am doing here as a medical oncologist?' His answer was, 'You bring the donor; I will give you whatever you want.'

But I still didn't get the message. Because this particular hospital where I was working at the time is next to a highway I told him—'You are doing cardiac bypass surgeries here, and you see a lot of trauma cases here; you must be using tens of units of blood every single day. All those patients don't need whole blood, in fact that may be harmful to them; they only need packed cells. So, when you are separating the blood, keep at least 6 bags of platelets aside for me. If I need it, I'll use them, if I don't need them, you only lost 6 bags of platelets for which you did not invest anything. You are just going to

---

4 NCCN guidelines are published by a network of leading cancer care centers within the U.S. related to best practices regarding cancer screening, treatment, and management.
5 Not SICH; he is referring to a different hospital.

throw them away anyway.' After all this, he still says—'You bring the donor; I will give you whatever you want.' So, that is the situation. If you cannot even educate the professionals, how can you educate the common man on the street?

I went back to the mother and said, 'this place is not conducive for leukemia treatment; you must take him to Dandaka.' But then she put me through the guilt trip—'I have a sick husband at home and I cannot leave him alone; if you treat my son here, at least my daughter can stay with him for a few hours and then I come and stay with him, so I can move back and forth. If I go to Dandaka, nobody will be able to take care of my husband. He is bedridden.' So, I said—'okay, but you have to understand the limitations that are here, and the outlook may not be good.' I was very honest with her. But she said, 'I am prepared for that; just do whatever you can.' So, I cut down my orders to the bare minimum. One of the orders was to infuse normal saline 100 cc per hour; and for 1 week, the 3 days I made rounds, not one single day did the patient have a running IV.

By the fifth day, the boy's uric acid level was up; it was a good 15. Even though he had a central catheter, he never got the IV fluids and the allopurinol I ordered. And his Mom came to me that day, insisting 'you treat my boy today.' I had to tell her, 'If I treat your son today, he will develop tumor lysis syndrome, his kidneys will stop working, then if he doesn't get dialysis he will die.' I told her, 'we need to wait a couple days and bring down the uric acid level, then I will start treatment.' But still, she insisted that I start chemotherapy that day. I had to remind her, 'I told you, right from the beginning, I told you this place is not conducive to leukemia treatment. You can still take him to a bigger hospital.' The point is, if I had had proper nursing care, I could have treated that individual; whether he would have survived or not is a different story, but at least I would have felt like I did my part. I couldn't do my part because there was no nursing care. And if you keep on compromising and compromising, and you continue to bang your head against the wall, at some point you stop and ask yourself 'Why am I doing this?'

And that is when I decided to start teaching sessions for the nurses. If you look at the vital sign sheets, every single day, the temperature is 98.4, pulse is 84, respirations are 18, blood pressure is 110/80; every single day. I said, very directly, if they are constant it means you did not check them; you are just writing in the numbers. I bluntly said that; not in a political way, I just bluntly said that: it means you are not doing it. Even after I said that a few times, nothing changed. And here, they don't even have vital signs sheet. They have a sheet, but it is always empty. The only time it gets filled out is when we apply to the Government to pay for febrile neutropenia. When you apply for that, you put the temperature points and we join those dots with a line and write the patient's name on it, and send a copy to the Government so that they approve the reimbursement. Otherwise, you can see on any of those wards, any of the patients, the sheet is not filled out. So, as a nurse, if you are not making the bed and not talking to the patient or not talking to the family, or not even taking vital signs… I am confused, what are you doing?"

* * *

Dr. Rashi arrives, takes her seat, and clinic begins in earnest. At one point, a cat enters the clinic and scampers toward the table. Dr. Rashi, a formidable woman, shrieks and pulls her knees up toward her chest. "I am *terrified* of cats!" she cries, and everyone in the clinic laughs. The skinny gray cat is shooed out of the clinic by the ayah who stamps her feet violently; it flees out the yellow shuttered doors and back into the hallway.

An elderly woman, wearing a pale orange and white sari that reminds me of a Creamsicle, supports her daughter's emaciated frame as they walk into the clinic. The mother sits on a stool and hands Dr. Rashi a thick stack of crumpled and folded medical records from a nearby hospital, where her daughter was enrolled in a clinical trial for relapsed chronic leukemia. Dr. Rashi patiently and efficiently sorts through it all, impressively piecing together a logical medical history from the jumbled heap of test results and scrawled progress notes in front of her.

"She is telling me that she sold all of her jewelry, all of their property to pay for her daughter's treatment," Dr. Rashi explains, translating for me. Even though the medications on the clinical trial were free, they still had to pay for transportation and their food—all other expenses.

"So what did you tell her?"

"I told her we would admit her daughter, do our best to see where her disease is, run the tests she needs. But I told her that her daughter is very, very sick. I am trying to prepare her for the inevitable."

As the woman rises to leave, she pulls up the edge of her orange sari to wipe the tears from her eyes.

A young boy with suspected rhabdomyosarcoma arrives next to the clinic. He wears a blue collared shirt and sits on a wooden stool supported by his father and uncle. His face is twisted into a grimace. "He's having pain," Dr. Rashi says to me, "and it will take a few more weeks, if everything goes smoothly, to complete all the diagnostic workup. So in the meantime we need to treat his pain." She writes out a prescription for morphine and directs the father to the pharmacy. The man returns shortly. Apparently, the pharmacy would not fill the prescription because he is missing his MHS card. Dr. Rashi is not impressed. "I don't know, but they should dispense it right? It doesn't matter. This child is in pain. I told them to go back to the pharmacy and demand it. I gave him permission to be rude. I told him if he has trouble to come back."

She pauses. "But he won't. Because they would rather dispense ten tablets, then have to deal with me, believe me." She laughs, full and throaty.

* * *

I'm tired after a long day at the hospital, and not really up for visiting Hameeda in the hospice, but I know it's the right thing to do. Staff at SICH and volunteers from the palliative care department are concerned that she is not getting appropriate care at the hospice, and the biggest concern is the quality of the food she is receiving. "It's too spicy! She can't eat it. And who serves someone sick that very rough rice? It needs to be soft!" they bemoan.

Concern is also voiced related to the quality of the nursing care and their availability in the evenings and nights. I am asked to deliver some baby powder, ten diapers, a bag of oatmeal, and retrieve the five fentanyl patches I delivered a few weeks ago, but which apparently have not been used because Hameeda is able to swallow tablets. The patches are expensive and the palliative care department wants them back.

Hameeda is sleeping when I arrive but awakens easily when I softly call her name. Her face immediately brightens, and I am glad I made the effort to visit. I deliver the powder, the oats, and the diapers, and a pink plush stuffed animal bear that I bought in Old City. She burrows her face into the soft pink fur and decides to name him Pinky. Her hands are covered with the orange-red swirls of mehndi[6]; she tells me she did it herself and I am appropriately impressed. I sit down on one of the plastic chairs by her bedside and feel something wet soak through to my right thigh. A catheter drains amber colored urine into a bag dangling from the side of her bed that is so full it looks about to burst. The major issue is her skin. Because she is paralyzed from her waist down due to the compression of her spinal cord, and because she is not being turned or moved frequently enough, Hameeda has developed large pressure sores on her lower back and feet. She can't feel them, but she can see the large black scabs and red ulcers forming on her lower legs.

"I am so missing my life," she sobs into her beautiful hennaed hands. "I *hate* this life! No legs, no life! I miss my food, playing, walking…," her voice trails off as she continues to cry.

There are no words. I put one hand on her shoulder, huddle closer, rest my other hand lightly on top of her head. I feel the springy mass of curls underneath, pushing up in protest—a body begging to be set free.

Reference

National Comprehensive Cancer Network (NCCN) Guidelines. (2023). Available at: https://www.nccn.org/home

---

6 Decorative, intricate patterns drawn on the body (usually on the palms, hands, and arms) with henna, a plant dye; commonly done before weddings and special events.

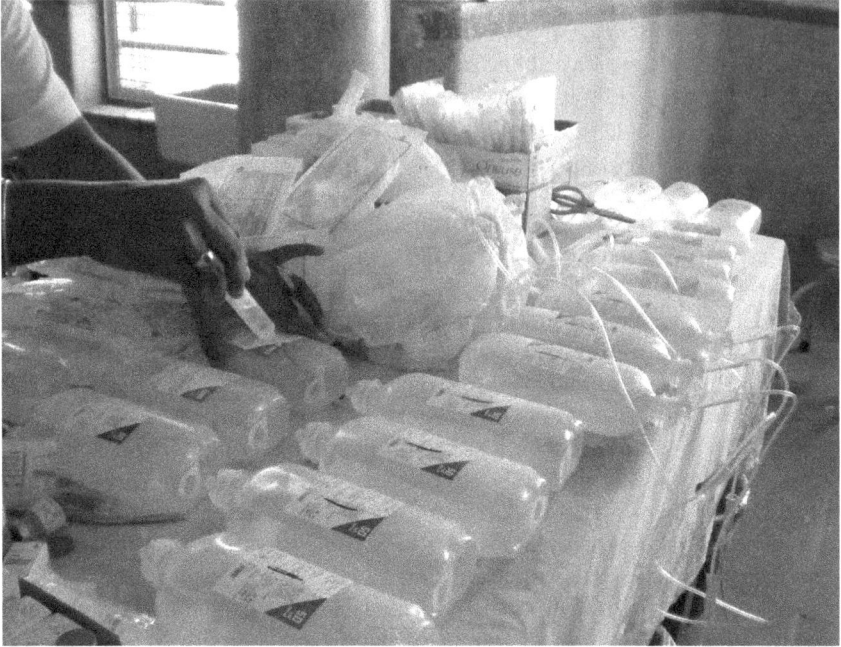

Figure 6.1 A nurse prepares medications and intravenous fluids, South Indian Cancer Hospital, Female Ward.

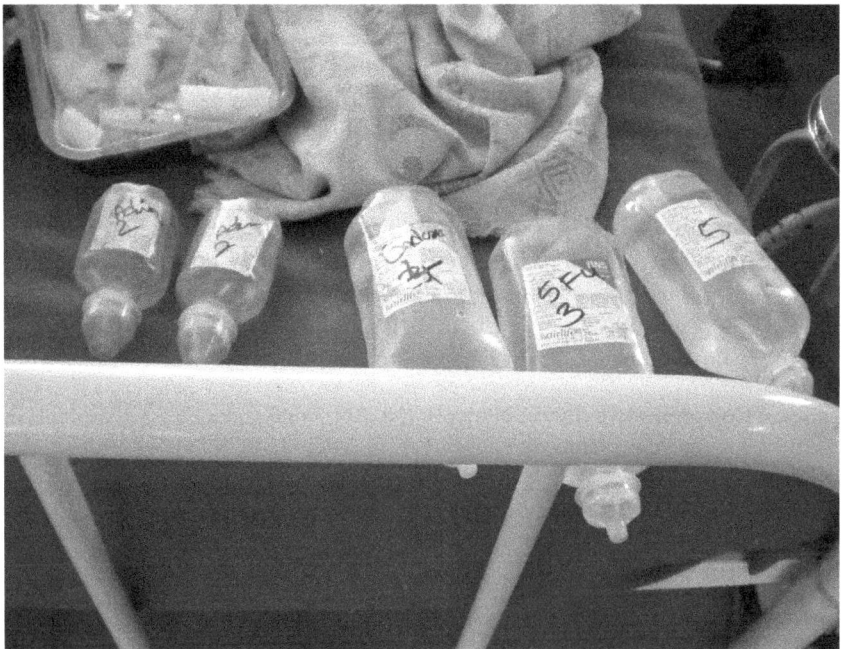

Figure 6.2 Chemotherapy treatments placed at the end of a patient's bed to be given later that shift, South Indian Cancer Hospital, Female Ward.

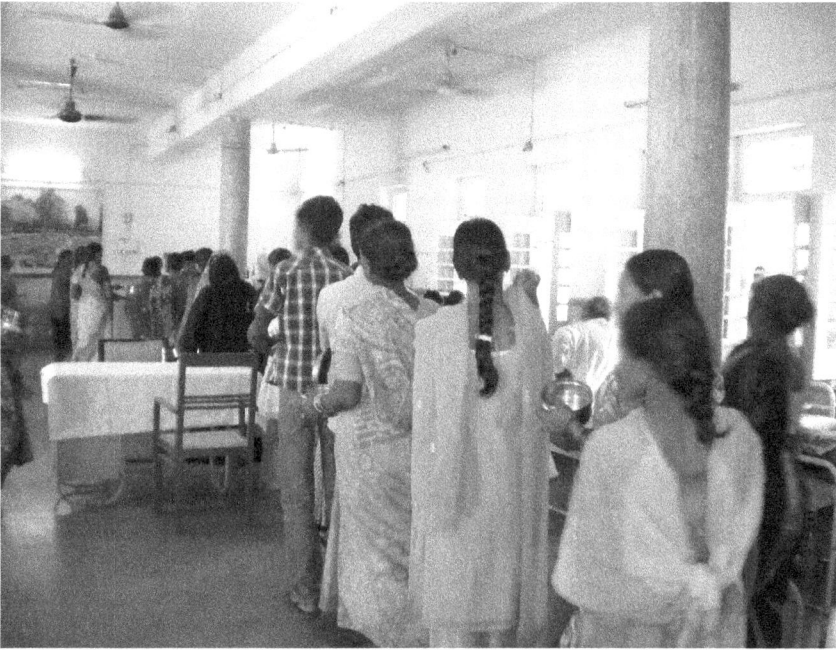

Figure 6.3 Family attendants queuing to receive the patient's daily meal of an egg and banana, South Indian Cancer Hospital, Female Ward.

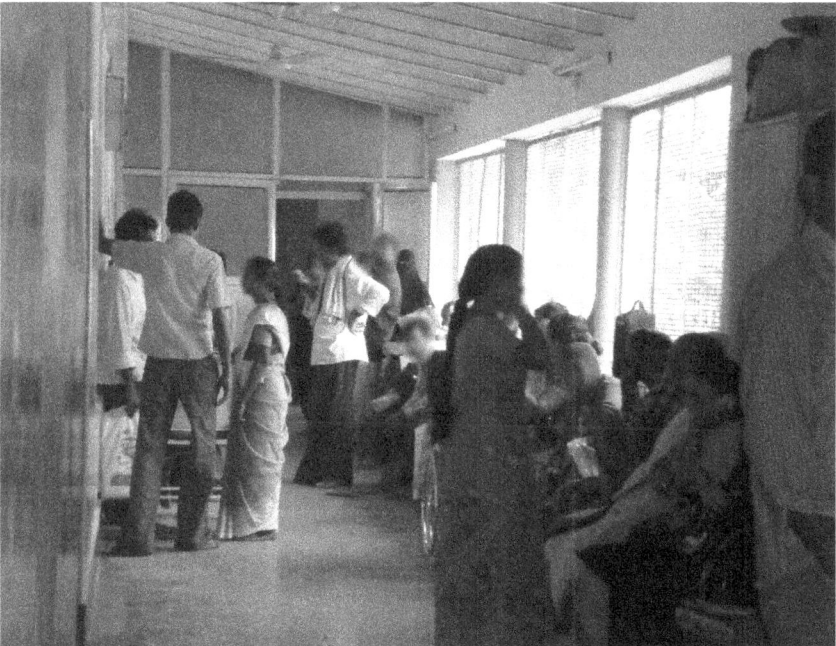

Figure 6.4 Patients and family members waiting to be seen, South Indian Cancer Hospital, Palliative Care Clinic.

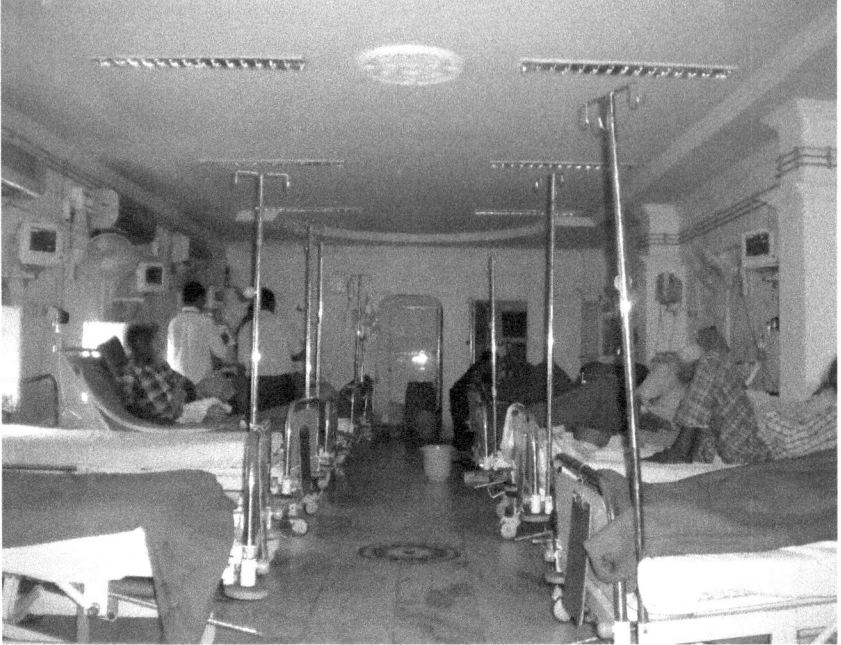

Figure 6.5 The Intensive Care Unit (ICU), South Indian Cancer Hospital.

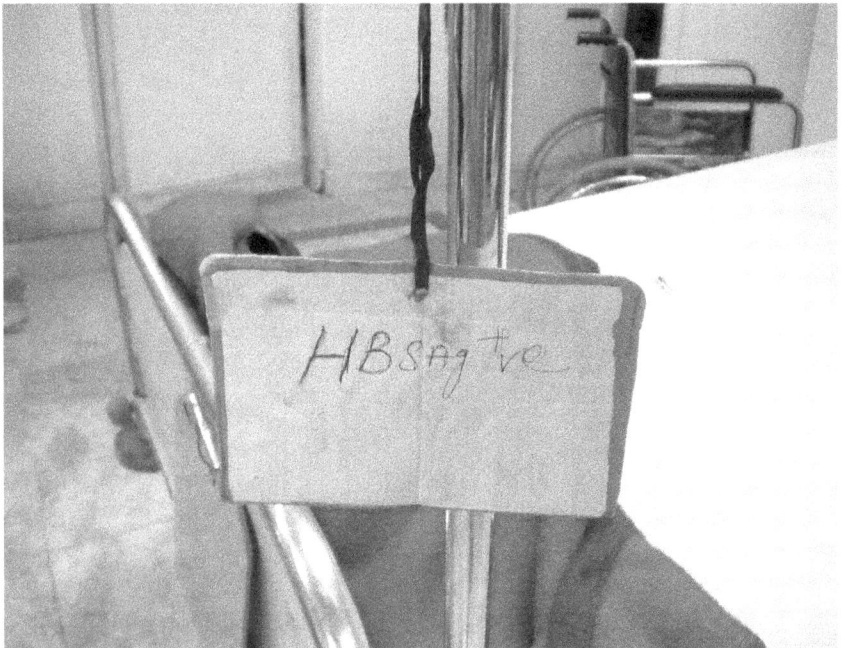

Figure 6.6 Sign indicating a patient's positive hepatitis B status, South Indian Cancer Hospital, Intensive Care Unit.

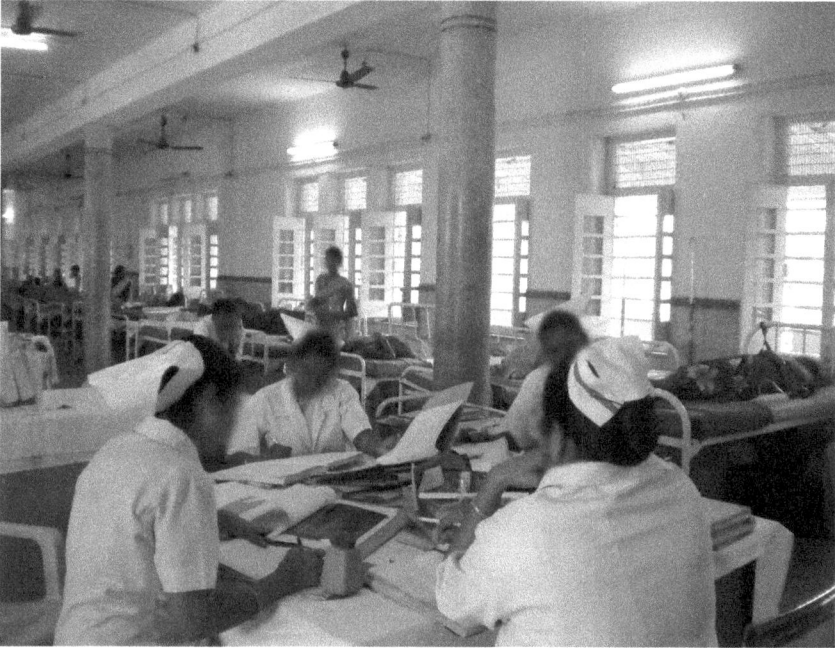

Figure 6.7 Nurses completing documentation, South Indian Cancer Hospital, Female Ward.

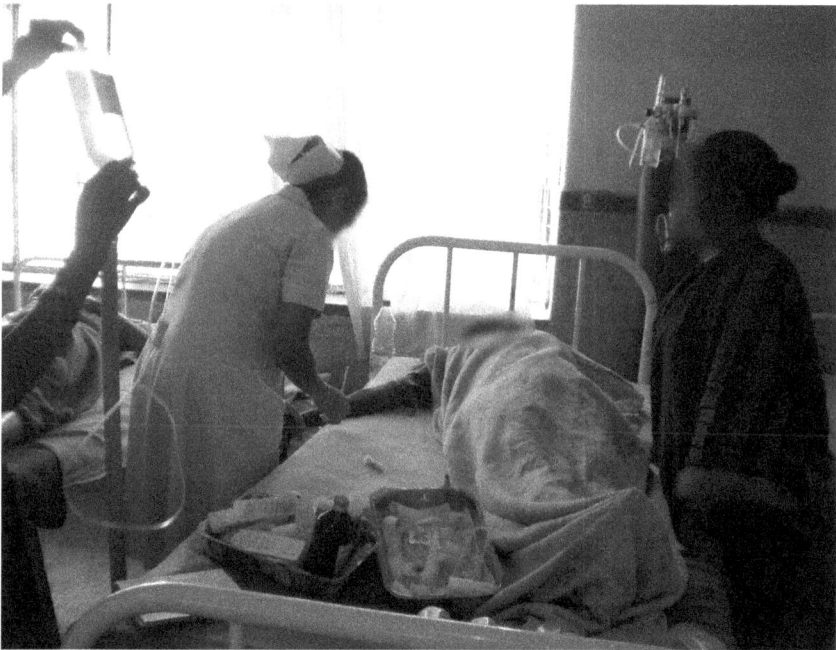

Figure 6.8 Nurse starting an IV to administer chemotherapy and medications to a patient while their family attendant watches, South Indian Cancer Hospital, Female Ward.

PART III

The Community

7 The Stigma That Cannot Be Washed Away

The Home Care Program

We want from day 1 after a patient has been diagnosed with terminal cancer, they should have a counselor, access to palliative care, to home care. In every hospital! They should have counseling for side-effects of chemotherapy, side-effects of radiation. They should know what will happen after radiation, what will happen if the disease recurs. They should know what to do if a wound starts, what can happen if they don't do proper dressings. Proper guidelines, proper knowledge, proper awareness of prevention, and early detection should be created to the people, to society, so that we do not see this sort of patient in such a horrible situation.

Jotika, health counselor, home care team

"We are here Madam!" Jotika calls out, slightly short of breath. Jotika is tall and moves with confidence; her thick dark hair hangs in a single braid down her back, skimming her buttocks as she walks. Occasionally, her left eye drifts laterally, refusing to synchronize with the movements of her right. She escorts me downstairs to the waiting van where I meet the rest of the home care team—two nurses, Leah and Menakshi, and the driver, Krishna. The driver, who is doing 40 days of puja (spiritual devotion), wears all black with an orange kerchief tied around his neck and his forehead is marked with orange and black horizontal lines.

This is the only home care team in Dandaka.[1] Even though families desperately need their help, some people do not want the team to visit; they worry—"what will the neighbors think if someone comes to our house, saying they are from a cancer hospital?" "They have the stigma that, 'cancer is contagious,' and neighbors will isolate them. So, they want our help, but they ask us to park our van a *long* distance away from their home," says soft-spoken Menakshi.

---

1 This was accurate to the best of my knowledge during the time of my fieldwork.

DOI: 10.4324/9781003413158-11

The first patient we see is a 36-year-old female with cancer of the tongue that has metastasized to her liver and lungs. The patient is stretched out on a bed with a massively distended abdomen and swollen lower legs. Her husband and two brothers are caring for her. Jotika takes the lead, and I am surprised when I learn she is a health counselor, not a nurse, given her impressive clinical acumen. Flipping through the various medical papers the family provides and piecing together information about the patient's complex course, Jotika thinks the patient may benefit from a paracentesis, but isn't sure if the patient's abdominal swelling is from fluid, which would be helped by draining, or from the tumor itself, which would not. She directs Leah, the nurse, to do an abdominal exam, which is inconclusive. The recent ultrasound report would provide some clarification, but it cannot be located.

Jotika calls to consult with Dr. Amit in the palliative care clinic and a decision is made to treat the patient with medications and reassess her in a few days. The team spends over an hour with the patient and family, Jotika expertly building rapport with the anxious husband and hovering brothers, who listen, rapt, to her every word, and whom she eventually gets to smile and laugh. The husband shows us the homeopathic treatments they are using; one smells like tea tree oil, and as he spreads it on a shallow saucer he explains its purpose: to warm up the room since today is a bit dreary and drizzly.[2]

As we are leaving, one of the brothers follows us back to the van, asking questions the entire way which Jotika patiently answers. "So many doubts, they have!" she says, sliding the door shut.

"That was the brother," Jotika explains, "he is concerned that the husband hasn't done everything for the patient and he is wondering if more chemotherapy or radiation would be helpful." I nod, thinking of similar conversations I have had with families in the U.S.

The home care team, being on the frontlines in the community, has seen some disturbing cases. They all agree the most upsetting was a woman with advanced breast cancer, who was not referred by the hospital, but by a concerned relative. When the team arrived, they were shocked by what they saw—a woman with a deep, severe wound, lying half-naked on an uncovered wooden bed, her chest crawling with maggots. Over 200, by their estimation. The woman was so weak she couldn't talk. Out of fear, or neglect, or likely both, no one in the family would touch her, not even to give her a glass of water. When the home care team finally did, the patient cried.

---

2 This was one of the few examples I observed related to homeopathic and/or Ayurvedic medicine during my fieldwork. Within the hospital setting, the emphasis was strongly on a traditional biomedical approach to care and I did not observe patients or family caregivers engaging in complementary or alternative healthcare practices or treatments or discussing these with clinicians; in fact, clinicians within the hospital seemed mostly dismissive of these practices, attributing them, at least in part, as a reason for late or missed diagnoses.

The patient's husband, a security guard in a central jail, explained initially it was a small, marble-sized lump, treated with some radiation. But afterwards, an ulcer developed and, according to Jotika, the husband didn't want to spend more money on treatment, thinking, "the cancer will not heal anyway, even if we spend a lot of money on her, it is not going to help." So instead he went and got medications for the pain, but never dealt with the worsening wound.

It wasn't just the extent of the patient's rabid disease that was traumatic, but how the woman had been ostracized by her family, due to lack of knowledge and fear, that really upset the team. The husband's sister apparently even told the patient, "you have done something wrong in your past life, this is the reason you are now facing this problem." After seeing this patient, the team really began to wonder—"how many people are out there in this condition? How many people are suffering like that, at home, alone? How many people live far away and don't know about SICH, don't know what is cancer, don't know about our home care service?" The team worked closely with the husband and he learned how to do a good, proper dressing; he called the home care team to tell them all the maggots were gone. The next day, his wife died.

* * *

Our next patient is a 40-year-old woman with lung cancer that has spread to the bone. "This is the fourth time we have seen her in a month," Jotika whispers to me as we walk down a narrow dirt lane in to a low-ceilinged one room cement block home that is occupied almost entirely by a bed and a rickety table. The woman's husband greets us warmly as we enter. He is slight and spry and moves about the small home agilely, his hennaed hair with its unnatural reddish hue giving him a distinctly leprechaun look. Again, Jotika runs the show. Sister Menakshi, who looks sickly herself—too thin and with a nagging cough—does not say a word, but records some things in a book as Jotika counsels the patient about her medications—apparently the patient has been constipated for four days, but has not been taking her laxatives as prescribed. The visit lasts about 30 minutes, and then we are on our way to see a 68-year-old paralyzed woman, Akanksha, with metastatic breast cancer that has invaded her bone, liver, and lungs.

Akanksha was diagnosed just four months ago, but did not receive any treatment because the cancer was so far advanced. Her hair is matted and disheveled and tied up in a loose bun, and she sits on a cement floor atop a folded square of purple and yellow blankets, paralyzed from the cancer that is squeezing her spinal cord. The cramped room is painted yellow and has blue shuttered doors that separate it from another small room where a man sleeps on a low bed. The patient's left arm, which is grotesquely enlarged, began to swell last night and the woman's son, thinking it was an adverse reaction to the morphine, stopped administering her pain medicine. She is now in horrible agony, writhing and crying on the floor. Jotika instructs the family to boil some salted water to sterilize dressings for her wound. While we are waiting for the water to boil, the elder daughter pulls up her sari blouse, and thrusts her chest toward Jotika. Jotika and Menakshi both do a mini-breast exam and have a long conversation with her in Hindi. I catch the words "cervical" and "gynecologist." She lowers her blouse and seems slightly reassured.

"She is worried about a breast lump," Jotika whispers to me. "Understandable," she says, her eyes traveling toward Akanksha on the blankets in front of us.

"Did you feel anything?" I whisper back.

"No, no," Jotika tells me.

"What did you tell her to do?" I ask.

"We told her she needs to be seen by a gynecologist, get a mammogram, get cervical cancer screening."

"Where can she do this, at SICH?" I ask. Jotika shakes her head.

"Probably not possible. Too far away. She will have to wait until a doctor comes around to the village. But even then, that will just be for a checkup," Jotika acknowledges.

Jotika directs her attention back to the patient whose tumor is pushing through the skin of her mangled right breast. Leah makes bandages by folding and rolling bits of cotton in to strips of gauze, tying them into little bundles, then dunking them in the boiling water. She carefully washes her hands, dons gloves, and then uses the sterilized gauze bundles to swab and clean the wound of drainage and pus. Another family member is instructed to pulverize five antibiotic tablets of metronidazole (Flagyl); the powder is then sprinkled on to the wound to help reduce odor and infection and then covered with a piece of clean cloth.

The rest of the time is spent talking with the family about the importance of taking the morphine regularly, and bowel and bladder and skin care. The family is clearly very poor, and I ask Jotika how they will pay for supplies and medicines. "We give them what we can, samples. We get some money, about 1,000 rupees (about $15 USD) a month that we can use to buy medicines and supplies for people who cannot afford them," she explains.

When Jotika instructs the family to administer a 5 mg tablet of morphine, the daughter errantly places it in the patient's swollen, weak hand, which is unable to manipulate the small pill. It predictably falls into the maw of blankets and has to be retrieved by the son. He places the tiny white tablet gingerly on his mother's tongue, a small, delicate act of communion. As we are leaving, the son follows us out, peppering Jotika with questions until the minute she gets in to the van. I am struck by Jotika's patience and presence; she is not anxious to leave, she gives her full, undivided attention to this young man whose mother will soon die.

Jotika calls our next patient to let them know we are on the way, but discovers that his family, frightened by the patient's rapid deterioration, has already taken him back to the hospital. "Ugh," Jotika hangs up the phone, clearly upset. She feels badly we did not get there in time. "We are only three for this *entire* city," Jotika says, extending her arms. "And the patients are so far away, one here, the next *way* over here. If only there wasn't so much traffic. Then we could see more patients," she says as the van bumps along, stopping short of dogs, cows, goats, autorickshaws, other cars, pedestrians. She slouches down, kicks off her sandals and presses her feet against the front seat. "We are helpless, we feel so bad, all these patients who need us and we cannot see." She sighs and closes her eyes. "God must save them."

***

The new admission lives south of City Center. She is a 56-year-old woman with recurrent rectal cancer who looks at least 70. The family lives down a narrow alley in a two-room cement block home with a doorway painted bright yellow with red flowers and a stone floor swept spotlessly clean. The woman lies on a low wooden plank bed covered with a few folded blankets. She is terribly cachectic; her marriage thali, the sacred gold chain she wears around her neck, looks painfully heavy on her thin and fragile frame. She lifts her head slightly when Jotika, myself, and Leah enter the room. The red undergarment she wears under her dark blue sari is visibly saturated with fluid, and the brown sari blouse that slips off her upper torso speaks to dramatic weight loss that does not require a scale to quantify. A small child, who looks about three, plays with a comb and a rusty knife, banging them against the end of the wooden bed until he is shooed away by the patient's husband.

The husband says he recognizes me from the hospital, but I cannot place his face, nor that of his wife. Jotika and Leah team up and take the medical history: the patient had done well initially after chemotherapy and radiation, but now the cancer has returned and she has a large, painful ulcerating mass and a colostomy. Jotika lightly touches the patient's arm, looks into her eyes, and the woman begins to cry. "She is worried about the burden she is placing on her family," Jotika translates. The grief and sadness in the woman's eyes bore through me; she stares at some indistinct point past all of us.

The couple has an adult daughter, disabled due to polio. Leah asks her to boil water and fetch some newspaper. I see the daughter scuttle across the stone slab floor, dragging her shriveled and impotent legs with her arms in an awkward, jerky, crab-like movement. The bandages Leah makes are put in a tiffin and then submerged in the boiling water, along with a set of forceps. Leah places some antibiotic tablets into the folds of the newspaper and grinds the pills into a white powder with a stone.

The power cuts just as Jotika and Leah begin to attend to the wound. The electric fan in the corner stops whirling and the one light in the dark room stops shining, forcing the husband to open the two shutter doors to the outside alley. He stands protectively in front of the door to shield his wife as much as possible from the prying eyes of neighbors. Leah tenderly removes the woman's undergarment revealing a lemon sized fungating ulcer emerging from the woman's rectum, white pus oozing from its center. The husband looks away briefly. Leah irrigates the wound multiple times, washing away the white and revealing a beefy, red, deep wound. The entire time Jotika talks comfortingly with the patient and her husband. After Leah is satisfied that the wound is clean, she takes the forceps, extracts a bandage sachet, cotton wrapped in gauze, from the now-cooled water, squeezes the excess water out against the side of the pot, applies a generous supply of the antibiotic powder from the newspaper and dabs it gently on to the patient's wound. She then carefully covers and secures the wound with a larger gauze pad, gives the woman a dose of oral morphine, and, with the assistance of Jotika and myself, helps her change in to fresh and dry clothes.

The woman slowly pushes herself off the wooden bed and shuffles over to where Jotika is sitting and making some notes. She begins to stoop to touch Jotika's feet in the ultimate sign of respect and deference, but Jotika grasps her thin arms and gently guides the woman upwards before she can complete the act. "This is my duty, it is not necessary," Jotika says softly, helping the woman back to her bed. The husband follows us out to the van and says goodbye to each of us. We walk by a group of people gathered around burlap bags, pulling at strings, cutting and piecing flaps together. Two puppies are curled together against the edge of the building.

"That's what she used to do," Jotika says to me sadly. "That was her job, the patient. She used to put together these jute bags, for vegetables, for groceries."

* * *

At the Dvipa University campus, where we stop for lunch, malnourished and sad looking dogs patrol the grounds hoping for scraps and then realizing none are forthcoming, curl in to tight, still balls to conserve energy. The driver takes a walk as he is fasting and will not be eating lunch. Jotika, Menakshi, and Leah generously offer me rice and curry they have brought from home in an amusing one-upmanship of culinary prowess.

"Here, you must have mine!" Jotika says, scooping an incredibly large amount of her rice and curry onto my plate.

"Mine too!" Menakshi chimes in, pushing an even larger portion of her rice and curry on to my already full plate.

Not to be outdone, Leah leans over, and though I try to stop her, empties the entire contents of her tiffin of tomato curry on to my rice. "Tomato curry, here, for you, Madam."

I laugh, knowing that refusal is futile. "You are going to make me very fat!" I exclaim as I begin to eat the equivalent of three lunches, grateful that all traditional Indian pants are made with drawstrings. They laugh with delight.

I try to tell the team "thank you," but am harshly reprimanded.

"No more 'thank yous!'" Jotika warns, looking genuinely offended. "Do not insult us! We are friends! 'Thank you this, thank you that,' it is not necessary!"

Mandal Outreach

A small crowd gathers in the lobby of South Indian Cancer Hospital—Jasmine, the hospital administrative coordinator; Marcus, a visiting doctor from Germany; Dr. Darshan, a palliative care doctor; Bishnu, a hospital social worker; Seetha, a new volunteer; and me. We all pile into a van that has been hired to drive us to a mandal outside the city limits. "Villages make up mandals, mandals make up districts, and districts make up states," Jasmine explains.

This outreach program is supported by the SICH Volunteer Society. Each Saturday, Bishnu, a soft-spoken, gentle, middle-aged man with a moustache, takes a two-hour bus ride to join community health workers in six villages, helping to identify patients in need of palliative care support. Before coming to work at SICH, Bishnu spent 15 years as a child labor activist, helping to remove children from day labor jobs and encourage parents to enroll them in school.

It's difficult for Bishnu to see children abandoned in the hospital by their parents, parents he knows are overwhelmed by their child's illness and competing financial demands and responsibilities. Parents faced with impossible choices: leave, and their child faces cancer alone; stay, and no one is working and there is no money. If both parents decide to stay at the hospital, the rest of their children typically drop out of school to work and earn income for the family. Bishnu's philosophy is that counselors must *think* first; they cannot become overwrought with emotion, despite the dire circumstances of the patients. If they do, it prevents finding solutions. "That is my rule," he says. "That I should not cry with patients. They tell us their problems so that we can search for some answer."

The landscape changes quickly once we pass beyond the city limits. The roads are empty, the sky is blue, the air smells clean, and it is quiet. I sit next to Seetha, a professional Indian woman interested in volunteering with the Society, who is accompanying the team on this trip to get a feel for the kind of work they do. She is warm and friendly and has spent a considerable amount of time working in the U.S., mostly in Chicago. When she makes reference to two children and a fiancé, I get the feeling she has a story to tell, something simmering just below the surface.

"I am divorced," she whispers, twisting her back against the van window so she faces me more directly. "It was an abusive situation and I had to get out."

I nod, strangely unsurprised by how freely she volunteers this sensitive information.

"It is complicated, and people here can be narrow-minded. I wouldn't talk to anyone else here about this," she says quietly, subtly tilting her head toward the others in the van.

"But then I met someone else," she continues, "and I was supposed to get married a few weeks ago. I was engaged to a doctor I met in the U.S. He is Indian, we dated for 4 years. He's divorced too, with children. He came to India to meet my whole family. We fixed the date, got everything arranged, and then he went back to the U.S. to finish his rotation."

I put her age at around my own, 38 or 39. Her fingernails are painted a pale lavender; she taps them nervously against her white cell phone.

"And then things got a little weird. He seemed unsure about things. We talked about it, but he said, no, no he wanted to get married. So, he comes here, to India, and we are in the car driving to the temple to get married and he is acting strange. I ask him, I say, 'Do you really want to do this? Are you okay?' And he says, 'Actually, no, I don't want to get married, I can't marry you.'" Seetha pauses and looks out of the van at the passing empty land caught frame by frame in the window. "We had to go there and explain to our families and it was terrible, everyone was there, everyone had arrived. That is a really big deal, here in India, getting married."

"Yes, I know," I say.

"And getting left, right before the wedding, well, that is a really, *really* big deal," says Seetha.

I think about how awful it would be to get jilted in the U.S., and then I multiply that by a thousand, which probably still grossly underestimates the intensity of the Indian matrimony factor. I think about the stigma of divorce in India and then add on top of that being left at the altar. The weight of it, this slab of humiliation, makes me feel a deep tenderness for this woman I have just met and an odd desire to protect her.

"I am so sorry that happened to you," I say. "That's terrible."

"So, I'm here today trying to distract myself, trying not to think about it anymore. He is back in the States and we've talked a few times, and you know what's crazy? Is that I want him back, I think I would still marry him."

She looks utterly exhausted, and I believe her when she says she hasn't slept well for days. She lets out a self-deprecating laugh. "I don't know why I am telling you all this. I just feel like I have to let it out, to talk about it."

"It helps to talk about it," I say. And I add, lowering my voice even more, "I don't advertise this here, but I'm divorced too."

I put my hand on her shoulder, trying to convey through this small gesture that she is not alone, that she will, somehow, get through this.

* * *

The van bounces down a dusty road to the first village, where we visit a 12-year-old boy who is paralyzed from the neck down due to a cervical fracture that no one seems to know how it happened.

"When we first came to visit him," Jasmine leans over quietly to tell me, "he was sleeping on the cement floor, they didn't have a bed for him, it was so sad. So, we donated a bed and a wheelchair."

The boy is wearing a turquoise collared shirt and gray pants. His limbs are thin and his hands are contracted in to twisted fists that lie limply by his sides. He has a quick smile and alert eyes that dart from person to person, taking us all in. An old yellow pillow wedged against the wall props him up in the donated bed. Despite being paralyzed for five years, he seems in good spirits and well cared for by his attentive family, whose concrete block home with a dirt floor is small and simple, but extremely orderly and decorated with colorful yellow and blue paint around the doorframe and swirly, colorful rangoli[3] by the entrance. The boy's mother says something, and Jasmine translates: "She is saying he was an excellent and bright pupil before he became bedridden. Now he cannot go to school, but his sister brings homes lessons from the teacher." I can't help but wonder if this is possibly reversible, if a surgical treatment would help this small boy. But the medical records are vague and unclear.

We visit an elderly woman with head and neck cancer who completed a course of radiation and is having trouble with mouth sores, and a 55-year-old woman with multiple myeloma who became paralyzed from the waist down four days ago. I am surprised by the passivity of Dr. Darshan. It is Marcus, not Dr. Darshan, who looks into the patient's mouth to assess the extent of the mucositis with the flashlight that he brought in his modified black doctor's bag. It is Marcus who checks the reflexes of the woman with multiple myeloma. When Marcus offers the reflex hammer to Dr. Darshan, he accepts it reluctantly and does a perfunctory test of the patellar reflexes—only of the left knee. He seems uncomfortable with an audience and perhaps equally uncomfortable doing a physical exam. As we walk back toward the van, I ask Jasmine about how families obtain morphine in the villages. "They have to come or send a family member to bring the morphine back from South Indian Cancer Hospital," she says.

"You can't bring it here to them?"

"Oh no," she says. "We don't have a license to do that. It is illegal." I wonder about the fentanyl patches I was asked to transport to Hameeda last week at the hospice but decide not to ask. Jasmine tells me it would cost a family member about 30 rupees and take about two and a half hours via bus to reach SICH from the village. And even then, there is the possibility they could travel all the way there only to discover the morphine supply has run out.

At the next village, we see a 35-year-old woman with HIV. The woman's husband reportedly died of a heart attack, but his death occurred outside the village and the exact circumstances are unclear. The implication from

3 Rangoli are decorative designs drawn on the sidewalk or in front of a home typically consisting of bright colors made from colored chalk, paint, sand, rice, or flower petals. They are meant to welcome Hindu deities and guests and are thought to bring good luck and prosperity.

the care team is that this case involved a relationship between the patient's husband and a same-sex partner. But I'm not sure if they have factual information that led them to this conclusion, or if this is an assumption related to a lack of knowledge about the various methods of HIV transmission or the general stigma surrounding HIV in India.[4]

The woman was diagnosed with HIV when she was three months pregnant with their second child; both of her children have tested negative. The patient looks well, says she feels fine, her tiny feet dangling a few inches from the ground as she sits on the white plastic chair talking with the team. Only her father knows of her diagnosis.

I think about the women in the village whose husbands have more freedom to roam about, how homosexuality is largely condemned and denied, but certainly still exists, and how women through arranged marriages are likely partnered with men unable to openly express their sexuality. I wonder if I, as a sexually liberated middle-aged Western woman, felt deeply uncomfortable trying to even find tampons in the city of Dandaka, how would a woman in this remote area go about buying condoms to protect herself and then convincing her husband to use them?

As if reading my mind, Marcus asks Jasmine about counseling the patient about safe sex practices now that she is a widow and could potentially have other sexual partners.

"The patient will get very angry if we talk about that," Jasmine says quickly. "She is widowed, so she will not get remarried, that is the rule."

"But, uh,…" he falters. "Is that rule ever broken?" he asks.

"No," Jasmine says definitively.

Marcus tries another approach. "But even if she does not get remarried, she may have a relationship with another person and so it would be important to counsel her…" he trails off. Jasmine shakes her head. "The community health worker knows the patient well. If she has the opportunity, they'll talk about it," says Jasmine firmly, her tone clearly indicating the conversation is over.

***

On the way home we stop at a dhaba, a roadside restaurant. Before we eat, Seetha and I seek out a sink to wash our hands. We walk through the outdoor seating area into the covered kitchen, but don't see a sink.

---

4 Much research has been done to understand and reduce stigma associated with HIV within India (and other countries). See Ekstrand, M. L., Ramakrishna, J., Bharat, S., & Heylen, E. (2013). Prevalence and drivers of HIV stigma among health providers in urban India: implications for interventions. *Journal of the International AIDS Society*, 16, 18717; Steward, W. T., Herek, G. M., Ramakrishna, J., Bharat, S., Chandy, S., Wrubel, J., & Ekstrand, M. L. (2008). HIV-related stigma: Adapting a theoretical framework for use in India. *Social Science & Medicine*, 67(8), 1225–1235.

"Here, we can just use one of these," Seetha says, grabbing a bottle of water from one of the picnic-style tables.

She carries the water bottle over to the edge of the cement wall. I hold out my hands and rub them together while she pours water over my palms. We switch, and I do the same for Seetha. In the surprisingly intimate act of washing each other's hands, I see the unmistakable light orange tracings of faded mehndi on her palms. She notices me noticing.

"That's the mehndi for my wedding," she says sadly, shaking the water from her hands. "It was all up my arms," she motions from her wrists to her shoulders. I don't say anything, and we start to walk back toward our colleagues. She turns to face me. "I had to go home and scrub it all off with nail polish remover." She pauses. "I got a terrible rash."

I imagine her hunched over a sink, sobbing, scrubbing and scrubbing the stubborn signs of marriage off of her skin with acetone, trying to wash it away, knowing that the stain of humiliation and shame will linger much longer than any mehndi.

National Service Scheme

I am asked by staff at SICH to prepare a basic talk about palliative care for social work students. Along with Jasmine representing the palliative care team, Swati, another hospital volunteer, and Nidhi, a tobacco cessation counselor whose glasses seem lost in the folds of her pudgy face, I travel to a rural district about an hour outside Dandaka. It turns out that the all-female audience is not, in fact, social work students. Instead, they are participating in a seven-day National Service Scheme (NSS) camp, a public service program conducted by the Ministry of Youth Affairs and Sports of the Indian Government whose primary aim is "personality development" through community service. As a special foreign visitor, I am asked to raise the flag at the daily morning flag-hoisting ceremony; as it unfurls flower petals unexpectedly shower down upon me.

After the class and lunch, we are shuttled down a two-kilometer dirt road to a small village where Nidhi is scheduled to give a talk about the dangers of tobacco use. When we arrive, residents are corralled in a dusty patch of earth in front of a cluster of low-ceilinged, one-room cement block homes. The NNS leader, a lanky, bossy, and beady-eyed man, aggressively orders everyone to clap in unison and return a salute that is disturbingly reminiscent of The Third Reich in an attempt to bring order to the chaotic mass of village women and children. Nidhi's lecture is off to a rocky start because the target audience—men who use paan[5]—are not there; they are working in the fields. Children from the village wearing tattered clothes with slick upper lips from runny noses and croupy sounding coughs swarm out of nowhere; I am awkwardly perched on a broken plastic chair the students insisted I sit upon, trying my best to be inconspicuous. I am not successful. The children crowd around me, pressing against my legs and arms, touching my odd skin and hair. I see only three girls; they linger in the back of the ring of children, shyly making eye contact, tentative as crocus blossoms. The children are creating such a ruckus that Nidhi is having a difficult time delivering her message—and I feel terrible that I am the cause—but she forges on.

When Nidhi has finished, the NNS students, who know we represent the palliative care program at SICH and who know I am a nurse, implore us to see some of the villagers who are ill. Swati agrees. Immediately, I panic, knowing I am woefully ill-prepared to provide any modicum of medical care in this village. We step over rivulets of sewage, past wandering goats and somber-faced villagers, mostly housewives and old men who watch us intensely from their doorsteps, to the home of a young girl who is significantly developmentally delayed—I am told she is chronologically seven, but behaviorally more like a three-year-old. "Consanguineous (intra-family) marriage," a student whispers to me as way of explanation.

One of the NNS students, wearing a light blue sweatshirt and clearly a leader in the group, picks up the girl who is sitting on the ground and

---

5 Paan: a stimulating preparation of betel nut, spices, and often cured tobacco that is chewed; when combined with tobacco, it is a contributing cause of head and neck cancers in many Asian countries.

explains that the child's grandmother, frustrated by the girl's inability to care for herself, beats her while the parents work all day in the fields. A neighbor, who has joined the crowd gathered outside the home, repeats something I do not understand while aggressively tugging at my arm.

"What is she saying?" I ask the student.

"She is begging you to take this child away from here. She wants you to take this child to your home, to a better place."

I am humbled and saddened, and all I can muster up is a lame, "I'm so sorry." I hate myself for being so selfish that in the midst of this tremendous suffering, this abject poverty, I am edgy and restless and all I can think is *please don't let me get sick here; please don't let me get lice or ringworm or a bad upper respiratory infection or tuberculosis.* The student in the blue sweatshirt cradles the small girl close to her face. She does not seem concerned about any of the possibilities I fear, and my self-loathing quickly morphs to envy: of her openness, her willingness, her courage.

The next patient we are taken to see is an elderly woman whom we find lying in the middle of the dirt road. She tells us she fell and broke her leg, and unable to move, she has remained in the middle of the road for an undetermined period of time. A student adds that the woman is the primary caregiver for her six-month-old grandson, who was also found crying in the street next to her. Neighbors occasionally bring her food and water. Swati looks to me for help. I run through a quick list of possibilities in my head: Stroke? Hip fracture? Fracture of the femur? Spinal cord compression from advanced cancer? Polio? Depression? I ask a series of questions: she can move and bend her legs without pain, there is no swelling, her sensation is intact, no bowel or bladder incontinence, no headaches, no back pain, no one-sided paralysis. Her legs seem strong on exam, but she feels weak. I ask about her family. She says her sons died two years ago, one from an accident—she is not specific—and one from tuberculosis. Everyone looks to me to explain why this woman cannot walk, but I have no idea why this poor woman is lying in the middle of the road. I promise to talk the case over with Dr. Madhu. We turn to leave, and the woman looks at us imploringly as we move further away from her, a motionless, inert bundle that becomes smaller and smaller as the distance between us grows.

In the van to return home, children bang on the windows and doors as the driver starts the engine. Each strike against the car by their tiny fists leaves a dusty, smudged imprint. I lean my head back against the seat and close my eyes, my heart too tired to break.

References

Ekstrand, M. L., Ramakrishna, J., Bharat, S., & Heylen, E. (2013). Prevalence and drivers of HIV stigma among health providers in urban India: Implications for interventions. *Journal of the International AIDS Society, 16,* 18717.

Steward, W. T., Herek, G. M., Ramakrishna, J., Bharat, S., Chandy, S., Wrubel, J., & Ekstrand, M. L. (2008). HIV-related stigma: Adapting a theoretical framework for use in India. *Social Science & Medicine, 67*(8), 1225–1235.

PART IV
Other Hospitals

8   Cash for Compassion

Triumph Cancer Hospital

The people who are paying cash, they have a separate wing altogether where you can see cleanliness and all those things; you have individual rooms once you get out of the ICU and all that. But if you have MHS [the government health insurance plan], the moment you walk into that section of the hospital, you see a big difference. There is no cleanliness; there is no hygiene, and they don't spend any money for people to clean that place and all those things, so that is where they save the money. Just because you are taken care of in a corporate hospital, it does not mean that you are getting 'corporate' level care. And not only that, say for example MHS pays 6,000 rupees for febrile neutropenia; you probably use up the entire 6,000 in 2 days if you go with the expensive antibiotics. In the corporate hospital, the hospitalization itself will cost you that much for 2 days or 3 days. So, that is the reason why they have a separate kind of environment for MHS people. Once the MHS money is used up, the corporate hospitals don't want those patients anymore.

Dr. Varun, volunteer oncologist

The heat has descended upon Dandaka like an oppressive wool cloak, and it is only mid-February. I wait for Rose, a senior nurse, in the busy lobby of the Block III building of Triumph Cancer Center, a collection of white, orderly buildings. The Center's roots and mission as a Trust hospital make it a unique hybrid—not fully a government hospital like South Indian Cancer Hospital (SICH) and not fully a private hospital like the multiple ones that have mushroomed within the city. The Trust, established by a former Chief Minister, whose wife died from cancer, is now overseen by his son, a well-known Indian film celebrity. Triumph Cancer Center provides care to MHS patients, as well as a handful of credit patients (those who have some sort of health insurance coverage, generally through their employers) and cash patients (those who pay entirely out of pocket). Because it is a Trust hospital, with a specific mission of service to the poor, the cost of out-of-pocket care is ostensibly cheaper than a traditional private/corporate hospital.

DOI: 10.4324/9781003413158-13

I notice a large purple and white sign prominently posted in the lobby that lists "Patient Rights and Responsibilities." It is very similar to a "Patient Bill of Rights" found in U.S. hospitals that delineates what a patient can, and should, expect when they seek health care at the particular institution.[1] There is an even larger purple and white placard titled "TARIFFS" that lists the price for different procedures and room rates. Prices are listed for single rooms with air conditioning, double rooms without air-conditioning, deluxe rooms, and standard rooms. A general wardroom costs 1,000 rupees (about $15 USD) a day, a day in the surgical intensive care unit is 2,500 rupees ($40 USD) a day. The most expensive room is the Super Deluxe A at 6,000 rupees ($85 USD) a day. Procedures are also listed: Pap smear, 220 rupees ($3 USD); X-ray abdomen, 200 rupees ($2 USD); Magnetic Resonance Imaging (MRI) whole body screening 10,000 rupees ($145 USD); Bone scan, 3,100 rupees ($45 USD); Master health check-up, 2,500 rupees ($36 USD); Blood culture, 1,000 rupees ($14.50 USD). The most expensive treatment I see listed is the Rapid ARC IGRT at over 2 lakhs: 2,45,000.00 ($3,562 USD). As I ponder what exactly a Rapid ARC IGRT may be, Rose gently taps me on the shoulder. I turn to see a woman resplendent in a sparkly bright green salwar suit with a warm, authentic smile and short cropped black hair. She wears, appropriately, glasses with light pink frames. She looks so friendly and kind I instinctively want to hug her. She immediately apologizes for being late. "I am supposed to be here at 8 am, but I got permission to come later today." She hesitates. "I had to go by the cemetery."

I wait.

"Today, last year, I lost my daughter. My only daughter," she says, her voice quiet and even.

"Oh, Rose," I lower my voice and put my hand gently on her shoulder. "I am so sorry."

"She was 25, there was an accident..."

She doesn't offer any more information, and I don't ask. Her sadness sits there, heavy in front of us, like a still and solid orb amidst the swirling activity and noise of the lobby.

"And then, 2 years back, I lost my husband. Cerebral malaria," she says and motions to the back of her skull with her small hand.

"Okay, let's go!" she says abruptly and cheerfully before I have a chance to suggest we should perhaps reschedule. We head off toward the High Dependency Unit (HDU), similar to an American postanesthesia care unit (PACU), where patients go immediately after surgery.[2] In the HDU, the ratio is two to three nurses

1 See https://www.opm.gov/healthcare-insurance/healthcare/reference-materials/bill-of-rights/.
2 At Triumph Cancer Center, patients transitioned from the Operating Theater (i.e., Operating Room), to the HDU, to the Surgical Intensive Care Unit, and then to the general wards. This set-up was in contrast to SICH, where patients transitioned from the Operating Theater directly to the ICU.

(depending if they have patients on ventilators or not) to six patients. The nursing supervisor proudly tells me that Triumph Cancer Center has 420 beds, and about 240 nurses, all of whom are CPR trained; here, all the nurses are required to wear name tags.[3] I am told patients come to Triumph Cancer Center from all over the State and the world—Kenya, Saudi Arabia, the U.S.—for treatment. Family members can stay on the campus at either the relatively inexpensive hostel or the more expensive lodge. Despite these options, it is still more than many families can afford, and so, similar to SICH, many poor families create makeshift camps in the landscaped roundabout in front of the hospital.

I am impressed not only with the cleanliness, but with the nursing documentation, which is considerably more patient-focused and pertinent than what I have seen at SICH. Some of the charting and orders are done electronically, but it is still largely a paper-based system, and I don't have to look far before I see a stack of the dreaded ledgers that the nurses are required to maintain.

The general wards are set up differently and organized by "cabins"—cubbies with a single cot and small bedside table partitioned by white curtains. Here, the nurse-to-patient ratio is more concerning: 17 beds and two nurses. Rose admits they are understaffed.

Rose takes me next to the Day Care Unit, an outpatient treatment area for patients receiving chemotherapy and other types of infusions. The unit is clean and orderly, but I notice there is no separate area to mix chemotherapy. Rose confirms nurses mix all medications, including chemotherapy, at the bedside: "Because the patients want to see! They are paying and they want to be sure they are getting the drug. Some of them are paying lakhs and lakhs for treatment and they are suspicious," Rose explains. I nod, concerned about the safety implications of this practice, but also cognizant of the constant vigilance required to avoid being cheated.

Throughout the hospital, I don't see many sinks, but I do see designated areas for the disposal of needles and syringes, and more nurses wearing gloves. I also don't see patients or family members being yelled at or shooed away. What I am particularly struck by is the stratification of care based on the ability to pay. Rose takes me proudly to the sparkling, brand new building exclusively for cash patients; the MHS patients are cared for in a separate area of the hospital that is darker and more cramped and reminds me more of SICH.

Rose interrupts our tour to ask me if I would like to attend a cultural program being held today at the hospital. The cultural program turns out to be a graduation ceremony honoring the 30 Bachelor's nursing students who have completed the four-year program from the affiliated Triumph College of Nursing. The program is a combination of traditional graduation ceremony with the requisite speeches and acknowledgments, talent show with group

---

3 This was an interesting distinction between SICH and suggests a different level of accountability and safety protocols. At SICH, I did not see any hospital personnel with an identification badge or nametag.

and individual dance performances, and beauty pageant with the graduates strutting in catwalk fashion across the stage to hip-hop music.

"Human values are the most important: human feelings, the human touch. Put them all into practice. Always be sympathetic toward your patients. Always get the patient's blessing," urges the liaison from the College of Nursing. "What will add value to your practice is compassion. Nursing makes the hospital. Have pride in your job. Have the interests of the patient in mind and remember you are an important part of this hospital," says the hospital CEO. The Chairman gets up and talks frankly about salaries: 7,000 Rupees ($100 USD) per month for BSc nurses, 6,000 ($87 USD) Rupees a month for those with GNM certificates. "The Institution will take good care of you," he assures.

The graduates are all female and they wear a dazzling array of sparkling and colorful saris; some walk toward the audience seductively, flipping the edge of their sari flirtatiously as they pivot and walk back to the group of giggling classmates. Others walk quickly and look uncomfortable being so clearly on display. Each graduate is given the microphone, which crackles and competes with the loud thumping background music, to make a brief speech: some recount benign escapades from living in the hostel; some rattle off a list of hobbies and favorite colors ("black with red"); many thank God for the opportunity to serve others. A surprising number make a public plea to be forgiven for any mistakes they made in clinicals or any offenses unintentionally brought to bear on their friends or family members.

After an hour with no obvious end in sight, I attempt to make a discreet exit. A girl in the audience calls out to me from the center of a row.

"Madam! Madam! You must stay!" she cries out. I hesitate and she calls out again.

"Okay!" I smile and sit down on one of the carpeted steps of the auditorium, as I don't want to disrupt the program by making my way back to the seat I have just vacated.

"No, no!" she says loudly, "here!" She stands up, offering her seat to me. I try to politely refuse, but she is insistent. She smiles as I squeeze myself back down the aisle, moving toward her and her now empty seat; she has moved on to the lap of her classmate. Her glossy black hair is pulled back into a waist-length braid and her frame is birdlike and delicate. I feel like a sweaty, pale giant next to her.

Her name is Beulah, and she is a GNM student in her last year of the program from Kerala. She tells me that almost all the women in the nursing program are from Kerala. "Of the 45 in the hostel (similar to dorms), 90% are Keralites."[4]

---

4 The greatest number of Christians in India lives in Kerala (making up about 20% of the population; see Pew Research Center, Religious Demography of Indian States and Territories, 2021); nursing has traditionally been viewed as a noble profession for Christian women, and consequently many nurses in India hail from Kerala.

"Why is that?" I ask. "It's a profession we like and want to do," she says. "And a chance to go abroad!" she smiles broadly, her brilliant white teeth gleaming.

Beulah wants to know why I am in Dandaka. When I tell her, she pops up suddenly, grabs my hand, and winds us down to the front of the auditorium. One of the senior students is having their minute of fame at the microphone, and I worry we are being disruptive and rude, but no one seems to mind. Beulah introduces me to the Principal and another faculty member from the College of Nursing who are sitting in the front row.

"You must speak! Say a few words!" the Principal insists.

"Oh, no, no, that's okay," I say, ill-prepared to give a speech.

"No, you must!"

After the last catwalk strut and mini-speech thanking God and asking for forgiveness, I take the podium. *How are you?*, I begin in the local language and the crowd erupts in laughter. I keep my remarks short: I tell them how impressed I am with their accomplishments, the important role they have in the lives of patients and family members, and how I am privileged to be here.

After I finish, a young man bursts on to the stage and begins breakdancing.

* * *

I wake the next morning feeling like taffy, moving slowly and uncomfortably through my morning routine in the early heat of the day. Back at Triumph Cancer Center, I am met by the effervescent Rose. She takes me by the hand to the New Ward Day Hospital, the outpatient infusion area for cash patients, briefly explains my purpose to the nurses, and leaves me in the capable hands of Sister Leta, a GNM nurse who has been working at Triumph for three months. The ward has a particularly charged energy today because they are preparing for a visit by the National Accreditation Board for Hospital and Healthcare Providers (NABH), which Rose explained to me earlier is a voluntary credentialing process for corporate and private hospitals in India. I understand how this can change and alter behaviors in profound ways. Back in the U.S., I remember new signs being posted, surprise protocols appearing, equipment moving, and documentation being buffed—all temporizing measures for a visit from the Joint Commission on Accreditation of Healthcare Organizations (JCAHO). I recall a physician from a prestigious hospital who once shared an interesting anecdote about his institution's approach to a JCAHO site visit: the hospital hired multiple moving trucks to drive extra equipment around the city for a few hours during the inspection in order to make sure hallways and exits remained clear as required by the regulations.

The Day Hospital's 17 beds are made with clean pale blue linens and partitioned with white privacy curtains. At the foot of each bed, a bottle of hand sanitizer is attached by a metal hook. I am heartened by the sight of this antiseptic effort, but I don't see it used by staff or patients during my visit. There is a lone sink in the cramped nurses' station. One of the floor supervisors stops by and conducts a brief in-service regarding hand hygiene. The five nurses assigned to the Day Ward circle around the tall man dressed immaculately in white, each animatedly demonstrating the preferred handwashing technique. It is a lively reenactment of handwashing, an elaborate and enthusiastic pantomime dance, based on the World Health Organization (WHO) 2009 Handwashing Guidelines posted by the sink. I am initially encouraged by this, but then discouraged when I observe only sporadic handwashing by the staff (none in over two hours) and definitely not between patients.

I notice certain things are similar to SICH: limited good, basic hand hygiene; an assembly line approach to care; the absence of clear, individual patient assignments; an incredible amount of documentation; and concerning chemotherapy administration practices. Other things are different: better staffing (six nurses for 17 patients); a more organized, cleaner, and less chaotic work space; less obvious crowd control (however, a security guard is stationed outside the ward door regulating entry); patients are identified by purple and white wrist bands issued when they are admitted; nurses are required to perform a full patient assessment on a special nursing form within 15 minutes of the patient's arrival on the ward, which includes vital signs and measuring height and weight; medications are more clearly documented; and overall, the nurses' role appears more defined—I don't see family members providing much personal care or ayahs or assistants performing what would traditionally be considered duties of the nurse. Interactions with patient and family members seem gentler, softer.

Attempts are made at quality improvement. Rose proudly shows me a special notebook for "Quality Indicators" that lists incidences of needlesticks, medication errors, accidental dislodging of IV catheters, and sentinel events. I flip through the notebook quickly and see hashmarks through all of the categories, suggesting no adverse events have occurred. It is unclear to me how long they have been keeping these records, and if the upcoming inspection was a catalyst for initiating this particular ledger. Rose is very interested in the Quality Improvement efforts in U.S. hospitals and is particularly intrigued by the computerized reporting of events that can be monitored for trends and evaluated to try to understand the root causes contributing to a problem. I am impressed that they are at least trying, even though the method relies solely on self-report and I wonder what incentive the nurses have for reporting errors in a hospital environment where I am told they can be fired easily.

I ask Rose if there is a written job description for the nurses, and if so could I see a copy? "Of course, I will get that for you,"[5] she assures me.

---

5 I was never able to obtain a copy of the job description. From my fieldnotes: "I'm sorry, but we are not supposed to give that out," the Nursing Superintendent explains when we stop by her office. The three nurses in the Superintendent's office begin to talk animatedly among themselves. "I would have to get permission, go through the proper channels," the

Sister Leta is a kind, gentle, and helpful guide. Her eyes dance above the blue surgical mask she wears, and her hair is slicked back into a neat bun, secured with a hairnet. "Come, I will tell you everything!" she says enthusiastically, showing me the documentation forms nurses complete when patients arrive on the unit. I am especially interested in the required pain assessment, which includes a 0–10 scale with faces indicating varying degrees of distress. Leta diligently fills out the scale for each patient but isn't sure what she would do if a patient reported severe pain, in the 7–10 range.

Leta wears the same pair of gloves for the majority of the morning; I see her change them once. Another nurse removes her gloves and cuts off the tips with a huge pair of scissors before throwing them in to the trash. "This way, they won't be reused," Leta explains.

I ask Leta about the allocation of nursing tasks and if they are given a particular patient assignment. "No," she says. "Different nurses do different things. One for the indent, one to take the admissions, one to give the chemo…" I notice that she is doing a bit of everything, all except for the computerized data entry. "But you…?" She interrupts me. "I am junior. I do everything!" she says cheerfully.

"Come, do you want to watch me mix the chemotherapy?" I follow her to the bedside, where she takes the plastic bag from the patient's husband that contains two boxes of oxaliplatin. "Family members purchase their medications here from the medicine store," Leta says. Leta has all of her supplies in a clean, plastic blue bin. She wears gloves (but not fresh ones), and the mask she has been wearing throughout her shift is pushed below her nose and mouth and dangles loosely around her neck. She squirts saline in to the oxaliplatin vials, agitates them, then draws up the medication with a syringe and injects it into a larger bottle of fluid which she labels with a black magic marker. I do not see her check the patient identification band, nor do I see her double check the medication with another nurse, recalculate the dose, or have the chart in front of her when she is hanging the medication. There is some residual chemotherapy in the second vial and it is given back to the family member who stuffs it in to his satchel.

The family members watch Leta like a hawk, and I recall Rose telling me that nurses have to mix the medication at the bedside because otherwise the family members—who have paid significant sums for the treatment—will be concerned that they are not actually being administered chemotherapy. There are no IV pumps, so Leta hangs the bottle to gravity and adjusts the flow regulator.

Superintendent continues. "That's okay," I say. "I don't want you to go to any trouble. Only if it is easy." More discussion in Hindi ensues. It is decided that the Superintendent will ask her supervisor for permission and then I can collect the document from Rose next week. After four attempts, I am unable to get a copy of the job description.

After the patient completes treatment, Leta hands the family member a survey. It contains 18 questions. There are five specific questions related to housekeeping, but only one for nursing services, which simply asks the respondent to rank nursing staff as "excellent," "good," "average," or "poor."

* * *

The MHS Block of Triumph Cancer Center is darker and more crowded than the Cash Block and contains approximately 100 beds, divided primarily among eight units that seem clean, orderly, and relatively private. I am escorted to the MHS Day Care unit, the government subsidized equivalent to the Cash Day Care outpatient chemotherapy Unit where I observed earlier with Leta. Here, I meet Nisha—a recent Bachelor's graduate from Kerala.

"I remember you! I remember you!" Nisha cries when she sees me, flashing a metallic smile. "You gave a speech to us!" she says, recalling the impromptu address I gave the other day at her graduation ceremony. She is the first person in India I have seen wearing braces and her innocent enthusiasm is contagious.

Nisha introduces me to a gaggle of nurses, both students and staff, who crowd around, all wanting to take their picture with me. It is flattering and funny. I notice, not for the first time, that as soon as the camera is turned on them, the nurses abruptly stop laughing and smiling, their faces instantly becoming serious and solemn. You'd never guess that seconds before, and immediately after, the camera clicks, they are giddy with unabashed joy.

Nisha takes my hand and leads me around the hospital, repeating, "Ask me any of your doubts! Anything!"

I do, and I learn that patients are required to have a family attendant present to receive care, similar to SICH, but the expectations of what the family member will do is very different. I learn that the staffing ratios are much better, and on the Day Ward, which has 16 beds, there are four nurses and three GNM students. Throughout the hospital, and specifically on the MHS Block, I look for evidence of similar patient interactions that I have witnessed at SICH: dismissive gestures, shouting, ignoring. I don't see it.[6]

Nursing students—both BSc and GNM—are everywhere, smiling, and curious, and eager. The GNM students wear white uniforms with blue and white checked collars—they look like picnic basketed clergy. The BSc students wear all white uniforms with a longer blouse and a special insignia

---

6   One of the goals during observations at Triumph Hospital, and other care centers in Dandaka, was to establish some basis of comparison with SICH related to patient-nurse interactions and care delivery models. While I did not witness harsh interactions between nurses and patients at Triumph Hospital, it is important to point out that I spent significantly less time observing at Triumph (and other hospitals) compared to SICH; it is possible these types of interactions did occur and that I simply was not present to observe them.

on the lapel. They crowd around, asking questions about my research; they genuinely seem interested and they want specifics.

When I explain the project to them, I get varying answers related to pain management and morphine. Most of the nurses tell me that morphine is "never" given on their ward—injectable or tablets—and that Tramadol (a weak opioid) is what is ordered for severe pain. They are all very careful to clarify that they would only give a medication "as per the orders of the physician." A few tell me they never experience any distress related to poor patient pain control, but at least one tells me differently—that she has witnessed patients in terrible pain and found it very difficult.

At one point, a supervisor comes on the unit and tells all of us to put on our masks. "To prevent cross contamination," Nisha gravely explains as she ties the blue paper surgical mask around the back of my neck. "She is telling us that we must all put on our masks and gloves." Apparently, a big emphasis of a NABH inspection is monitoring for infection control, although I find the emphasis strangely misinterpreted as some practices I have observed, such as donning gloves without washing hands or failing to change gloves between patients, defeat the purpose.

I ask Nisha where I can wash my hands, as I have not seen a sink anywhere on the unit. "Here, come," she says, grabbing my hand and leading me off of the ward, around the corner, to an adjacent ward where I am given an extremely generous squirt of hand sanitizer. I rub it in to my palms and some of the viscous liquid drips on to the floor.

I still am curious if there is an actual sink. "Yes, come, come," Nisha says, pulling me around yet another corner, into the break room and into a miniature sized bathroom where a curious small red cube of soap sits on the sink counter. She watches me intently as I scrub my hands.

When it is time for me to leave, Nisha walks me to the front entrance, gives me a firm embrace, and a flash of her endearing metallic smile. "I love you!" she says and then waves me goodbye, promising to keep in touch.

Desino Cancer Hospital

They [private hospitals] are no better. A doctor has total and complete control over what happens to a patient, you are completely at the doctor's mercy. Your test results may or may not be accurate, you may or may not get treatment. You have to beg for it, even people who have money.

Kate, SICH volunteer

Because it is a corporate hospital, there is no chance of shouting on patients. Here [SICH], we can take that privilege because it is a government institute! In private hospitals we cannot shout because people are paying; the hospital supervisors won't let us shout on patients.

Sister Deepa, general ward nurse

Desino Hospital is a new, private hospital dedicated exclusively to cancer care in arguably the poshest area of the city. The name strikes me as a little odd for the name of a cancer hospital, *desino* being Latin for end. The lobby is rather cramped and crowded, similar to Triumph Cancer Center; however, the atmosphere is much calmer, and it's also significantly cleaner. Notices about patient privacy are posted prominently in the hallway.

I meet with Dr. Pavan, medical oncologist and friend of Dr. Rashi's. "Rashi never calls and asks for anything, so this must be really important," he says. "How can I help you?" He is extremely kind and I explain my research briefly. "I'm spending most of my time at South Indian Cancer Hospital," I say, "but I thought it would be helpful for me to see a private cancer hospital, and how the nurses work here."

"Certainly," he offers. "Let me call Sister Anna, she's the nursing superintendent for the hospital. I'm sure she can help you."

"And what will you do for lunch?" Dr. Pavan asks, concerned. I tell him not to worry, I ate a late breakfast and I live close by.

Sister Anna enters Dr. Pavan's office wearing a white uniform with a blue smock and a paper mask tied tightly around her face. She has a small white cap on top her head. She looks far too young to be a nursing superintendent, but it turns out she has been a nurse for almost 14 years. Right away, Desino has the feel of an American hospital in the way that Triumph Cancer Center and SICH do not. It is not just that the facility is shiny and new, it's that it is busy, but with a calmness and efficiency to the busyness that I have not witnessed elsewhere.

Anna worked overseas in London before being recruited to Desino Hospital when it opened two years ago. On our tour, she proudly shows me the 11-bed surgical ICU and tells me a pediatric ward and medical ICU will be opening soon. The nurse-to-patient ratio is much better here: one nurse to four or five patients for all shifts, and in the ICU, it's one nurse to one or two patients, depending on how sick the patient is. Nurses have regular staff meetings and professional development training, and the hospital tracks certain aspects of quality control in the ubiquitous ledgers—things like medication errors, needlesticks, and the amount of time that elapses between when a patient arrives and when they see a nurse or doctor. But it's unclear who reviews all of this information, and even less clear what they do with it. Unlike SICH, family attendants are not required for a patient to get treatment. In fact, only one attendant is allowed per patient, and they are definitely not allowed to sleep in the hallway.

A financial counselor explains that about 70% of the patients who come to Desino pay cash; the hospital does not accept MHS patients. The remaining patients are credit patients, meaning that they have some sort of employee or insurance plan that pays a portion of their bill. I ask him if he is able to show me the list of prices for certain procedures or medications. He tells me he cannot give me such a list, as it is so variable based on the treatments ordered, but he does show me a red and white binder. In it are loose-leaf papers which list the cost of certain items: 24 hours in a "general ward," which is like an infirmary—cubbies divided by white curtains—costs 1,200 rupees ($17 USD). A deluxe private room runs upwards of 4,000 rupees ($58 USD) per day. A bed in the surgical ICU is 4,600 rupees ($66 USD)—almost twice that of Triumph Cancer Hospital.

The financial counselor laughs when I ask him what a typical hospital bill may be, but to humor me, he pulls up a spreadsheet on his computer screen that lists all of the patients, pending bills, and outstanding balances. I quickly scan the computer screen—the highest I see is about 75,000 rupees ($1,090 USD). "We collect a deposit up front," he explains, "and then daily collect some of the outstanding balance." He explains that sometimes things get more complicated when a patient needs unexpected care and the bills escalate, and the family is not prepared. I notice that blood tests, like to check a potassium level, cost more if you are staying in a deluxe room than in a standard wardroom.

We meet with the head pharmacist who assures me that immediate release morphine tablets and injectable morphine are available at Desino, although it seems that fentanyl patches are more commonly prescribed. "Most commonly we give Tramadol or Voveran for pain on the wards, this controls pain well," Anna tells me. "We only use morphine for when the prognosis is not good." She says she certainly has witnessed patients in pain and has given injectable morphine a few times on the ward but cannot be more specific.

Anna takes me all over the hospital—they have an MRI machine and even a PET scanner, and a large radiation department. I notice another big difference too—not only are things quieter and more orderly, but it is cooler—the entire building has air conditioning.

As nursing superintendent, Anna is actively involved in the hiring of new nurses. I'm curious if private hospitals have a more clearly outlined job description for nurses, so I ask if one exists and if she may able to share it with me. I was never able to get one from Triumph hospital, but Desino, as an even more Westernized hospital, perhaps has one. But Anna looks a little confused.

"Is there a document, maybe a letter, that describes the role of the nurse? What they are expected to do for their job?" I try to clarify.

Anna nods. "Human resources I think has that." She picks up the phone in her office, makes a hushed call. "They are free now, they have had their lunch."

We walk back upstairs to the human resources department. Four men are crowded in a room filled with folders and computers. The Manager of Human Resources sits with his back to everyone, hunched over a tiffin of rice and curries. The assistant manager listens to my story and my request for a copy of the job description of a nurse, but he is clearly concerned about interrupting his boss's lunch. He talks in hushed tones. "Madam, please sit. A few minutes, please." He directs Anna and me to chairs in an adjacent room. I start to feel guilty, as this is becoming a much bigger production than I intended, and I am certain Anna has other things to do.

A little later, the assistant manager returns. He is carrying a small glossy purple booklet. It is the employee handbook. He lets me look it over; it looks fairly generic but there is an entire section called "Job Descriptions" which says an employee will be given one for their specific position. I point to it. "Is it possible for me to get a copy of this, the job description for a nurse?" He and Anna then launch into a tangential and detailed conversation about nurses being on three-month probation when they come, the references they check, the entire hiring process, the difference between in-charge nurses and staff nurses.

"Well," I find my break, "I'd love to see a job description for a staff nurse if you are able to share it." He looks uncomfortable and begins telling me about the test nurses are required to take before they are allowed to work at Desino. Anna already showed me a copy of this document: 25 rather odd and concrete questions that one could argue tell you little about the competence of a nurse,[7] questions such as: "*What is the medical term for cancer?*" and "*How many types of insulin are there?*" But I am encouraged that the test

---

7   The questions for Desino Pre-Employment Exam for Nurses [all sic]: (1) What is the Normal range of Vital Signs?; (2) List out few emergency drugs?; (3) What are the Colors & Gauges of IV Cannula?; (4) What are the important observations during emergency?; (5) What is medical term for cancer?; (6) How frequent a cannula to be changed?; (7) What is the time duration for changing a urinary catheter?; (8)How many types of insulin?; (9) What one is long acting insulin & which one is short acting insulin?; (10) What are the types of I/V fluids?; (11) What is the time duration for changing a nasogastric tube?; (12) What is UTI?; (13) What is URTI?; (14) What is another name for BP apparatus?; (15) What are the medicines used for steam inhalation?; (16) What are the nursing measures for rise in temperature?; (17) How will you assess the pain of a patient?; (18) How will you assess dehydration?; (19) What is the minimum time duration for a blood transfusion?; (20) What you will do if a patient has blood transfusion reaction?; (21) What is CPR?; (22) What is the rate of compressions and rescue breaths in CPR?; (23) How will you check the position of a nasogastric tube?; (24) What is BMT?; (25) What are the job responsibilities of a nurse?

includes at least one question about how to assess pain, and another, the final question, that asks, "*What are the job responsibilities of a nurse?*"

Anna explains that a potential new hire nurse has to get at least 15 questions correct—a 60%. I seize on the last question, perhaps too enthusiastically, and tell Anna that that is exactly what I am interested in knowing: does she know how nurses typically answer this question about their job responsibilities?

"Oh yes, they'll just write 'to take care of patients' or 'give nursing care,' something like this," she says. "Oh," I say, disappointed.

I slide the glossy booklet across the desk back to the assistant Human Resources manager. I decide to try one last time. "Do you think it is possible to see a copy of the job description for a nurse?" He looks at Anna and then back to me.

"Well, it is not really written down," he finally admits. "It is more oral," he explains. "From the in-charge, then told to the nurse."

"That's interesting. Why is it oral?" I ask.

"Well, madam, if it is written down, then if the nurse is asked to do something not in that written document, she will not do."

Pillalu

There's this mentality in India that if you have less, you'll do more. Or if you don't have it, you'll find another way to do it. Like if you don't have garbage cans then there won't be garbage…There was an event where someone threw some garbage out of the ward on to the street. And it was caught and someone complained. So, I asked, 'where are the garbage cans?' And I was told the garbage cans had been removed, because then there wouldn't be any garbage; people would have to find another way to dispose of their trash. Apparently, the garbage area was so messy and dirty they just decided to get rid of the bins entirely…A Western mentality would be, 'well, maybe we need more garbage cans.' But the Indian mentality, is, 'if you don't have it, then you won't need it, or 'if you have less, you'll figure out a way to make it work.' I don't know where that comes from, but it's rampant.

Jennifer, SICH volunteer

A fragrant, late spring breeze fills my bedroom, billowing the blue flowered curtains. My simple room is modest, but I never get tired of the view: the swaying palm trees, the bright white stucco, orderly joint family home abutting against our apartment building with the multitude of healthy green potted plants neatly lining the balconies of different family units; the Spanish tile of the roof below, the mosque in the background, the tangle of satellite towers and dishes further in the distance, like a small city of white suction cups on tall metal toothpicks. It's so hot now that I don't even have to turn on the geyser for warm water to bathe. It gushes out hotter than warm, all on its own.

When I leave for the hospital, Ruma and Joanie are still fast asleep in their shared bed, like batteries—head to toe, toe to head. I am continually amazed at how I find people sleeping in India, in the most improbable of places and positions, and so soundly: women dozing on the backs of motorbikes in hot, honking, impossibly congested traffic; babies fast asleep on crowded, jolting, stifling buses; men snoring alongside busy thoroughfares.

Pillalu is the massive women and children's government hospital that looms almost menacingly next to SICH. It is a much more well-known hospital than SICH, so much so that each day it is the landmark I give to the autorickshaw driver. I have been dreading observing at Pillalu because I have heard multiple disturbing stories about what it is like inside, and I have prepared myself for the worst. Along the road, leading up to the hospital, hundreds of people crowd around the counters of small medical shops, push toward chaat (snack) carts splattering and steaming with crispy dosas, soft idlys, and spicy vadas, and haggle with merchants selling a variety of brightly colored plastic toys. Men squat alongside roadside barbers for a morning shave, stray dogs with spear-like ribs nudge and poke in piles of trash, and mothers holding infants and toddlers brave the on-coming and constant mad flow of erratically driven motorbikes, autorickshaws, and chauffeured cars with equanimity. By the entrance to the main lobby, in a small sliver of shade, I watch a steady stream of people approach the hospital entrance. They share the same look as the patients who come to SICH: barefoot, weathered, exhausted.

A security guard carrying a wooden stick stops most of them, refusing to let them pass. Some produce pieces of paper, ostensibly proof they are allowed to enter; others argue for a few minutes and are ultimately allowed to proceed; others are simply turned away with little discussion. Some people, determined not to be deterred, try a second time; they walk away, wait a few minutes, and then when the guard is distracted make a run for the front door. One elderly woman wearing a green sari and carrying two heavy plastic bags, tries this tactic, but is caught by the security guard who grabs her upper arm and forcefully pushes her away. Another younger woman's sneak attack is thwarted when the security guard grabs the bun in her hair and physically drags her away from the hospital entrance. I am allowed to enter without question.[8]

The Emergency Service Room (ESR) is a small, nine-bed triage unit where pediatric patients are evaluated and stabilized before either being formally admitted to another ward or discharged. The staffing is three to four nurses on days, two on evenings, and a luxurious four on nights. I am so surprised by the night staffing, I clarify it twice: apparently, like most Emergency Departments, all hell can break loose at 2 am. I am greeted warmly by the head nurse and senior nurse and a group of enthusiastic nursing students. The students seem a bit unanchored; they do not have specific patient assignments, designated nurse preceptors, or a clinical instructor nearby. I ask them why they decided to become nurses.

"To serve others!" some chorus. "It is nice to help people!" one calls out. "My sister is a nurse!" another volunteers. "To give blessings to others," one says flatly. Many are from the state of Kerala.

The head nurse calls for the security guard posted outside the ESR while the physicians make rounds. "They can only have one family member present for rounds, to hear the information," the charge nurse explains. I try to imagine how difficult that must be for parents, knowing how helpful it can be to have an extra set of ears to process complex and stressful information.

Suddenly, the mother of an infant starts to wail; her son has stopped breathing. A team of doctors and nurses quickly gathers around the child's bed and they attempt to resuscitate the baby, unsuccessfully, for over 20 minutes. The security guard also is there: he positions himself solidly between the parents and their dying child.

* * *

---

8   Yet another example of how my status as a white foreigner provided unfair and unearned privilege in terms of access to space and individuals.

The ESR is in the newer building of Pillalu; the older portion of the hospital stretches out across the street. I am told the hospital—the only maternal and pediatric government hospital in the state—is sanctioned for 400–500 beds, but the current census is over 1,000 patients. I believe it; people are everywhere, camped out in the concrete courtyard of the hospital in the unrelenting sun, lining the cramped corridors, piling up along the stairwell, squatting in every conceivable corner.

In the main hallways, garbage is piled in dark corners and the public bathroom swims under a few inches of brown murky water with floating bits of trash. The smell of urine and unwashed bodies is stronger here, but I've also noticed it becoming stronger at SICH as the daily temperature climbs. Some of the wards are disturbingly cramped and dirty, while others are remarkably clean.

"Come! You must see the twins!" two of the nursing students cry and grab me with their tiny hands. They lead me through a convoluted maze of corridors to a special newborn unit. The gruff nursing supervisor is not pleased I am there and reprimands the students sharply. She says something to the students about me going into the room alone.

"Go, go!" they say.

"It's okay? I…"

They swing open the door and push me, solo, into a small room. At first, I think there has been some mistake as I don't see anyone, or anything. Then, abruptly, an unusual shape pops up from the bed. I see two girls with shaved dark hair wearing pink dresses. But the head is all wrong; it is entirely too large and elongated. It takes me a bit to process what I am seeing and then I understand—they are conjoined twins, fused at the occiput (back of the skull). They adeptly clamor over the rails of their shared bed and come toward me, locked in a painful looking backbend, twisting and twirling so each can get a good look at me.

My shock is quickly followed by anger. No wonder the nursing supervisor was upset.

I stay for a few awkward minutes. The girls seem smart; they understand English and tell me they are nine years old.

When I exit their room, I see the nursing supervisor. The students have disappeared.

"That is very, very sad," I say. The nurse tells me the girls have lived most of their life in this small room at Pillalu, abandoned by their parents.

"Sometimes the media will come, journalists," the nurse says sadly. "They take pictures. And worse." She pauses. "I don't want them to feel like an exhibition." She tells me they were unable to be surgically separated at birth because one would die.

"Do they have to stay confined in this room?" I ask.

"Yes, mostly, especially during the day. If they come out, they will be a spectacle. Everyone staring. But in the evenings and at night, when it is quieter, they come out here," she gestures in the hallway, "and they walk around a bit."

***

The next day, I return to see the twins, this time with a few toys—some bubbles, a big colorful picture book, and a magic marker craft set. The gruff nurse supervisor seems happier to see me this time, perhaps convinced I am not there to ridicule or harass the children. The girls are lying in their bed and when I enter they swing themselves out onto the floor in a highly coordinated, and clearly well-practiced, fluid motion. "See!" the nurse says proudly, "that is how they manage."

An ayah in the room with the girls sees the toys, shakes her head, and mutters, "waste" but the girls are delighted. They like the bubbles but have a hard time manipulating the wand, and the oversized picture book is a big hit, but they both want to look at it at the same time, which is physically impossible. I make a mental note to get a second one. They are happily drawing with the magic markers when the ayah abruptly begins to gather up the toys and lock them in a metal cabinet in the corner of the room. It's the same scenario I have witnessed before: supplies given, then mysteriously sequestered away.

This time I intervene. "No," I say firmly, "we are keeping these out so they can play with them." The ayah doesn't argue when I place them back on the bed.

***

One of the general pediatric wards, a 16-bed unit, with five empty beds, is oddly quiet. Three nursing students sit together, looking incredibly bored while two staff nurses oversee the changing out of mattresses, which is a dusty task. It's not readily apparent to me which mattresses are new and which are being replaced. A physician sits at a front table, a green cloth surgical mask tied tightly around his face, assessing children brought in by parents.

I ask the students if they are enjoying their clinical rotation at Pillalu and they are quiet.

"This is a government hospital, mandatory rotation," one finally says, with an air of resignation.

The staff nurses are both very friendly and have had many years of government service at Pillalu. They are interested in my research and I ask them a few questions about pain control in the hospital.

"Do you ever give morphine?" I ask.

They shake their heads: no. They do not give morphine.

"Do you think that pain is controlled well here, in general?" I ask. Both nurses shake their heads. One becomes visibly distressed, on the brink of tears.

"No, no," she says. "And that is very sad because the first duty of the nurse is to control pain."

***

"We are all caught in the loop, here in India," Joanie says, gathering up a load of laundry to put in the washer and making a circular motion with her index finger in the air. She is angry with Fathima who hasn't shown up for three nights in a row to cook and apparently is not answering her phone.

"And I gave her 3,000 rupees for her medicine. What to do with these people?" she asks beseechingly. "They are so unreliable! And I'm the only one who can misbehave and yell at them. You can't talk to them," she says referring to my abysmal Hindi, "and Ruma's always still at the office." She sighs dejectedly. "And wait until I tell you about this, Virginia, you'll be mad and want to puke," Joanie says walking into the kitchen. She holds up a plastic bin of grains. "Bugs! She's been cooking with grains infested with bugs!"

"Really?" I ask skeptically.

"And we told her the food wasn't tasting right!" Joanie says, incensed. She is so passionate, shaking the container of rice up and down that I start to laugh, I can't help myself.

"It's not funny, Virginia!" Joanie admonishes.

I get control of myself. "How did you figure that out?" I have learned to ask for specifics.

"Well, Ruma was cooking last night, I didn't feel well, I had a migraine, and she saw it."

"Hmm," I say noncommittal.

"And we've *got* to keep her from putting the vessels in the sink!" she calls out from the kitchen. "I told Fathima don't make a mess if you can't clean it up!"

Fathima returns the following evening and serves us chai, and even spoons a sample of what she is cooking for dinner into Joanie's eager mouth, like a baby bird. It's hard to reconcile this intimate gesture with the harsh words Joanie had for her yesterday. I wonder at the perverse pleasure that seems to come from both criticizing and complimenting maids, cooks, drivers. It's a strange and foreign equation to me: as if occasional benevolence has a price and intermittent kindness gives the right to be cruel.

* * *

The power cuts around 2 am and I wake up hot and sweaty. The ceiling fans are still and the apartment is stifling, stagnant. Even Ruma and Joanie can't sleep and there is murmured restlessness.

When I return from the hospital later in the afternoon, the power is still out. Joanie greets me at the front door.

"Virginia! Still no lights," she sighs. "It's depressing."

"Has it been out all day?"

"Yes, this is what happens. During this season, all this load shedding."[9] She paces around in her pajamas, her hair pulled up in a sloppy ponytail, her round moonlike face shiny with perspiration.

---

9 "Load shedding" is an energy conversing strategy to unburden an overly stressed electrical grid that involves cutting power on a rolling basis to different sections of the grid. However,

"It's like living in a primitive land." She pauses. "Although that would probably be better, because we'd be in a cave and it would be cooler!" We both laugh. She places her palms on the framed picture of the goddess Lakshmi that hangs outside my bedroom door. "Spare us the horror tonight! Please!" she implores, appealing to the deity. "I couldn't sleep all night, I am so irritable," Joanie admits. "I called my Mom at 5 am, cried and sobbed to her about everything and then I finally fell asleep!"

I decide I better eat my yogurt before it all goes bad in the fridge, which is only operational for a few hours a day now.

"How are you feeling?" I ask Joanie, as I spoon out the pink strawberry yogurt from the plastic container. She has not been feeling well the past few days.

"My chest is still really congested," she says, and I can hear it in her raspy, froggy voice.

"What antibiotics did they give you?" I ask. She shakes out an assortment of tablets from a small white paper bag. Some are antibiotic tablets, along with an antacid, lactobacillus (a probiotic to maintain "good" gut bacteria), and a decongestant. I hold up the Augmentin, the antibiotic, pills. "Here, these are the really important ones," I say.

"These are supposed to make me better?" she asks.

"Yes, but you need to take all of them even if you start feeling better."

"Oh, I hate going to the doctor," Joanie says. "They are so habituated to seeing ill people, they have no empathy, no empathy at all Virginia. The woman at the counter says, 'give me 300 rupees and sit over there.' They just don't care."

"Why is that?" I ask, intrigued. "And I'm sure you went to a nice place," I add, knowing Joanie most likely went to a private clinic and not a government facility.

"Oh yes! We drove so far away, too far for me to even go to a follow-up. Shilpa took me there. But it doesn't matter. That's just how it is here; people are so used to seeing these things. Imagine if I were someone who was really sick, 'here pay 3,000 rupees and then go figure out how to get yourself admitted to the hospital!' Ahh, going to the doctor makes me feel *exponentially* more sick! It's true Virginia, I just cannot bear it," she says emphatically, and falls back on to her bed.[10]

I was told by one local that this is not actually true, and power outages were not due to load shedding. His theory was that the power company simply turns off the power until people are entirely frustrated and agree to pay more for their electricity, and that they do this routinely each summer as the temperature rises.

10 In this instance, Joanie's economic status did not seem to result in higher quality or more compassionate care. I found it interesting that Joanie specifically mentions a lack of empathy, and attributes it to desensitization of clinicians and acknowledges that this lack of empathy can contribute to patients feeling even worse. I did not accompany Joanie to the clinic and thus did not directly observe the interactions between her and the clinical staff, but her perception that empathy was lacking, regardless of money expended, seems noteworthy and provides further evidence of the complex contexts that can influence the delivery of patient care.

References

Kramer, S. (2021). Pew Research Center, Religious demography of Indian States and Territories. Available at: https://www.pewresearch.org/religion/2021/09/21/religious-demography-of-indian-states-and-territories/

U.S. Office of Personnel Management. Patients' Bill of Rights. (2023). Available at: https://www.opm.gov/healthcare-insurance/healthcare/reference-materials/bill-of-rights/

PART V
Conclusions

9   How Life Shines Through

There's no one dealing with the big, underlying issues. You see how filthy this place is, how dirty the corridors are. It's unhygienic, but it's not really about how often the floors are washed. Family members have nowhere to stay, no-where to sleep. They do the best they can, but there is nowhere to wash their hands. They use the little bit of water in the drainpipes. The government needs to address the underlying problem, and no one is doing that. The social format needs to change.

Dr. Varun, volunteer oncologist

The population of stray cats has exploded in the apartment building ga-rage. They are scrawny and wiry and poke around for morsels of sustenance amidst the ever-changing collection of refuse and recycling that accumulates and then disappears in the strange subterranean junkyard.

Before I left for a palliative care conference in Nepal, I fed them a can of tuna and a can of sardines donated by Paul. The day I did it, Hasan, the watchman's son, saw me struggling to open the lid of sardines and quickly provided a can opener and then watched in fascination as I spread the food on the side stairwell for the meowing crowd of skinny and hungry cats. They devoured the food in seconds.

Now, as I make my way downstairs in the early morning and see the kit-tens weaving among the piles of trash, looking up at me expectantly, the simple gesture seems terribly misguided, cruel even. I won't be here to feed the cats every day, and even if I was—I don't know where to get more tuna or sardines easily. Did I torment the kittens by giving them one good meal that I cannot provide again in any sustainable way? And let's say I could fig-ure out some way to feed them regularly, does that make sense? What if I do feed them tuna every day and they miraculously become bigger and healthy? I have no way to spay or neuter them, so they will continue to multiply, and more cats will emerge that run the risk of being malnourished and weak and neglected. Have I contributed to the problem by trying to "help?"

A feeling of absolute hopelessness washes over me as the kittens rub against my legs, meowing persistently and loudly. I want to build them a

DOI: 10.4324/9781003413158-15

shelter, set up permanent feeding stations, fund a team of veterinarians to establish mobile spay and neuter clinics, conduct educational campaigns with residents about responsible and ethical pet ownership. But how would I even begin to go about this? Would people care? Would anyone support me? How long would it take, and how many animals would suffer in the meantime?

I take a deep breath, exhausted before the day has even begun. I step around and over the kittens and make my way down to the end of the lane where I will catch the next auto that whisks me away to the hospital, where I know immensely larger and more complex challenges await, along with the struggle of knowing how to help.

* * *

It's impossible to move quickly and the hospital feels like the inside of an oven. It is really, really hot. I sit on the white plastic chair in the palliative care clinic, my thighs sweating through the cream-colored leggings I am wearing under my turquoise kurta. I've given up trying to coordinate colorful outfits as the temperature climbs. The heat makes it annoying to manage a dupatta, and I don't want to wear extra jewelry.

I notice the clinic is noticeably quiet and less crowded.

"This is very common. It's too difficult to make the journey in the heat, people get too tired, so they don't come," Pradeep explains. Abhipsa, the other palliative care nurse on duty today, doodles on a notebook, swirly, flowery designs she makes with a freshly sharpened pencil. Everyone looks wilted.

Abhipsa and Pradeep are interested in the conference I attended in Kathmandu about expanding palliative care services in Nepal. I tell them about the idea of developing a program where nurses in Nepal could prescribe and dispense morphine more independently.

"The idea is to help give access to morphine to people who live far away from hospitals, or cannot get to a pharmacy, or when a doctor is not available," I say. "Like with the rural outreach program that you run. Do you think something like that would work here?" I ask.

"No, that would never work here," Pradeep says quickly, without hesitation.

"Why not?" I ask, curious.

"Too many problems. If something goes wrong, it would be on our heads," he says. "They would want large prescriptions, for more than 10 days and then what if they misuse the tablets? That would be our fault."

He doesn't even want to entertain the idea.

* * *

Jasmine meets me in a small conference room that after weeks of writing and obtaining the appropriate signed and stamped letters, I finally have official permission to use for my remaining interviews. She shows me the schedule she has typed up to satisfy Suresh, the guardian of the room, whom I have privately nicknamed Napoleon. He is a short, stocky man with no sense of humor who has made accessing the room exponentially more complicated and frustrating, insisting on additional approvals, signatures, and assurances before unlocking the room each and every time. It got a little better, but not much, after I was advised to pay him additional money "for his trouble," which I reluctantly did.

"See, here, madam," Jasmine says pointing to the paper, "Here, I have said you will use the room from 10 am to 3 pm, even though you may only need it 11 am to 2 pm. Better this way," she says conspiratorially. We sit down at the table, and I provide some updates about the project. I show her on my Arizona Highway calendar the target date I hope to be finished with all the interviews. She is intrigued by the glossy photos of Arizona.

"This is where you live?" she asks, pointing to May, a photo of Dominguez Butte at Lake Powell.

"No, more like here," I flip forward to July which shows a rainbow arching over the Tortolita Mountains dotted with saguaro cacti. I show her more iconic pictures of saguaro cacti and she is intrigued by the details of these curious plants: that it takes about 50 years for them to grow one foot, and that they only grow in a very special and unique part of the world.

"Just like you are special!" she laughs. She laughs even harder when I tell her they are a protected species, and if they must be uprooted, they have to be cared for in a special "cactus orphanage," or nursery, until they can be replanted.

"Not like India," she says moving her hand in a fast sideways motion. "Chop, chop, chop, we just tear it all down."

"Well, we used to do that, and that's why they are protected now."

"It wouldn't matter here, we would still chop them down," she says.

I tell her that the light in Arizona is beautiful, and that people come to paint and photograph the area at different times of the day and year to try to capture the fleeting beauty.

"I used to paint," she says suddenly.

"I didn't know that. I can see how you would be an excellent artist, you have a gift for color, for beauty," I say, motioning to her perfectly coordinated amber salwar kameez with a multicolored dupatta and matching bangles. She smiles.

"Yes, before I was married. Watercolors, oils. So many paintings. Now, no time."

I think how the cultural expectations and duties of marriage and motherhood have constrained Jasmine, how if she had the opportunity to truly spread her wings and fly what she could do. She speaks English, Hindi, and the local dialect fluently. She is socially sophisticated, bright, and curious.

"There were all my paintings, after I got married, they were in my parent's house, but they all were destroyed, all lost."

"Oh no, what happened?" I ask.

"They moved. They didn't think about all the paintings hanging up, there was so much dirt and dust…" her voice trails off. I think about all of her creative expression lost forever because of others' carelessness, haste, or ignorance.

"That's terrible, to lose all of your creative work, I'm so sorry," I say. She nods, sadly.

"Maybe when your children are a bit older, you'll have more time to paint again?" I offer feebly.

"Maybe," she says. She does not sound convinced.

"When did you get married?" I ask.

"Ah, that is a very long story," she says. "I got married when I was 16." Jasmine goes on to tell me how she was forced to marry her first cousin.

"I said no, but my father didn't speak to me for ten days. There was *so* much pressure from my mother-in-law, my father's sister. She is old and there is no one to take care of her. My husband is an only child," she says. "It happened so fast, just like this, check, check, check." She ticks imaginary boxes in the air.

"I wanted to study more, and they promised after I got married I could keep studying. But that didn't happen. I cried for two or three years. My life closed then."

She is silent and looks out the window.

* * *

I want to check in with Sister Deepa before her presentation today, and I find her on Male Ward I with three other nurses in the break room, eating.

"Hello, Sisters! I'm sorry to disturb you," I say, pushing open the break room door.

They smile and gesture for me to enter. "Virginia, just a little, come eat," they say. I squeeze in around the small table. Sister Chaaya hands me a tiffin lid heaped with rice and curd and tops it with an idly and delicious mint, tomato, and coriander curry. A young girl wearing a pink T-shirt and braids sits on the bed propped against the break room wall, scooping rice into her mouth.

"This is my daughter!" Deepa says proudly.

"Ahh, did she come to hear your class?" I ask.

"Yes," says Deepa again, proudly. "She has summer vacation from school for a few days."

I realize what a big deal this is, for Deepa to teach a class to her peers. In 2003, Deepa traveled to Mumbai for a special training course about breast cancer and postoperative care. Apparently, the hospital nominated her for the program, but she had to foot the entire bill for attending the conference. She found the training very helpful and had hoped to come back and teach her colleagues what she learned but was not given the necessary support by hospital leadership to do this. When she shared this with me, I promised her I would try to make it happen.

But it wasn't easy.

When I first proposed the idea—that Deepa teach a class to the nurses—I was told she could not get permission to reserve the auditorium: "She is a simple staff nurse, not Bachelor's, not a head nurse. She must teach with you."

"Okay," I had said, more familiar now with the bureaucratic hurdles and process. I wrote a letter requesting permission for a jointly taught nursing class, had it signed by Dr. Madhu, then Jasmine helped me get it signed and stamped by the Director—a two-day process—then took it back to the Nursing Superintendent for her final approval and signature—another two days—then made a copy of the document and took it to Suresh to reserve the auditorium, who was skeptical and wanted more documentation that the class had truly been approved by the Director before he would finally book the auditorium.

"You are not hungry?" Sister Pooja asks, looking at me with concern when she sees my tiffin plate is not yet empty. I explain that the heat has reduced my appetite. They all nod in understanding.

"Are you married?" Pooja asks.

"Not yet. I have to work on that when I get back home," I say laughing.

"That's why you don't have any problems!" Pooja says. "Everytime I look at you, I wonder, how are you smiling all the time? How are you always active?" Pooja leans in closely, scrutinizing my face for the answer. "What are you eating?"

"What am I eating?" I repeat, smiling.

"Ah!"

"Well, right now, lots and lots of mangoes!" They are in season now, stacked in golden pyramids at every street corner.

"Only mangoes?" they all laugh.

"Right now, many, many mangoes. They are delicious!"

After we have finished eating, it's time to get down to business and Deepa pulls out multiple pages of handwritten notes stapled together. She asks me to review the information and I do; it is extremely complete and well organized. "This is excellent," I say, and I mean it. "You will do a great job. I'm so happy you are presenting today!"

As I am leaving, Sister Chaaya stops me and gently slides the pink bangles off of my left wrist. She shuffles them in her hand and reorders them—skinny, fat, skinny—and then slides them back on to my wrist and pats my arm with a warm smile.

***

Deepa's presentation is scheduled to begin at 12:30 pm, but by now I know the drill and don't panic even when 1:15 rolls around. The Nursing

Superintendent is there, sitting in the front row of the metal black chairs. Her small, elfin feet dangle childlike a few inches above the auditorium floor, her white stockings bunched up slightly around the ankles. With her wizened face and kind expression, she looks like a smiling walnut.

If Deepa is nervous, it is not obvious. She does a fantastic job and makes it a point to talk specifically about common sexuality concerns of female cancer patients, which I was not expecting. She surprises me again at the end of her presentation by leading us through a ten-minute breathing and exercise session, which is a little bit yoga, a little bit range of motion, a little bit meditation. We start by wiggling our eyebrows. We hold our arms out by our sides and move our eyeballs back and forth. We do a series of deep knee bends and gyrate our hips like we have Hula-Hoops. The nurses eat it up.

Any doubts I had about the Nursing Superintendent's receptivity to Deepa teaching the class dissipate when she is the first to start clapping enthusiastically, saying, "This is her first time!" Afterwards, she pinches my cheek and presses two pieces of candy into my palm.

"Was my talk good?" Deepa asks me shyly when we are cleaning up.

"Yes!" I say giving her a hug. "More than good! it was excellent. You are a very good teacher, your thoughts are well organized. And everyone really responded well to the mini yoga session."

"Yes, we need that. There is no time to exercise here, the sisters need this to release tension," Deepa says wisely.

"You did a very good thing today, giving her confidence like that," Esha, the translator, says to me later, privately. She came not to translate, but just to help; I get the feeling she is lonely at home. Esha smiles—I find her curiously tiny teeth with the large front gap completely endearing. "That is what will change the culture here."

***

I bring a batch of attendance certificates[1] to the hospital and ask Deepa to sign them.

"*Me* madam?" she asks doubtfully.

"Yes, yes. You taught the class, so you must sign the attendance certificates!" I say.

"Okay," she says, embarrassed, yet obviously pleased, taking the black pen in her hand.

One of the nurses on the ward hovers close by as Deepa signs and then returns her certificate. The nurse squeals with delight and clutches it to her chest. "This is my first certificate!"

---

1 After each class, formal certificates of attendance were distributed to the nurses, which were highly valued by attendees.

As Deepa signs her name in careful cursive at the bottom of each certificate, she turns to me and asks, "What is the process to reserve the auditorium for teaching a class?"

"Oh, I'm so glad you are interested in this!" I say enthusiastically. "I think it would be great if you teach more classes, and maybe some of the other nurses will want to teach too." I detail the entire process, realizing as I articulate it just how many steps are involved. Without help and support, I fear she won't be able to do it. After I leave will anyone help her reserve the auditorium? Arrange for snacks? Distribute certificates of attendance? I am saddened to think that this may be the last class Deepa teaches.

It's been almost nine months, but a nurse approaches me as I am talking to Deepa and asks the questions I hear in my sleep: "Had your breakfast?" "What did you eat?" "Where do you stay?" "You cook your own food?" "How much money did you make at your job in the U.S.?"

I try to answer patiently, because I know I won't be hearing these questions for much longer and in that strange way of nostalgia, I will miss them.

***

The heat hangs like a yoke. It is 108 degrees and everything feels hazy and slow. Everyone is desperate for rain.

I find Dr. Rama in the simulator viewing room in the basement of the hospital; I want to personally deliver a copy of the letter I am giving the Director that acknowledges her help during my fieldwork. The room is cool, one of the few air-conditioned places in the hospital. When I comment on the relief from the heat, Dr. Amit says laughing, "it's for the machines, not the people!"

A few inches behind the large glass window a woman lies on her back, the lower half of her body completely exposed, her legs spread apart, a urinary catheter emerging from the brown folds of her vagina. The machine, establishing a plan for her radiation treatment, swings around her pelvic area. The small viewing room is crammed full with eight people of mixed gender, and I get the feeling most of them do not have a patient-related reason to be in the room; they are, understandably, simply trying to escape the heat. It is hard to reconcile that in a society where contact between the sexes is strictly regulated, where males and females don't even kiss in Indian shows and movies, and where modesty is so highly valued, that no one seems particularly concerned that we are all staring straight at the woman's genitals.

***

It is my last official day in the hospital, and I have invited all of the nursing staff to a presentation of the preliminary findings from my research. I'm nervous about how it will be received.

Jasmine and Esha are there to help, as well as Sisters Deepa and Asha who volunteered to help organize snacks for the session: cool drinks and biscuits.

Jasmine opens the auditorium, twists the key in the huge padlock that bolts shut the door, and we go through the motions that have now become routine: turn on the computer, Esha will wipe the dust from the keyboard with her pinky finger and look dismayed, we will sweat and sweat until the air conditioner kicks in. The session, which is supposed to start at 1 pm, will start after 1:30 pm. I relax into the predictability of it all.

I am curious how the dynamics will play out today because it is the first time—to my knowledge—that the government nurses, pediatric nurses, and palliative care nurses have all come together, despite all always being invited to each class. There is some palpable tension as members of the different factions choose to self-segregate by the seats they select in the auditorium. Bharati from pediatrics and Daya from palliative care sit together off to one side, giggling like schoolgirls behind pieces of paper they hold in front of their faces.

Esha translates and I discuss my observations—even some of the more delicate ones—about handwashing, shouting at patients, wards left unattended. The 40 nurses that have gathered listen, silent and stone-faced. Occasionally, I see confirmatory nods. No one looks particularly upset or surprised by anything I've said.

"Please tell me what you think," I ask the nurses after I have finished. "Did I make mistakes? Does this sound right to you?"

The nurses sit quietly, politely, smiling, but no one says anything. I try again.

"It's very important that I understood everything properly. I may have made mistakes. You don't have to say it is okay to be nice! You can tell me the truth!" They titter and laugh, but still nothing.

I try again. "Do you agree with what I said? Does it sound right?" A few head nods. Daya raises her hand. She says that I was accurate in saying that there are three distinct groups of nurses. Another nurse chimes in and says that, yes, they really want better facilities, especially to mix chemotherapy. Daya adds that when a nurse is absent, it has a big impact because of the short staffing and that this is particularly hard on head nurses.

"Anything else?" I probe. Silence. But it doesn't appear to be an angry silence.

"Did anything I say make you mad? Angry at me?" I ask.

More tittering and laughter. "No, no!" they chorus and shake their heads.

"Is there anything I'm missing?" Some more laughter and rapid conversations in Hindi.

"You! We'll miss you!" one of the nurses from the ICU says.

"Thank you! That is very kind," I say. "Anything else I'm missing?"

"A husband!" they call out. I burst out laughing and blush, which makes them laugh even harder.

"How did you feel here? What do you think of South Indian Cancer Hospital nurses?" they ask, looking at me intensely.

"You were very kind to me, always feeding me! I'll miss you," I say. "Also—I think you have a very difficult job," I say slowly, working to choose my words carefully. "You see many patients each day who are very, very sick. I think you should consider meeting each month, rotate who gives a small talk to teach each other about a topic of interest, be able to support each other."

More nodding. "Almost all of you are very worried about exposure to chemotherapy, and I think this is a serious issue that needs to be addressed so it can change."

"How?" Sister Asha asks.

"Well, I don't think that's my place to necessarily say *how* it changes, because you know the system best. But I think it can change."

"We can't do anything, we are government nurses only!" another nurse says.

"I disagree," I say. "I think you are a powerful group of nurses. You run the hospital! You have more power than you realize, and I think if you come together you can find creative solutions."

The Nursing Superintendent is quiet, and at first I fear I have offended her. But then she smiles and leaps up to present me with a lovely gift from the nursing staff, a metallic replica of City Center encased in plastic which lights up with the turn of a switch. A flurry of picture taking ensues; the nurses crowd around, hugging me, kissing me, shaking my hand.

"When are you coming back?" they ask. "When will you be back?"

"Hopefully soon," I say.

"You are most welcome to come back any time," Agnes says solemnly, holding my hand.

"We love you!" one of the head nurses tells me as she slides two studded golden bangles on to both my right and left wrist.

"Thank you, thank you, you are very kind!" I say, overwhelmed by this spontaneous and unexpected outpouring of affection.

Deepa discreetly presses a beaded necklace into my hand. "For you," she says and hugs me. Sister Meena waits until the very end, after everyone has left and she begins to cry.

"After so many years, no one has come. And you come, and we learn so much from you. You are so kind, so soft. We are very rough!" she says.

"No, I don't think so," I counter gently, touching her shoulder.

"No, we are! But you taught us how to behave, how to do things," she says. "I'll miss you, madam," she says and leans her head against my shoulder.

My heart aches for these nurses, and for all of their frustrations, disappointments, challenges. But with Meena's head resting gently on my shoulder, it all evaporates and is forgotten, at least for a brief moment.

***

Hameeda's curly, dense hair is clipped back by a sparkly purple plastic barrette in the shape of a ribbon. She has lost weight. Marcus and I are there to help take Hameeda outside, one of her few requests—besides fried chicken. I notice that her stuffed animal Pinky has been joined by another, larger, pink stuffed bear, which she has named, curiously, Bull.

Unfortunately, the hospice wheelchair is a decrepit piece of equipment with a missing right leg, requiring Hameeda to wedge her paralyzed and swollen extremity precariously against the blue leather strap that connects the side panels of the wheelchair to prevent it from dragging on the ground. There is nowhere to easily hang her urine collection bag, but undeterred and determined, Hameeda ties it to the arm of the wheelchair. Vasudha, the fearless social worker from the hospital, arrives with a friend to provide extra manpower in case we need help moving Hameeda. We are quite the entourage—me, Marcus, Vasudha, and her friend—all accompanying Hameeda out in her wheelchair stroll. It is not easy going. The gravel road out of the hospice is bumpy and full of potholes, and despite Marcus's careful and steady navigation, I watch Hameeda's paralyzed leg like a hawk, fearing it will slip off the blue leather strap and get inadvertently caught in the wheel. As we approach the main road, Marcus hits a particularly bad divot, and the other leg falls off the wheelchair with a clatter. None of us can fix it, so Vasudha and I manage to reposition Hameeda's swollen feet so they rest awkwardly on top of each other on the blue strap.

The main road, although not as bad as the entrance in to the hospice, is still riddled with hazards. At one point, Vasudha asks Hameeda if she would like to go to the park. I think it sounds like a lovely idea, until Vasudha says it's too far to walk, we'd need to take an autorickshaw.

"An auto?" I ask, confused, trying to figure out how four of us and a paralyzed young woman will manage an auto.

No one else seems bothered by this idea, but the nurse in me has visions of trying to maneuver Hameeda into an auto, ripping out her catheter, bursting a pressure sore blister. I wait for someone to come to this conclusion too, but no one does, so I say, tentatively, "I wonder if that may be a bit difficult with the wheelchair…" I trail off. The plan is thankfully abandoned.

Suddenly, Hameeda squeals with delight; she has spotted a white and yellow blossom that has fallen from an overhead tree on to the pavement. I cannot believe she has noticed it amid all the commotion, the traffic, and the falling apart wheelchair. Marcus stops pushing the wheelchair and goes to retrieve it for her. She grabs the delicate blossom and holds it up to her nose, breathing in the fragrance. "So, so nice!" she gushes. "I love flowers!" she exclaims. She pushes it toward me and I, too, breathe in the delicious scent. It smells like a magnolia, and reminds me of sultry, summer nights back home.

For the remainder of the walk, we all work to gather as many flower blossoms as we can find, and there are a surprising number on the road in almost pristine condition. The delicate pink, white, and yellow blossoms pile up gently in Hameeda's lap, and Vasudha playfully tucks one behind her ear, the petals peeking out behind waves of curly hair.

    Evening settles, carrying on its dusky shoulders the sounds of a neighbor-hood ending its day—children crying, pots and pans clanging, the mournful sing-song call of the vegetable cart vendor, and the man on a bike collect-ing newspapers and cardboard. Marcus pushes Hameeda back toward the hospice along the uneven and difficult path, and I watch her, this young woman—whose body has betrayed her, whose family has abandoned her, who may die alone, a slow, agonizing death—as she laughs and lifts up flower blossoms and lets them fall softly back into her lap, over and over again.

    And I think, how true, the words I heard last week from one of the volun-teers in the palliative care clinic, trying to make sense of suffering that simply makes no sense:

I marvel at how life shines through.

10 The Similarities in Our Differences

Frequently, I was asked by nurses in India, "Is this the same in your home?" At the time, everything seemed so different I stumbled over the question. With further reflection, I have come to more fully appreciate the similarity of our experiences and our responses to them. The concerns of nurses at SICH are ones my American/Western nursing colleagues and I also face and deal with in ways that are sometimes productive and sometimes not. We struggle to help patients who have limited resources and can feel underappreciated and misunderstood as a profession. We sometimes feel powerless and at the mercy of individuals (usually male) in positions of higher authority and can experience a sense of helplessness in witnessing human suffering. We must cope with difficult and demanding co-workers, patients, and family members, and the frustration of working in what is still too often considered a low-status job. However, we also experience and celebrate similar successes—the patient who survives therapy and still keeps in touch years later; the tremendous personal satisfaction in comforting a dying patient; and the camaraderie of working with like-minded colleagues who view caring for the ill as a calling, not only as a way to pay the bills.

After returning from the field and reviewing my data with clearer eyes, I was frankly surprised at how many parallels I could draw between nursing challenges and realities in India and those in the U.S. Clearly, patients with money and influence don't only receive preferential treatment in India. Ask any U.S. nurse who has been pulled aside by their supervisor and told about the "VIP" (Very Important Person) patient who will get the private room, the next coveted Magnetic Resonance Imaging (MRI) slot, and care only provided by senior physicians, no medical trainees.[1] The U.S. also has egregious disparities in who receives health care and who does not; our

---

1 While socioeconomic status can certainly improve access to care and the quality of care received, it is not foolproof. Recall the comments from Kate, Joanie, and Dr. Varun regarding the difficulties of receiving care and navigating the medical system in India, even for patients with connections and affluence, as well as Dr. Rashi's concerns about the care provided to patients on the "paying wards" of SICH.

DOI: 10.4324/9781003413158-16

emergency departments are filled beyond capacity with patients suffering from unmanaged, chronic illness who lack adequate health insurance—patients who are disproportionately poor and people of color.[2] In rural areas of the U.S., patients lack access to cancer care too, often having to travel hundreds of miles to a specialized treatment center. Nurses in the U.S. can also achieve emotional distance by focusing on indirect aspects of patient care, disappearing behind computer screens to document in a labyrinth of electronic health records that require them to click, and click and click... and click. Family members are needed to provide care and advocate for patients in the U.S., too, especially in settings such as nursing homes or other long-term care facilities, or with home hospice where a full-time family caregiver is required, and expected, to provide a tremendous amount of care to a dying person, including toileting, giving medications, and managing tubes and drains.

Nurses in the U.S. aren't always well educated about pain and symptom management either. Entire supplementary curricula have been designed to address this deficit and teach nurses—as well as physicians and other healthcare providers—basic skills about pain management and caring for terminally ill

2　Structural racism not only makes it more difficult for individuals to access health care, but if they are able to access care, clinicians may "neglect, disbelieve, or actively discriminate against patients"; see *Medical News Today: Racism in healthcare: What you need to know, 2020*, for a succinct general summary of research studies (primarily U.S. focused) documenting how racism negatively impacts health outcomes related to pregnancy, mental health, emergency care, chronic illness, overall life expectancy, and pain control. Specific to cancer care, see the *U.S. National Cancer Institute summary of cancer disparities, 2022*. Within the nursing community of the U.S. significant attention is being directed toward understanding and dismantling structural racism within health care. For example, the updated *National Institute of Nursing Research's 2022–2026 Strategic Plan* specifically addresses social determinants of health (i.e., social factors that influence health outcomes) and the impact of structural racism on health equity; conversations within the American Academy of Nursing are largely focused on policy and leadership imperatives related to these topics; see, for example, the 2022 September–October issue of *Nursing Outlook*, which includes a number of articles related to racism in nursing practice and research. Specific to pain research, see the three-part series, *Confronting Racism in Pain Research (2022) in the Journal of Pain*. Of note, the majority of medical literature about racism and health care is focused in the U.S. A 2022 global scoping review of "Racism in healthcare" by Hamed et al., *BMC Public Health* found no articles about the topic published before 2001 and a sharp uptick in the number of articles published per year in 2019 and 2020 with an increase of 65% from 2018 to 2019; the majority of the 213 identified articles were U.S. based (67%), followed by the UK and Canada (7%); only one identified article focused on India; it describes discrimination of Indigenous communities within Kerala, conducted by researchers in Australia, George et al. (2020). "'Everything is provided free, but they are still hesitant to access healthcare services': Why does the Indigenous community in Attapadi, Kerala continue to experience poor access to health care?" *International Journal for Equity in Health*. Understanding the manifestations and impact of structural racism in the delivery of health care in low- and middle-income countries is a critical area of future research.

patients.[3] But many nurses still do not receive this type of training (which can be expensive and time-consuming) and there are countless studies about the myriad ways the U.S. healthcare system and clinicians fail to meet the needs of seriously ill patients and families, particularly in regards to effectively communicating prognosis and managing pain.[4] Shortages and stock-outs of morphine and other important pain-relieving opioids is also not a unique scenario to India, and are happening with increasing frequency now in the U.S.[5]. In U.S. hospitals there are also complicated and difficult dynamics between nurses with seniority and new graduate nurses, permanent employees, and contract nurses (e.g., "travelers" or per diem workers), night shift and day shift employees, nurses who work in the intensive care unit (ICU) and those who work in outpatient clinics. Perhaps stigma regarding cancer is not as prevalent in the U.S. as it once was, but it is all too commonly experienced by patients suffering from mental illness, substance use disorders, or obesity. Employees in the U.S. also seek government jobs for stable benefits and job security, and we have all, at some point, interacted with unhelpful or dismissive government officials and bureaucrats—why should we expect it be different in other countries?[6]

But some aspects of care in India were quite different and more nuanced and deserve a closer examination. Let's start with how nurses entered the profession in the first place.

How Nurses Become Nurses

In the U.S., women, and an increasing number of men, are commonly drawn to nursing because of an interest in the biological sciences, health, and wellness; the flexibility to practice in a variety of different settings and with

---

3 A well-known curriculum designed to help nurses learn palliative care skills is the End of Life Nursing Education Consortium (ELNEC) curriculum. It has been adapted for various patient populations and care settings, and international trainings are offered. See http://www.aacnnursing.org/ELNEC

4 There are many studies and reports that support this claim, including the landmark SUPPORT study, Connors, A. F., Dawson, N. V., Desbiens, N. A., Fulkerson, W. J., Goldman, L., Knaus, W. A., ... & Hakim, R. (1995). A controlled trial to improve care for seriously ill hospitalized patients: The study to understand prognoses and preferences for outcomes and risks of treatments (SUPPORT). *JAMA, 274*(20), 1591–1598, and more recent reports issued by the 2015 Institutes of Medicine: Dying in America: Improving Quality and Honoring Individual Preferences at the End of Life and Relieving pain in America: A blueprint for transforming prevention, care, education, and research.

5 Issues related to medication availability are also discussed within the Introduction. See Hospitals are confronting a new opioid crisis: an alarming shortage of pain meds, StatNews, 2018; the U.S Food and Drug Administration (FDA) Shortages website (injectable morphine is listed as "currently in shortage," April 7, 2023).

6 My first job as a new nurse was in a U.S. government hospital. While many employees were dedicated public servants, I was appalled at the limited effort put forth by some employees, and even more appalled when I realized they would keep getting raises and were highly unlikely to ever be terminated.

different types of patient populations; the ability to make a positive difference in the lives of others; and competitive salaries and opportunities for professional advancement. In contrast, many of the nurses I met at SICH (and they were almost all female, with only a few exceptions) did not voluntarily choose to become nurses. They had their education curtailed (commonly due to marriage) and were forced into nursing against their wishes, often by a family patriarch desirous of the income and stability of a government job.

Nurses I met told me they experienced intense family pressure to enroll in nursing, or stay in nursing, even when they were miserable and hated the training. Most entered training at the tender age of 15 or 16, overwhelmed and repulsed by the intense realities of bodily care they encountered. "I didn't know what I was getting in to," was something I heard often from nurses when they told me about their early days of training. It doesn't take much imagination to see how a nurse may approach patient care differently if they feel pushed into a profession of service they did not want to enter in the first place. The limited degree of decision-making power women experienced in both their natal and married homes was very real for the nurses I interviewed and knew during my time in India.

Relatedly, most nurses ended up at SICH not out of a desire or specific interest to work with cancer patients, but because of logistical reasons, such as the need to relocate to the city of Dandaka after marriage or as a transfer from another government hospital to qualify for a promotion. Many came from lower-middle class families that did not have the financial resources to hire additional household help, and therefore had immense domestic responsibilities. When nurses told me their schedules (up at 4:00 am, cooking breakfast for a large extended family, an hour-long bus commute to work, returning home, cooking dinner for a large extended family, etc.), I became exhausted just listening to them. For some, I think being at the hospital served as a respite—a time to connect with other women, relax, and take a break from their work at home. As Dr. Madhu explained to me during the earlier days of my fieldwork:

You know, Virginia, average Indian women—like Radha, Abhipsha, Jasmine—they have so many responsibilities with their families and home-life. It is their job to prepare all the food; they don't have money for cooks and maids. All the food must be freshly prepared; they make breakfast, then as soon as they finish breakfast they are thinking about lunch, then they must make lunch, then tea, prepare dinner, then plan for breakfast the next day. The kitchen is always active. Before one meal ends, they are chopping vegetables for the next one. It's a woman's job to prepare the meals and the food, and if that is not happening, then people wonder if something is wrong.

The Actual Work of Nursing

The actual work of nursing that I observed in India was vastly different too. With few exceptions (the palliative care and home care nurses being prime examples), nurses delivered very little hands-on care, and a major focus of work involved clerical duties and completing rote, mechanized tasks. "This is routine work, we come, we give chemo, and we go" was a phrase I heard in various permutations from many nurses. Nurses were often reduced to scribes, diligently hand recording in a dizzying array of ledgers mundane details of supply inventories and patient census that had little to do with actual patient care. I was told this emphasis on documentation was related, in part, to the residual influence of British colonialism, which stressed bu-reaucracy and detailed recordkeeping. There also seemed a clear protective factor in engaging in this type of "clean" paperwork, as it created significant distance from the messier elements of bedside care. More senior nurses were assigned documentation and administrative tasks, while more junior staff mixed and administered medications and chemotherapy. Sometimes when I asked nurses at SICH what they found most difficult or challenging about their job, I was provided with extremely concrete, and unexpected, examples. For example, one experienced nurse described mathematical calculations for chemotherapy as the most stressful part of her job as an oncology nurse. This answer surprised me, given the preponderance of human suffering all around, and reflects what many nurses felt was their primary obligation and task—to administer chemotherapy.

Status and social ranking was a key determinant in the degree, and type, of engagement with bodily fluids and personal care. For example, I was told ayahs ("sweepers") were commonly delegated to perform fecal disimpac-tions, place urinary catheters, and shave genital regions prior to surgery on the general wards.[7] Contract ward nurses were more likely to be inserting intravenous (IV) lines than higher status government nurses who sat at the front desk and did paper work. The reticence of nurses to engage in intimate aspects of patient care is complicated but can be traced to deeply entrenched views linking this type of "polluting" work to low-caste individuals and the moral risk of engaging in intimate care with nonrelated members of the op-posite sex.[8] The avoidance of "polluting work" was painfully apparent in the sad case of Hameeda, the orphaned, Muslim girl whom the nurses at SICH

---

7   Recognizing the significant role in patient care assumed by ayahs and ward boys, some ini-tiatives have been undertaken to provide them with additional training. See "Now, certified courses for ward boys, ayahs," in DNA India (2013), which, of note, includes the subtitle "Ward boys and ayahs will no longer be insensitive toward patients as they will be trained to take better care of the ill." See also innovative programs affiliated with academic institu-tions in the U.S., such as the University of Utah (2013/2014), Ward boys in Gujarat, India: Doing much more than meets the eye; and Teaching the ward boys in Gujarat, India, which describes the implementation of a successful five-day, 30-hour training course for ward boys focused on professionalism, communication, infection control practices, basics of patient care, and stress management.

8   See the excellent paper by Nair & Healey, 2006. A profession on the margins: status issues in Indian nursing in https://archive.nyu.edu/bitstream/2451/34246/2/profession_on_the_

essentially refused to care for after she became bedridden and incontinent. While the specific cultural context of gender relations and the caste system may be unique to India, proximity to bodily fluids and intimate patient care needs based upon status is not. For example, it would be highly unusual for a physician in the U.S. to help clean an incontinent patient, and sometimes also uncommon for nurses, as this task is often delegated to lower paid and lower status unlicensed patient care assistants. In other words, as one's status increases, so generally does the distance from the bedside and the body, regardless of where you practice.

Given that family members generally occupied the lowest status rung within SICH, it is not surprising that they engaged in the most bodily care. I was simply amazed at how much direct patient care was delegated to, and assumed by, patients' family members within the hospital.[9] Sons, daughters, wives, and husbands who had no medical training, and limited support, administered medications; monitored chemotherapy; changed wound dressings; emptied catheters; fed, mobilized, toileted, and bathed patients; and suctioned away respiratory secretions. It was up to family members to advocate for their loved ones, and almost all patients were required to have a family member present, all day, every day, to be eligible for treatment in the hospital.

When I observed in the ICU, I was particularly puzzled when Adishree—an exceptionally bright and dedicated nurse—went out of her way to leave the unit, go in to the corridor, and locate a patient's family member simply so they could help a patient sit up. It was confusing to me that Adishree wouldn't just go ahead and do this herself. The clear, normative default, with

---

margins.pdf, which provides historical perspective related to the delegation of personal care tasks by Indian nurses to family members, ward boys, and ayahs:

> Disputes were frequent between western nurses, who strongly felt that the nobility of nursing lay in a willingness to tend to every need of the human body, and their Indian students, who often felt that their experience of life within the hospital and society would be much easier if bedpans and baths could be delegated to sweepers and ward-boys...Issues of caste and pollution thus clearly formed part of the daily experience of the average Indian nursing student, who strove to distance herself from the "polluting" aspects of the work, which had negative caste and class associations...Commentaries on nursing produced by observers and by nurses themselves are so strongly infused with an awareness of caste and pollution that it must be acknowledged as a valid impediment to professional progress.
>
> (p. 12)

9 The strategy of relying on family members to provide care to hospitalized patients is not unique to India, and is described as a common scenario in other LMICs, such as Bangladesh. See Hadley, M. B., Blum, L. S., Mujaddid, S., Parveen, S., Nuremowla, S., Haque, M. E., & Ullah, M. (2007). Why Bangladeshi nurses avoid 'nursing': Social and structural factors on hospital wards in Bangladesh. *Social Science & Medicine*, 64(6), 1166–1177; Zaman, S. (2009). Ladies without lamps: Nurses in Bangladesh. *Qualitative Health Research*, 19(3), 366–374; Zaman, S. (2013). Silent saviours: Family members in a Bangladeshi hospital. *Anthropology & Medicine*, 20(3), 278–287.

some notable exceptions observed with the pediatric, palliative care, and home care departments,[10] was that family members delivered all hands-on care. This, in turn, determined when, and how, family members could share space with the nursing staff. When I asked Adishree why some family members were allowed to enter the ICU and others were harshly admonished when they dared to cross the threshold, she told me family attendants had to be invited in to do something specific: "*If there is a job to do, like ambulation [helping a patient walk], then we will go out and ask the family to come in so they can do it, and then they can leave.*" Once a family member had completed a specific patient care-related task, their presence was generally seen as problematic and a hindrance.[11]

This different sense of professional obligation as a nurse showed up in many forms during my time in the field: in the missed opportunities to help or comfort patients or family members; in the lack of recognizing ways to advocate for patients (even in the small ways that were feasible) and the reluctance to take action to help patients once a potential solution was identified; in the ease with which wards were left unattended, often for hours at a time; in the manner in which family members and patients were spoken to or ignored; and the general demeanor of the nurse in the delivery of care. While these findings may be surprising to Western-trained nurses, it is important to acknowledge practical and systemic barriers that likely altered nurses' sense of what they were supposed to do and how they could realistically do it. For example, consider public transportation, which was erratic and time-consuming. Most nurses depended on public buses to get back and forth from their home to the hospital and were at the mercy of unreliable transportation. This created problems in arriving to work on time and made leaving work—regardless of whether the next shift had arrived or not—acceptable. Political tensions (which reached a flashpoint during my time in India) commonly resulted in citywide transportation bandhs (strikes) and made commuting to work even more unpredictable. It is hard to be accountable for a ward full of 70 patients when it's impossible to get to work on time.

I heard, and observed, many instances of compromised patient care (at least through Western eyes). Stories nurses shared with me were terribly sad, haunting, and unsettling. Some of the more disturbing and dramatic events happened during night shift when nurses essentially shuttered themselves in back rooms away from patients. At the time, I didn't understand why this was happening and it distressed me, as leaving patients unattended in a U.S.

---

10 I attribute these differences in large part to the strong leadership and advocacy of Dr. Rashi and Dr. Madhu who provided essential support to the pediatric, home care, and palliative care nurses at SICH and in important ways made their difficult work somewhat more manageable.

11 To a lesser degree, this sentiment is evident within U.S. hospitals when nurses and other healthcare staff may become distressed or irritated if patients have large numbers of family members at the bedside and if they are seen as disrupting the clinical workflow.

hospital is a serious and punishable offense.[12] Were the nurses simply exhausted, having had no time to sleep during the day? Did they not see it as a problem to leave the ward unattended, knowing family members were there to provide some level of assistance? Or were they afraid of being harmed in some way? This last possibility was not shared with me during my fieldwork, but occurred to me when I later read descriptions of nurses on night shift and their vulnerabilities and fears related to sexual harassment or assault from ward boys, family members, or other hospital workers.[13]

Knowledge Deficit

A number of nurses shared that when they began working at SICH it was very difficult for them to see dying cancer patients. Many nurses believed, reinforced by their experiences at the hospital, that cancer is invariably fatal and always presents in advanced stages, and that pain is inevitable and largely unmanageable. This sense of futility that the patient would not survive no matter what they did was often cited as a major detraction from their job and a disheartening aspect of their work. Given the reality that most patients presented to SICH with incurable, late stages of cancer, and the fact that morphine was not always available or administered, this attitude was not unfounded.

On the whole, the nurses I observed had a very limited role in pain and symptom management, which is traditionally a core function of a nurse, and arguably more so, a cancer nurse. Even when a patient was in visible pain, nurses often minimized or dismissed the pain as not a legitimate concern. While nurses were quick to verbalize their knowledge deficits related to chemotherapy, they did not seem to have the same appreciation for their lack of knowledge related to pain and symptom management. Many nurses told me inaccurate information about managing pain (e.g., insisting that anti-nausea medications were analgesics) and two nurses told me they had administered placebos to help determine if a patient's pain was "real" or psychological. With the exception of the palliative care department and home care team, and to some degree on the pediatric ward, nurses at SICH did not routinely assess or ask patients about pain and relied upon the patient or

---

12 "Patient abandonment"—leaving patients without access to nursing care after you have assumed responsibility for them—is a serious allegation of nursing misconduct that can result in disciplinary action and loss of one's license to practice.

13 See Nair and Healey:

> Sexual harassment is an unavoidable experience for many of them [nurses in India] and it happens at the hands of not only superiors and doctors, but also the ward boys, relatives of patients and other workers in the hospitals. Nurses on night shifts are more vulnerable. This is an indicator of the low status of women in society, as well as often a reminder to women about the deviance of being seen in a public space at night.

(2006, p. 3)

family member to advocate for themselves if pain was a problem. Administering morphine and managing difficult pain was simply not part of the role of a nurse on the general wards.

Even with nurses who had undergone additional palliative care training, there were often misunderstandings related to appropriate opioid dosing and schedules, disproportionate fears about addiction, or viewing pain primarily as psychological. Despite the keen emphasis on documentation, there were sometimes concerning safety issues in how morphine was dispensed and accounted for. Only members of the palliative care team routinely administered IV morphine, the fastest way to achieve rapid pain relief, and they were available during limited clinic hours. Any morphine administered on the general wards was in oral form, the tablets dispensed by family members who had previously obtained prescriptions from the palliative care department (or rarely, their primary oncologist). After patients were referred to the palliative care department, the palliative care team then assumed responsibility for pain management—this was then, in turn, delegated to family members. It was also my experience in talking with patients and family members throughout the hospital that they rarely knew what medications they were taking for pain; they understood the tablets were for pain, but did not know the name or any specific details of the drug.

Morphine was actually more readily available (at least 10 mg immediate release tablets) than I expected due to the tremendous efforts of a dedicated group of hospital employees. However, there were still gaps in supply and staff developed a system of work-arounds to cope with shortages ("stock-outs") of morphine. In many ways, SICH was ahead of the curve with pain management, as it was the only hospital in the entire city during my fieldwork (including the swanky private hospitals) that had any sort of reliable supply of morphine. But morphine still had trouble reaching patients in need and seemingly trivial bureaucratic difficulties, like having the correct postage and envelopes, could make or break the difference in patients' obtaining morphine.[14]

The role of the nurse was both paradoxically rigid (in the general wards, defined primarily by chemotherapy administration and documentation) and blurry, and this influenced how pain for patients was addressed. For example, other health care providers at SICH were actively involved in pain assessment and management for patients, in ways that would traditionally be thought of as the purview of the nurse. Social workers, both in pediatrics and palliative care, assessed and offered specific recommendations for managing pain with patients and saw this as an important part of their job. In practice,

---

14 For a fuller discussion of micro and macro-level barriers related to opioid availability at SICH, see LeBaron, V., Beck, S., Black, F., Maurer, M., & Palat, G. (2014). An ethnographic study of barriers to cancer pain management and opioid availability in India. *The Oncologist, 19*(5), 515–522.

this overlapping of roles related to pain management seemed to supplant the nurse as the primary healthcare provider responsible for assessing and alleviating symptoms.

Fear, Power, and Stigma

Fear and distrust, underpinned by complex power dynamics, and the desire for control permeated the institution and influenced all interactions. Patients feared they would not get proper medical treatment, become a drain on family resources, and be abandoned at the hospital. Family members feared the social stigma of having a diagnosis of cancer in the family; worried how they would manage transportation back and forth from their village to the city for the patient's treatment; and were afraid patients would give up hope and their will to live if told their accurate diagnosis and prognosis. Nurses feared family members would blame them and become angry if a patient experienced a bad health outcome; worried they would develop cancer themselves; and were troubled by the consequences of exposure to chemotherapy. Nurses, understandably overwhelmed by the uncontrollable aspects of their job that constantly engulfed them and the social constraints they encountered as women and nurses, sought refuge in aspects of care and day-to-day life in the hospital that they *could* control: documentation, crowd control, and what, and when, and with whom, they took tea breaks and ate lunch.

Issues of power and hierarchy[15] showed up again and again—between physicians and nurses, government nurses and contract nurses, nurses and Class IV employees (ward boys and ayahs), nurses and family members—and manifested in all sorts of ways, but particularly related to communication and space. One of the most overt examples occurred when I was observing in the ICU and chastised for unknowingly using a bathroom designated for "Class IV" employees; I was immediately taken to a different, separate bathroom for higher status employees.

---

15 See Das et al.'s (2022) ethnographic work, 'We are nurses – what can we say?': Power asymmetries and Auxiliary Nurse Midwives in an Indian State. *Sex Reprod Health Matters*, 29(2), 2031598, for a rich discussion of structural healthcare system power dynamics, particularly related to gender, that constrain nursing practice and quality patient care in India and recommendations to support empowerment of nurses within India. Many of their findings related to power dynamics and interactions between nurses and patients corroborate results presented in this book. Importantly, Das et al. propose that "in order to improve auxiliary nurse midwives (ANM's) performance, the power asymmetries that are entrenched in the health system and everyday functioning of health facilities need to be addressed," and frame their data collection and analysis within "Expressions of Power," including "power over, power to, power with, power within," as described in VeneKlasen, L., Miller, V. Power and Empowerment. In: L. VeneKlasen, V. Miller, Editors. A new weave of power, people, and politics: The action guide for advocacy and citizen participation. The authors also provide a helpful justification as to why they chose not to disclose the Indian State where the research was conducted, a decision I made as well.

The strong emphasis on hierarchy and discrimination related to race and class can be historically traced to the influence of British colonialism, "status anxiety," and divisions that evolved as nurses were trained in India,[16] and entrenched beliefs of the caste system that assign individuals an immutable social rank from birth. These contexts were often the primary drivers impacting the delivery of health care. Kate, the American volunteer with Indian roots, offered this explanation of the relationship between status and health care during my fieldwork:

> *First of all, since it's a government hospital the patients don't have any money. And in India, if you don't have money you are completely expendable. So, their lives are already not valued. And on top of it, it's conditioning since childhood for the entire population of India to believe in this caste system, to believe that if you are of a lower caste and have no money you are worthless. You are actually less, so what's the point? That's the mentality. And we come in from the West thinking this is a valuable person, they're not getting proper treatment. But here it's not viewed that way. It's viewed as, what's the point? Like, we don't want to help them when they're healthy, let alone when they're sick when there's even less of a point to helping. It's hard to wrap my mind around it.*

Nurses were fearful of contagion, especially from highly stigmatized diseases such as HIV. The one available hospice in Dandaka during my fieldwork refused to accept patients with HIV, not an uncommon stipulation of hospices in LMICs. Patients with blood-borne diseases, such as HIV and hepatitis B, were often labeled and identified in public ways that did not protect patient privacy. During one observation in the palliative care clinic, a 37-year-old woman with HIV was seen to have her ascites (an abnormal collection of fluid within the abdomen) drained before traveling to Bangalore to an ashram that accepts patients with HIV. She was dreadfully sick, with a belly so swollen from fluid she looked nine months pregnant. From my field notes:

> *It was all over her chart, 'HIV positive' and everyone was talking loudly about it, not seeming to really care who heard. There was a big show of double gloving [putting on 2 pairs of gloves, ostensibly for more protection]. Daya actually recoiled when Pradeep tried to touch her arm with the glove he used with the patient. After the patient left there was a heated debate at lunch about HIV patients – I didn't catch all of it – Pradeep translated for me and said that Sarah insisted only HIV positive staff care for HIV positive patients in the U.S. I was going to correct her, but Pradeep told me not to.*

16 See Nair & Healey, 2006, *A Profession on the Margins: Status Issues in Indian Nursing*; and *Indian Sisters: A History of Nursing and the State, 1907–2007* by Madelaine Healey, Routledge, 2013.

Many nurses told me during my fieldwork they feared family members would physically assault them if a patient died unexpectedly or experienced a bad medical outcome on the ward. This fear had the quality of an urban legend (i.e., nurses told me they worried this would happen, and had heard of it happening, but no one could provide a specific example of when it actually *did* happen), but it was a very real fear. Sister Agnes told me family attendants can get very "demanding" when a patient is not doing well on the ward, especially if the doctor has not adequately discussed prognosis with the family: "*The family, they don't understand, we are helpless. They become aggressive, the attendants. They don't know about the prognosis, so they become aggressive on us.*" According to Agnes and other nurses I spoke with, this aggression could take the form of verbal harassment—or escalate to a physical attack: "*Sometimes they'll come and they'll try to beat us also. The attendants will be both angry and in grief.*"[17] As a consequence of this fear, nurses tended to withdraw and say little to family members after the death of a patient as a precautionary measure. This may explain, at least in part, the reluctance of the palliative care team to engage with the family whose young daughter died, or the security guard at Pillalu Hospital who positioned himself between the hospital staff and the dying child's parents. Nurses felt it was better, smarter, and ultimately safer for them to communicate as little as possible and minimize contact with family members in these situations. One of the SICH general ward nurses explained the challenge of knowing how to interact with dying patients or bereaved family members:

I cannot find words to tell them. I don't know how to console them… They keep on shouting at us, but in some cases, we are helpless, we cannot speak anything; in that time, I don't even find words to say. I cannot tell anything to the patient's attendants or to the patients. I remain very calm due to the suffering. I have a kind of depression. I don't say anything. I only do the formalities…In such time, whatever we talk will be taken wrongly. The patient's attendants will be suffering. Whatever we talk, they will get agitated. We know why the patient has died, but the attendants don't know why the patient has died. They think that the patient was good till now and he has now died; this nurse might not have given injection and all. They think that. But we know why the patient has died, if it is cardiac arrest, or did he die suddenly. We know that. They do not know. So, even if we talk something, it will be counted as wrong. That is why it is better to remain silent.

---

17 While I did observe frequent instances of family members repeatedly attempting to get nurses' attention, I did not witness any events where patients or family members verbally or physically attacked nurses. This fear is not unique to India. As one example, a scene in Abraham Verghese's novel, *Cutting for Stone*, about an Ethiopian mission hospital in the 1960s describes a nurse fleeing the ward after a baby dies, terrified the mother will seek retribution. See also Pyone et al. (2019) for a discussion of the experience of Auxiliary Nurse Midwives in Pune, India, and their concerns related to personal safety (as well as transportation difficulties, lack of resources, limited supervision and training opportunities, and challenges related to gender and social norms.)

On the whole, nurses seemed reluctant to get "too close" emotionally and physically to patients. Getting attached to patients who were inevitably going to die was painful, and there was not much reward for doing so, nor any formal structure of support. Nurses who did emotionally invest relayed how painful it was for them when the patients ultimately died. Recall the heartbreaking story told by Sister Bharati about the little boy who tried to find her as he was dying, despite his swollen shut eyes.

SICH (as are all healthcare institutions around the world, I would argue) was a factious organization. It took me a while to figure it out, but there were complex power dynamics at play between three distinct groups of nurses in the hospital: government ward nurses (who wielded the most power with tremendous job security); contract ward nurses (who had less power and were vulnerable due to less job security and worried about getting fired or dismissed); and contract nurses who worked in the palliative care and pediatric departments (who were most typically bullied by the first two groups, as they did not fall under the jurisdiction of the nursing superintendent, and were instead supervised directly by physicians). Tensions ran particularly high between the government/contract ward nurses and the pediatric and palliative care nurses. The former were envious of the professional development opportunities afforded the pediatric and palliative care nurses, and the latter were envious of the job security, higher salary, lighter workload, and benefits of the government nurses.

These power dynamics manifested in the delegation of space, where and with whom nurses ate their meals, and the organization of special events. For example, I was told that the ward nurses had "chased" the palliative care and pediatric nurses out of the communal hospital nurses' lounge, and consequently the pediatric and palliative care nurses did not share meals with the other ward nurses. In the beginning, I bungled moving among these three distinct groups, sometimes creating awkward situations. When the government nurses invited me to the hospital Christmas party, I understood it to be a hospital-wide event and casually mentioned it to the palliative care nurses, who I assumed were also invited—but who were not.

The only time I saw these three groups of nurses come together during my fieldwork was at the concluding seminar I gave when I discussed my preliminary findings; at this meeting, the groups voluntary segregated themselves with their seating choices and the general tension in the room was palpable. Even among nurses in the same group there was occasionally conflict. Generally, this involved nurses who were frustrated by what they perceived to be a laissez-faire attitude of their colleagues and superiors and an unfair distribution of workload.

Broader, macro-level, sociopolitical tensions also exacerbated complex power relations and divisions among the hospital and nursing staff. For example, during my fieldwork, a separatist movement within the State became reactivated,[18] and hospital staff and citizens of the city aligned themselves

---

18 This is purposefully not discussed in detail within the book in an effort to help disguise the State in which the fieldwork occurred.

between two distinct geographical allegiances. Not only did this political activity cause microlevel disruptions (transportation problems, businesses closed, rallies in the hospital lobby, etc.), but it served to clearly and deeply divide individuals along political lines and exacerbated preexisting tensions and prejudices between the groups.[19]

Nurses also had complex relationships with physicians. Most often, I sensed and observed a feeling of collegiality—particularly between general ward nurses and physician postgraduates (recall the cooperative interactions between general ward nurses and physicians during the nursing strike described in Chapter 2) and between the pediatric and palliative care contract nurses and their respective supervising physicians, with whom they had a close relationship and felt were generally supportive. Largely, nurses were extremely deferential to senior/attending physicians (e.g., standing up when they entered a room) and were expected to follow their instructions without question. Occasionally, though, government nurses pushed back and reprimanded physicians, usually lower-status trainees or residents, for a variety of transgressions (recall the incident from Chapter 3 when a nurse yelled at the doctor for telling family members to put blood products in the ICU refrigerator). In fact, one senior physician confessed to me while I was observing on the wards, "I'm scared shitless of the government nurses!"

Interactions and relationships between nurses and family attendants were also complicated and could shift depending on the needs of the nurses. At times, the dynamic was clearly adversarial, but at other times there was a sense of reciprocity and mutual benefit and trust. From my field notes:

> *The evening duty nurse has not arrived yet, but we leave the unit and 47 patients. Naveena hands a set of keys to a woman sitting at the end of a patient's bed on our way out.*
> *Is that a patient attendant?*
> *Yes.*
> *And you give her the keys? I am surprised.*
> *Yes, she will return the keys to us tomorrow morning.*
> *Wow. You must really trust her. I am curious if she handed over the keys to the medicine cabinets. Are those the keys to the ...*
> *Naveena interrupts me. Just the cabinet, with our uniforms, medicines, fluids...*
> *She is vague.*

19 For example, one senior nurse alluded to the fact that individuals from one geographical area involved in the political debate were "socially backwards," as women from the region frequently presented to SICH with cervical cancer—a highly stigmatized cancer (mis)associated with sexual promiscuity. I was told by another nurse that because of the political tensions, a new nursing organization had been created to specifically represent the interests of nurses aligned with the separatist cause. These political riffs added one more dimension to the complexity of divisions that already existed to stratify and fracture the nursing staff.

The keys are supposed to go back up in the metal cabinet upstairs,
but we're tired, so we just leave them with her.

These complex power dynamics underpinning race and class also manifested outside the hospital. For example, the extensive matrimony section
of the *Hindu Times* listed dozens of grooms-seeking-brides and brides-
seeking-grooms, all clearly delineated by caste, and many referencing the
fairness of a potential betrothed's skin.[20] At home, similar to nurses' treatment of family attendants, I witnessed my flatmates simultaneously trust—
and mistrust—Lakshmi and Fatima. Throughout my fieldwork, I remained
uncomfortable with the power dynamics involved with employing a cook
and a housekeeper, and found the constant negotiation, coordination, and
"required" supervision confusing and exhausting. I was often asked to "supervise" Lakshmi and Fatima to prevent theft or other unclear, potential
transgressions. From my fieldnotes:

Joannie calls me at the hospital.
  Your phone is switched off!
  Yes I've been working all day, doing interviews, I can't have the
phone on. What's up?
  You need to be home this evening, for the maid and cook to come.
  Okay. I'll be home.
  I have to work at the office till 10 pm.
  Okay.
  You must keep vigilance, Virginia. You cannot stay in your room.
You must keep vigilance.
  Why? Did something happen?
  No, but don't give it a chance.

Communication

There are numerous examples in the book of harsh interactions, or simply
no interaction at all, between nurses and patients, ayahs and patients, nurses
and physicians. Some of these instances may seem exaggerated, or even unbelievable, to a Western audience.[21] One of the most thoughtful responses

---

20 Fair/light skin in India has traditionally been considered highly desirable, and many products stocked in pharmacy shops or beauty treatments are advertised with the promise to
lighten one's complexion; during my fieldwork, I recall seeing a specific deodorant marketed
to lighten the skin under the armpits. In response to mounting criticism about its role in pro-
moting "light" as "ideal," the extensive line of beauty products in India, "Fair & Lovely,"
changed its name in 2020 to "Glow & Lovely."
21 This relates to the idea of "culture as what we no longer see," as discussed later in this chapter. Mayra et al. (2022) discuss differing responses from participants who viewed a picture
of a birth in India that displayed practices such as the midwife pinching the laboring woman

to this difference came from my interview with Jennifer, the volunteer from Australia with family roots in India. Here, she addresses what she views as the main factor behind these patterns of interaction:

I ask myself, 'why do the nurses feel they have to communicate that way'... I feel like the nurses that work in pediatrics aren't making much money...they're also struggling. They aren't that much better off than the patients, sometimes. Not to say that they're at the poverty line, but when you know how much they're making a month, and they're having to live with six people to a room themselves, or four nurses to a room or in a hostel... that's a lot of stress. I also wonder if it's just a way to cope, because how does a nurse do what she does? If you ask me, the nurses here experience daily trauma with what they see. If I had to deal with daily trauma, and I wasn't taught healthy coping strategies, I may also do that. I don't think they know that connecting with patients may actually benefit them rather than protect them, so I think they try to protect themselves by keeping everyone at arm's length...And India, in general, is very hierarchal. Like, the doctor is a doctor, and what the doctor says, goes. Anyone that has a bit more status than you has way more than you. There's tremendous disparity between the poor and the rich and anything in between. There's always someone poorer than you, or that has less than you. I think it's related to simple economics, who has more money...Who deserves to tell the ayah what to do? Well, the nurse does. Or, the ayah earns more than the patients, so the ayah yells at the patients when they misbehave. As in, 'you didn't clean up!' or 'two of your family members came in here when you know only one is allowed!' or 'you wore your shoes!' I think patients are fearful, afraid of misbehaving, because they do get yelled at. But then, you know, they need to maintain some order! I'm always trying to flip the coin and say, well, so if they didn't do that, then what

---

with forceps. The authors found the perception of the mistreatment of the woman varied between Indian nurses and midwives and nurses and midwives from other countries:

A difference is noticed in the perception of participants from India and elsewhere in terms of perceiving the severity of mistreatment that the woman in the picture is subjected to. This could be due to the difference in people's conditioning and exposure to the culture of violence, progress in the discussions about mistreatment, the level of efforts made to ensure respectful care and women's varied expectation of quality and respectful care in different contexts and countries that the participants come from. Indian participants' perspectives convey normalisation of mistreatment to an extent where, unless the act of abuse is extreme, it is side-lined. A participant from India even perceived that the picture shows good quality care while another felt some amount of shouting at the woman during childbirth is completely justifiable, as women are unable to hear through the pain and follow the instructions during childbirth.

(p. 9)

would happen? There might be chaos. There's a reason why they're doing what they're doing… I think it has to do with whoever has the money, has more power.[22]

There was the strong sentiment that others with lower status than one-self would respond best to harsh or direct communication. There was a repeated assumption, told to me by physicians, nurses, and ayahs alike, that patients and family members, who were primarily illiterate and poor, were unable to understand instructions. The only way to effectively communicate with them was to repeat things over and over again, generally in a loud and harsh manner—or eventually, to ignore them. There was a general mentality, by and large, that because patients and family were incapable of understanding, it didn't really make sense in an environment of limited resources and time to expend the energy to try to explain things to them.[23] In a crush of people, it was easier and faster to yell and get it done.

---

22 See Das et al. (2022) for a discussion of similar power dynamics between contract and government nursing employees as well as difficult interactions between nurses and patients: "*We have to deal with the male family members; you'll often find us shouting at them in frustration—maybe using bad language … (ANM, Facility B).*" Of note, Das et al. (2022) and Mayra et al. (2022) both discuss, similar to Jennifer, this idea of "trickle down power dynamics." One participant from Mayra et al. referred to this phenomenon as a "domino effect" where one care provider learns how to abuse from another, and this peer influence slowly turns everyone into an abuser. From Das et al.: "we observed that Auxiliary Nurse Midwives (ANMs) perpetuated the disrespect they faced in the facilities. We found that ANMs behaved toward the community as the managerial cadres behaved with them, with a perverse 'power over' expression dominating their actions. We observed many instances where ANMs asserted a sense of superiority over, and condescension toward, patients, reproducing the patriarchy they were subjected to themselves… ANMs sometimes explained to us how 'no matter how much we make them [the community women] understand … poor things, they are illiterate and don't understand.' There were many instances where ANMs' interactions with women were disrespectful and abusive, mainly verbally. Sometimes disrespect was also manifested in the way the women were handled physically by the ANMs. The ANMs did not consider their behaviour abusive; they justified their actions by saying that "this is the only language they [the community women] understand." From Mayra et al. (2022):

> Being voiceless in planning care provision leads to an assertion of power over women who are further down in the social hierarchy as this participant shared: "They take these women for granted. They feel I am taking care of you and I have this power over you to provide care to you, so you have to listen to me. This is my territory and you are bound to listen to me."
>
> (WB02, p. 6)

Also from Mayra et al. (2022)—reminiscent of Dr. Varan's plea at SICH to "change the social format"—this similar participant quote: "the hierarchy is knock on. Everybody is abusing the other who is lower in status than them … we need deep cultural change" (GL05, p. 8).

23 It is possible that the passive response of ignoring patients or family members reflected a similar goal to "avoid conflict through acquiescence," as seen in the practice of Chinese nurses in Tang's study (2007, p. 822) or as a way to gain some sense of control in chaotic

"Village people don't understand even when they are told multiple times," one pediatric nurse told me, summing up the general mentality of the staff. I found it interesting that no one seemed to ask *why* they weren't understanding, or to consider if the message was delivered differently, perhaps they would. This approach seemed to create a vicious cycle—as patients and family members were ignored they became more desperate, repeatedly approaching the nurses station and asking the same question, or more aggressively pushing through a crowd of people. Although there did seem to be a clear understanding of the genuine hardships patients faced, it didn't seem to translate in to a parallel appreciation for how to mitigate the effect of these hardships—for example, how to effectively educate patients unable to read about cancer treatment side effects or how to properly take their medications.

Nurses acknowledged their brusque communication style with patients and family members, and some (like Sister Meena) seemed uncomfortable with it at times, but felt it was justified and necessary, given their limited education, large crowds, and general "ignorance." Western volunteers with strong roots in India also felt that communicating in ways that Westerners may perceive as rude was more effective than being gentle and polite. On more than one occasion, I was told to stop saying "please" and "thank you." Jennifer freely admitted her style was rougher and more direct, and that she sternly reprimanded nurses when they did unsafe things, like recap used needles or didn't use aseptic technique when accessing IV lines. "It's what they respond to, it's what they are used to. The Australian way is just too gentle," Jennifer told me. Kate, an American volunteer, also came to a similar conclusion:

And I actually learned at this point, we've [Westerners] been conditioned to be respectful and not overstep our boundaries, but I think

---

situations. An article in *The Economist* explains a biographer's take on the reluctance of Sonia Gandhi to speak publicly: "Demanding responses from leaders is a 'Western-minded concern.' Ordinary rural folk expect 'silent' communication" (*The Economist*, 2013, p. 52). While obviously the context is different (political versus healthcare communication), it raises an intriguing question about the expectations of communication from the patients' point of view. Future research should explore this pattern of provider-patient communication from the patient/family member perspective; perhaps it is not as distressing to patients and family members as it may initially appear to Western-oriented eyes.

Similar to results reported by Tang et al. (2007) about ethical concerns of nurses in China, "the nurses told of many situations in which a patient or the relatives did not understand them, and conflict arose that interfered with care" (p. 816). Nurses at SICH described significant tensions between themselves and family members, as also reported in studies of nurses in Tanzania, Malawi, Iran, and China (Häggström et al., 2008; Maluwa et al., 2012; Shorideh et al., 2012; Tang et al., 2007). The findings reflect the frustration nurses experienced when they felt family members did not respect their nursing skills, questioned their judgment and interventions, or ignored the rules.

now I understand that here it's respected if you push it, and you can just say what you mean and be blunt. They don't respect people here for being polite or being too nice, or keeping quiet.

I also saw this communication pattern play out outside of the hospital, in the complicated dynamics that accompanied interactions between those who hired domestic help and those who performed the work. Joanie and Ruma were often, from my perspective, flat out rude to Fatima and Lakshmi—but this did not seem to ruffle any feathers, except mine. Tom, a visiting surgical resident from the U.S., also had a similar experience. He lived with an Indian roommate, and they had two housekeepers:

I don't get it. My roommate kicks back [Tom stretches back in his chair, putting his arms behind his head to illustrate] while these two women dust and clean around him, and I'm scurrying around trying to help them, straightening things up. And I almost think they respect him more for being an a—hole.

These different norms related to communication and interpersonal relationships are important for global health practitioners and clinicians to understand, as they underscore inherent power dynamics and ways of interacting that influence not only day-to-day life, but how nursing care is conceptualized, delivered, and received.

Perceived Powerlessness

Over and over again, I heard the phrase "we are helpless" from nurses when they talked to me about challenges related to their job. There was a clear sense that as a collective group, they felt they had little ability to influence change or improve conditions at SICH. Often when talking about difficult patient care scenarios, nurses would simply explain, "what we can do, we do." This expressed sense of powerlessness and helplessness is consistent with the experience of nurses practicing in other resource-limited settings where they witness the consequences of limited resources; struggle to cope with overwhelming aspects of their job with minimal supervisory support; deal with the frustration of thwarted attempts to advocate for their patients; and engage in contentious interactions with family caregivers and co-workers.[24]

---

24 See the following for discussions about the ethical challenges nurses encounter practicing in resource-constrained contexts: Harrowing, J., & Mill, J. (2010). Moral distress among Ugandan nurses providing HIV care: A critical ethnography. *International Journal of Nursing Studies, 47*(6), 723–731; Maluwa, V. M., et al. (2012). Moral distress in nursing practice in Malawi. *Nursing Ethics, 19*(2), 196–207; Shorideh, F. A., et al. (2012). Iranian intensive care unit nurses' moral distress: A content analysis. *Nursing Ethics, 19*(4), 464–478; Tang,

One SICH nurse, responding to my question if it was difficult for her to witness patient suffering, said this:

> *Difficult. So sad. Helpless. We can't help. They are helpless. What can we do? We cannot do anything....At that time we feel [vairagyam]. We can't do anything, we cannot do anything; helpless, that is all... What can we do?*

The local word the nurse uses in this quote essentially means giving up due to loss of hope. My translator explained:

> There is no good way of putting it in English in one word. It is the feeling of resigning to one's fate and just going through the motions because one feels like they must. Living life, but not really living it.

Sometimes, this sense of powerlessness as a nurse was accompanied by the fatalistic outlook that nothing would ever change at SICH, or in India in general.

At times, there existed a surprising dichotomy between the nurse as a "helpless" passive observer and their willingness to act independently. For example, giving medications to a symptomatic patient without a written order when the doctor was unavailable was a common occurrence during off-shifts. Additionally, nurses (especially in the palliative care clinic, pediatric ward, and community/home care setting) demonstrated significant autonomy in performing procedures such as paracentesis, opioid dose titration, and in writing prescriptions—things that are generally outside the scope of most nurses in the U.S. Despite these activities, however, nurses generally told me they felt disempowered and helpless. This may be because these activities largely went unnoticed, sometimes occurred surreptitiously, or were unappreciated or not acknowledged by colleagues with more power.

I felt this powerlessness, too, multiple times, within and outside the hospital. A personal reflection from my fieldnotes, after a particularly difficult day of observing in the hospital:

> *On the ride home a beggar with a left arm hanging limply, grotesquely disconnected from his shoulder socket, moves from stopped auto to stopped auto begging for money. I am ashamed to realize I am relieved when traffic resumes before he can approach me. And I wonder if that's what the nurses feel in the hospital—the stimulus is just too overwhelming so you have to stop, you have to block it out. You just*

P. F., et al. (2007). Chinese nurses' ethical concerns in a neurological ward. *Nursing Ethics*, 14(6), 810–824; Häggström, E., et al. (2008). Nurses' workplace distress and ethical dilemmas in Tanzanian health care. *Nursing Ethics*, 15(4), 478–491.

*can't take it anymore—so much suffering, so much need, so much sad-
ness, so much overwhelming despair and hopelessness. You just hope
it keeps moving, and doesn't stop in front of you. Maybe in a situation
where you cannot do anything, you simply do nothing.*

Influence of Religion

I was caught off guard by the Christian emphasis in a government, public
hospital and the evangelical agenda of the nurses, but I shouldn't have been.
Historically, Christian missionaries have been responsible for training nurses
in India and there is consequently a strong link between Christianity and
nursing in India. This is particularly true in the predominantly Christian state
of Kerala, where having at least one family member who enters the nursing
profession is seen as an important requirement in fulfilling one's perceived
Christian duty of service to the sick and vulnerable. The majority of nurses at
SICH (and other hospitals I visited) identified as Christian, a smaller percentage as Hindu, and only a few as Muslim. Divisions between Christian and
non-Christian staff and patients were sometimes unnoticeable and at other
times extremely obvious. For example, a few nurses made specific reference
to the "fact" that Muslim patients, specifically, would react more violently to
a patient's death or a poor medical outcome.

Just as I was asked frequently about my meals and my appetite, I was
asked with equal fervor about my religious well-being: where I went to
church, how often I prayed, if I had a Bible—and this often drilled down to
specifics; not just if I prayed, but specifically, how many hours a day. I tried
to dance lightly around these issues, with varying success. Trying to explain
I considered myself spiritual, not religious, did not generally go over well,
or seemed to cause significant confusion. An American physician at another
government hospital in Dandaka had a similar experience and confessed to
me he simply told the staff he was Jewish, even though he was not, to avoid
the conversation altogether.

Christian nurses told me during interviews that their greatest job satisfaction involved an opportunity to "do service to God" through caring for the
sick. This sense of gratitude and acknowledgment of a higher religious calling
sometimes appeared incongruent with behavior I observed on the wards, and
some of the nurses who talked to me most fervently about religion treated
patients and family members in ways I personally found challenging to reconcile with their professed faith. At other times, providers spoke of the privilege of caring for the ill in a spiritual context, and congruence was obvious in
the interactions I witnessed between nurse and patient.

Making Do and Getting By

Everyone affiliated with SICH talked about the stress and frustration that accompanied a serious lack of resources. Lack of protective equipment, medications, and basic supplies created significant distress for the staff. This was

particularly true for those who had previous exposure to higher-resourced environments such as private hospitals, or had worked abroad, and were aware of alternatives. Physicians and nurses shared poignant and harrowing stories of serious supply shortages. I was told frequently about the challenges of obtaining blood products to support critically ill patients or of not having essential chemotherapy drugs available to continue a cycle of treatment for a patient. Nurses had to make tough decisions about when to use a finite amount of a resource, such as gloves. Pradeep once told me: *We don't have enough gloves, so we have to decide when to use them, and when not to. We don't use them with every injection. If we will be doing a lot of injections we'll put on a pair of gloves and keep using that one pair.* Lack of material resources combined with extremely ill and poor patients often resulted in unfortunate and potentially fatal outcomes, as Dr. Rashi shared:

> *Now, you talk about morphine shortage. But we have chemotherapy shortages, we have shortages of IV fluids; at any given point there is a shortage of some medicine. Right now there is no daunorubicin in the hospital, for which we treat acute myeloid leukemia… We haven't had L-asparaginase for 2 months. So, we've had to send patients away, saying we can't treat you anymore.*

There were times, however, when I wondered if the lack of supplies provided an acceptable excuse for not engaging more with patients, as there were elements of nursing care (such as repositioning a patient in bed or helping a patient into a wheelchair or back to bed from a stretcher) that did not require special equipment or supplies, but that were still left undone. There were also times when supplies *were* available, but not used; for example, soap and running water were available, but hands were not washed. These instances may be due, in part, to a knowledge deficit or lack of awareness, but it may also have something to do with differing cultural perceptions of safety.[25] Throughout my time in India, I observed many examples, both within and outside the hospital, that seemed to highlight an overall different tolerance to risk than I was accustomed to. On the busy streets, families of three or four, often with very young children, could be seen riding on one motorbike, typically without helmets, and sometimes carrying objects such as large mirrors, propane tanks, or animals. Within the hospital, the close proximity of chemotherapy administration and exposure to cytotoxic agents in spaces where nurses consumed food, combined with inconsistent handwashing, made meal times, from my perspective, a stressful and potentially dangerous affair. However, the nurses I knew during my fieldwork did not express or demonstrate concern about the risks related to this set-up.

---

25 There is a large body of literature related to the many complex dimensions of cultural perceptions of risk in differing contexts, for example, related to financial decisions, genetic testing, or response to climate change and natural disasters. An interesting area of future research may be to explore this concept from the perspective of the delivery of nursing care.

Another serious resource deficiency involved the number of nursing staff. A common refrain from the nurses at SICH was that "heavy workload" created significant stress and decreased job satisfaction. "Because of heavy workload, we have no time to be with patients" was a mantra I heard frequently. This was commonly said with a sense of resignation and acceptance and was sometimes used by nurses to mitigate expectations of patients and families and exert control over patients and their care. While it is obviously true that the nurse-patient ratios were untenable on the general wards, sometimes as much as one nurse for over 50 patients, at times I wondered if the nurses actually *wanted* better ratios, as it may imply they would need to provide more direct care. From my observations, there were multiple "missed opportunities" to provide support and care to patients and family members, and this was most clearly evident when I observed on units at SICH (such as the ICU) where the nurse to patient ratio was a much more reasonable one nurse to three or four patients, or the Paying Ward where there was one nurse for two patients. Interestingly, even when nurses had the time to provide more direct and personalized care, they often choose not to (or it was not expected they would), even in the face of visible and obvious patient distress. When I tried to better understand this phenomenon, I was often simply told "there is no time." Many nurses blamed the lack of time to be with patients on the requirements related to documentation, but when pressed, most admitted this took only an hour or two of their total shift.

Pervading everything was the specter of abject poverty and the glaring disparity between the "haves" and "have-nots." All of the nurses recognized the dire financial situation of the patients who came to SICH, and many took measures to help patients who were hungry or needed basic supplies. Despite this, there did not always seem to be a parallel awareness of the tremendous vulnerability of the patients and family members, or the lack of options available to them.

To Advocate or Not—That Is the Question

The biggest assumption I brought in to the field that required critical reexamination was the idea of the nurse as advocate. American/Western nurses are inculcated with the concept that they are the patient's voice, their advocate.[26] We are taught it is our ethical duty to represent and fight for the best interests of our patient, regardless of the consequences.[27] One of the greatest compliments I ever received as a nurse was from a young, chronically ill patient who told me, "Thank you for being my voice when I couldn't speak for myself." I expected nurses at SICH to struggle in advocating for patients, but I expected

---

26 See the American Nurses Association (ANA) Code of Ethics, which among its provisions states, "The nurse promotes, advocates for, and protects the rights, health, and safety of the patient." Within the 76-page 2015 document, "advocacy" is referenced 29 times.

27 A high-profile example of patient advocacy despite adverse consequences occurred in the U.S. in 2017 when an emergency department nurse was roughly arrested for refusing to allow police to draw a blood sample from an unconscious patient; this incident was highly publicized and praised as an exemplar of the nurse's role in patient advocacy.

them to want to do it. My fieldwork suggests that they did not see it as important, did not want or know how to do it, or felt the risks were too great—or perhaps a combination of all. When I asked nurses in interviews who is most responsible for advocating for patients, the question frequently created confusion and required lengthy clarification before the nurse responded[28]; almost all answered it was the job of the family member. This was consistent with what I observed, especially on the general wards.

Times during my fieldwork when nurses (or others) appeared unaware of potential alternative courses of action and ways to advocate for patients reminded me of a placard I saw prominently posted in the small SICH medical library: "*Your Eyes Do Not See What Your Mind Does Not Know.*" I found the sign meaningful in its reference to the challenge of "seeing" alternatives if they are unknown, which often seemed to be the case at SICH; most nurses behaved as though they simply did not know other ways of providing care. These instances reminded me of a discussion in one of my medical anthropology courses related to the "best" definition of culture. After a lively debate, the esteemed professor simply said, "Culture is what you can no longer see." This conceptualization of culture seems particularly relevant in helping to contextualize normative choices made by nurses and others at SICH and why outsiders (including myself) could find it jarring or unusual.

Every nurse in every hospital knows their equivalent of the "Orange Attending" physician that intimidated Preeti and other nurses at SICH. And when faced with these individuals, some nurses put themselves on the line and fiercely advocate for patients—others do not. A few nurses at SICH did share stories of attempts to advocate for patients which ultimately resulted in frustration when their input was dismissed and rebuffed. One group of nurses told me they sometimes tried to question a doctor's order about giving chemotherapy to very ill patients whom they feared would not tolerate the treatment. They were intimidated to approach the senior physicians, so instead would ask the medical residents first—even though they knew this group of junior doctors had less decision-making authority.[29] In the end, no

---

28 Given the difficulties nurses had understanding the term advocacy, I was curious if the term appeared, and how frequently, within documents that may be more relevant or familiar to nurses in India. The 32-page International Council for Nurses (ICN) Code of Ethics (2021) states, "Nurses are patient advocates and they maintain a practice culture that promotes ethical behaviour and open dialogue," and makes reference to "advocacy" 11 times. The Indian Nursing Council publishes a Code of Ethics and Professional Conduct (only available as a hard copy for purchase; in 2013, I purchased the 2006, First Edition) references "advocacy" once in the 15-page document: "The nurse advocates special provisions to protect vulnerable individuals/groups" (p. 6).

29 This is not unique to SICH. It is generally less intimidating for nurses to approach more junior physicians (postgraduate residents or fellows) or advanced practice nurses (nurse practitioners, clinical nurse specialists) than senior attending physicians, and it is often expected that nurses will not "jump the chain of command" related to patient needs. How personality traits, structural factors, organizational culture, and disciplinary training influence a nurse's ability or desire to advocate for patients is a key area for future research.

one listened to them. One nurse hinted at being angry at this, but the clear consensus was: "The doctor has ordered it [the chemotherapy], and we must give it compulsorily."

For the most part, neither nurses nor other healthcare providers at SICH viewed patient advocacy as one of the central duties of the nurse. Letting go of this expectation effectively removed the nurse from the often sticky position of feeling caught between the interests of the patient and the orders of the physician—a scenario that can create significant distress for nurses in American hospitals. There are a number of reasons why this may be. First, nurse training in India does not emphasize advocacy as a key aspect of nursing practice, as it tends to do in the West. Second, there was a lack of nursing role models to demonstrate how and when to advocate, and junior nurses were not socialized to advocate for patients; in fact, they were sometimes reprimanded by senior nurses for doing so. Third, the existence of significant power differentials between nurses and physicians made it highly unlikely for the nurse to want to risk questioning the doctor's orders, especially for contract nurses with less job security. Fourth is the reality that it doesn't make practical sense to expend energy advocating for therapies or resources that are simply unavailable. Other structural challenges inherent to the institution also made advocating for patients difficult or impossible. For example, nurses on the general wards rotated from ward to ward every three months; this seriously compromised continuity of patient care and a sense of allegiance to being part of a collective unit or team. Problematic and dangerous nurse-to-patient ratios also made it nearly impossible for most nurses to move beyond the technical and routinized aspects of care, let alone advocate for individual patients.

At times, I wondered if one must inherently respect a patient/person before feeling an obligation to advocate for them[30]; this idea is particularly salient within the context of the caste system, where lower status individuals are inherently deemed unworthy of respect. Advocacy can be a risky endeavor, and in many ways, nurses make themselves vulnerable by advocating for patients.[31] I also wondered if advocacy was viewed differently by nurses at

30 After returning from the field, I read a study by Negarandeh, Oskouie, Ahmadi, and Nikravesh (2008), in which 24 Iranian hospital nurses were interviewed to understand their conceptualization of patient advocacy. Interestingly, the nurses in the study echoed this hypothesis, explaining that advocacy could only take place when there was respect for the patients' individuality and their inherent human dignity, and that respect was a necessary requisite for establishing trust between the nurse and the patient and his or her family (Negarandeh et al., p. 461).

31 In her qualitative study of 15 adult nurses working on medical-surgical wards, Snowball (1996) found that nurses must have a sound professional identity, high levels of self-esteem and self-confidence, a therapeutic relationship with the patient based on a sense of shared humanity, a work environment that fosters a culture of care, and feel they can make an impact within the health care team, to assume this "risk" and engage in advocacy behaviors. Nurses at SICH generally lacked these crucial factors, and this may have greatly impacted their willingness and ability to advocate for patients.

SICH since other providers (e.g., social workers, ayahs, ward boys, family members) assumed many traditional nursing responsibilities. When many perform "nursing roles," does this somehow dilute the nurse's responsibility for patient advocacy and lessen the degree to which the nurse feels able, or obligated, to advocate for patients? Or, conversely, when others frequently observe nurses engaged in tasks not compatible with their training (such as cleaning or recording inventories in logbooks), does that diminish the general expectation of the nurse as advocate?[32] These are intriguing and important questions that could be springboards for future research. Another provocative, yet important, question is to more critically examine whether nurses are actually obligated to advocate for patients, or more specifically, are nurses in the context of resource-constrained hospitals such as SICH obligated to do so? While many assert that advocacy is a key component of ethical nursing practice[33] not everyone agrees and there is a body of literature that challenges this assumption.[34]

Concluding Thoughts

This book is not a comparison of cancer care in India to that in the U.S./West. Rather, it is an examination of how health care is experienced by the poor compared to the affluent; those marginalized by society to those with power and influence; those who have the means to access quality care to those who do not. It is an examination of how nurses, hospital staff, patients, and family members navigate and seek access to limited resources within a complex web of contexts-within-contexts, one where the intricate hierarchical system of health care (e.g., surgeons above internists, physicians above nurses, government nurses above contract nurses, etc.) is superimposed upon the ancient undercurrent of a caste system, dictating a person's inherent worth and value. Seen in this light, many of the interactions that may seem confusing, shocking, or incongruent during my fieldwork swing more sharply into focus. Overall, it seemed more important (and frankly often in the nurses' best

---

32 This concept is often referred to as "task shifting" and can be a helpful response to short-staffing and a way to more efficiently deliver patient care by optimizing a broader range of individuals' skills. An unfortunate side effect of such an approach, however, can be to create role confusion, diminish opportunities for nurses to work to their full potential, or result in the inappropriate assignment of tasks. For example, within Mayra et al. (2022), they discuss a "task shifting" approach which involved nurses and midwives being inappropriately assigned to the fire-extinguishing service. Also recall the experience of the student nurses in the ICU being assigned the task of cleaning equipment versus learning patient care skills.

33 Gaylord, N., & Grace, P. (1995). Nursing advocacy: An ethic of practice. *Nursing Ethics,* 2(1), 11–18; Jameton, A. (1984). *Nursing practice: The ethical issues.* Englewood, NJ: Prentice Hall; Love, M. B. (1995). Patient advocacy at the end of life. *Nursing Ethics,* 2(1), 3–9.

34 Edwards, S. D. (1996). What are the limits to the obligations of the nurse? *Journal of Medical Ethics,* 22(2), 90–94; Willard, C. (1996). The nurse's role as patient advocate: Obligation or imposition? *Journal of Advanced Nursing,* 24(1), 60–66.

interests) to reinforce and maintain the status quo of the power hierarchy, both within the hospital as well as in greater society, versus working to meet the needs of patients and family members.[35]

After returning from the field, I more clearly see that the same core problems exist in India as in the U.S.; they are simply packaged differently, in ways that are more, or less, familiar. These common realities are likely amplified by unique social and cultural complexities that impact nurses at SICH and in India: issues related to gender relations and domestic/marriage responsibilities; lingering effects of the caste system; the influence and legacy of British colonialism; the incredibly high volume of patients with very advanced disease; and the challenges of providing care in an environment where basic infrastructure is often lacking. But the reality is that nursing is hard work, whether it's in Delhi or Mexico City or rural Virginia. Issues of power and privilege are universal. At the end of the day, "nurses cannot treat patients with respect and dignity when they themselves are not well treated."[36] We must ask ourselves: is it fair to expect nurses to advocate for patients when no one is advocating for them? Is it right to expect nurses to put themselves at risk without giving them the basic tools to protect themselves on the job? We ignore the plight of nurses at our own peril, as we may find ourselves deeply regretful when it is we ourselves in the hospital bed, vulnerable and hurting, in desperate need of care.

Afterword

Since my fieldwork, the palliative care program and oncology services at SICH have undergone significant expansion, including the allocation of dedicated inpatient palliative care beds. Dr. Madhu continues to lead the

---

35 See Mayra et al.'s (2022) findings related to gender-based discrimination for women giving birth in India through interviews with nurse midwives in "Why do some health care providers disrespect and abuse women during childbirth in India?", *Women and Birth*, 35(1), e49–e59, that has relevance for the findings of this book. The authors explain, "The way she [the patient] is treated by care providers in the labour room while giving birth is an indication of how the society and her family values and treats her" (p. 6). This finding resonants with the experience of many patients with cancer I observed at SICH. Mayra et al. also state:

> Poverty increases women's vulnerability to disrespect and abuse. It is a cross cutting factor, which is associated to her caste and socio-economic status. Respondents opined that poor women have no option but to seek care in public hospitals…[and from one participant], 'When we think about abuse of women in health care, we need to be very clear that in societies where abuse is normal it's going to be very difficult to change that in a health environment.
>
> (pp. 5–6)

> See the authors' figure which depicts factors influencing disrespect and abuse of women during childbirth across various levels of the social-ecological model.

36 See Maluwa et al. (2012). Moral distress in nursing practice in Malawi. *Nursing Ethics*, 19(2), 196–207, 204.

palliative care program and has received numerous accolades in recognition of her and the team's work. The palliative care clinic nurses now see an even higher volume of patients, many of whom are referred earlier in their disease trajectory, allowing the team to provide better and more comprehensive symptom support. Opioid availability has improved, and more opioid formulations are available with greater consistency. Sponsorship of the home care palliative outreach program was assumed by a new nongovernmental organization which increased the number of vans, some of which specifically focus on community-based pediatric palliative care needs. Dr. Rashi has since left SICH to pursue work in a corporate hospital in Dandaka, and new leadership directs the pediatric ward and services.

Change has been slower to arrive on the general wards. Nursing Superintendent leadership has transitioned multiple times and the nurses still struggle with limited supplies, staffing, and personal protective equipment. No general ward nurses are teaching classes and it remains unclear if any of the recommendations (see Appendix) have been adopted.

Hameeda continued to decline in the local hospice but became exceedingly lonely and in the last few weeks of her life returned to SICH. She died on the general wards while being cared for by members of the palliative care team.

August 2023

References

American Association of Colleges of Nurses. End of Life Nursing Education Consortium (ELNEC). Available at: http://www.aacnnursing.org/ELNEC

American Nurses Association (ANA) Code of Ethics (2015). Available at: https://www.nursingworld.org/practice-policy/nursing-excellence/ethics/code-of-ethics-for-nurses/

Connors, A. F., Dawson, N. V., Desbiens, N. A., Fulkerson, W. J., Goldman, L., Knaus, W. A., ... & Wilke, S. M. (1995). A controlled trial to improve care for seriously ill hospitalized patients: The study to understand prognoses and preferences for outcomes and risks of treatments (SUPPORT). *JAMA, 274*(20), 1591–1598.

Das, P., Ramani, S., Newton-Lewis, T., Nagpal, P., Khalil, K., Gharai, D., ... & Kammowanee, R. (2022). "We are nurses–what can we say?": power asymmetries and Auxiliary Nurse Midwives in an Indian state. *Sexual and Reproductive Health Matters, 29*(2), 2031598.

Edwards, S. D. (1996). What are the limits to the obligations of the nurse? *Journal of Medical Ethics, 22*(2), 90–94.

Gaylord, N., & Grace, P. (1995). Nursing advocacy: An ethic of practice. *Nursing Ethics, 2*(1), 11–18.

George, M. S., Davey, R., Mohanty, I., & Upton, P. (2020). "Everything is provided free, but they are still hesitant to access healthcare services": why does the indigenous community in Attapadi, Kerala continue to experience poor access to healthcare? *International Journal for Equity in Health, 19*(1): 105.

Hadley, M. B., Blum, L. S., Mujaddid, S., Parveen, S., Nuremowla, S., Haque, M. E., & Ullah, M. (2007). Why Bangladeshi nurses avoid 'nursing': social and structural factors on hospital wards in Bangladesh. *Social Science & Medicine*, 64(6), 1166–1177.

Häggström, E., Mbusa, E., & Wadensten, B. (2008). Nurses' workplace distress and ethical dilemmas in Tanzanian health care. *Nursing Ethics*, 15(4), 478–491.

Hamed, S., Bradby, H., Ahlberg, B. M., & Thapar-Björkert, S. (2022). Racism in healthcare: A scoping review. *BMC Public Health*, 22(1), 988.

Harrowing, J., & Mill, J. (2010). Moral distress among Ugandan nurses providing HIV care: A critical ethnography. *International Journal of Nursing Studies*, 47(6), 723–731.

Healy, M. (2013). Indian Sisters: A History of Nursing and the State, 1907 – 2007. Routledge/Taylor & Francis Group: New York.

Indian Nursing Council. Code of Ethics and Professional Conduct (2006). Available for purchase: https://indiannursingcouncil.org/publications

Institute of Medicine, Committee on Approaching Death: Addressing Key End of Life Issues (2015). *Dying in America: Improving quality and honoring individual preferences at the end of life and relieving pain in America: A blueprint for transforming prevention, care, education, and research*. National Academies Press: Washington, D.C. Available at: https://www.ncbi.nlm.nih.gov/books/NBK285681/

International Council of Nurses (ICN). The ICN Code of Ethics for Nurses (2021). Available at: https://www.icn.ch/sites/default/files/2023-06/ICN_Code-of-Ethics_EN_Web.pdf

Jameton, A. (1984). *Nursing practice: The ethical issues*. Englewood, NJ: Prentice Hall.

LeBaron, V., Beck, S., Black, F., Maurer, M. & Palat, G. (2014). An ethnographic study of barriers to cancer pain management and opioid availability in India. *The Oncologist*, 19(5), 515–522.

Love, M. B. (1995). Patient advocacy at the end of life. *Nursing Ethics*, 2(1), 3–9.

Maluwa, V. M., Andre, J., Ndebele, P., & Chilemba, E. (2012). Moral distress in nursing practice in Malawi. *Nursing Ethics*, 19(2), 196–207.

Mayra, K., Matthews, Z., & Padmadas, S. S. (2022). Why do some health care providers disrespect and abuse women during childbirth in India?. *Women and Birth*, 35(1), e49–e59.

Mele, C. & Victor, D. (2017, September 1). Utah nurse handcuffed after refusing to draw patient's blood. *The New York Times*.

Morais, C. A., Aroke, E. N., Letzen, J. E., Campbell, C. M., Hood, A. M., Janevic, M. R., ... & Campbell, L. C. (2022). Confronting racism in pain research: A call to action. *The Journal of Pain*, 23(6), 878–892.

Nair, S. & Healey, M. (2006). A professional on the margins: Status issues in Indian nursing. Available at: https://archive.nyu.edu/bitstream/2451/34246/2/profession_on_the_margins.pdf

Negarandeh, R., Oskouie, F., Ahmadi, F., & Nikravesh, M. (2008). The meaning of patient advocacy for Iranian nurses. *Nursing Ethics*, 15(4), 457–467.

Nursing Outlook (September-October 2022); 70 (5); 681-774.

Porecha, M. (2013). DNA Special: Now, certified courses for ward boys, ayahs. *DNA India*. Available at: https://www.dnaindia.com/india/report-dna-special-now-certified-courses-for-ward-boys-ayahs-1861601

Pyone, T., Karvande, S., Gopalakrishnan, S., Purohit, V., Nelson, S., Balakrishnan, S. S., ... & Mathai, M. (2019). Factors governing the performance of

Auxiliary Nurse Midwives in India: A study in Pune district. *PLOS ONE, 14*(12), e0226831.

Rees, M. & Biggers, A. (2020). Racism in Healthcare: What you need to know. *Medical News Today*, Available at: https://www.medicalnewstoday.com/articles/racism-in-healthcare

Ross, C. (2018). Hospitals are confronting a new opioid crisis: An alarming shortage of pain meds, *StatNews*. Available at: https://www.statnews.com/2018/03/15/hospitals-opioid-shortage/

Shorideh, F. A., Ashktorab, T., & Yaghmaei, F. (2012). Iranian intensive care unit nurses' moral distress: a content analysis. *Nursing Ethics, 19*(4), 464–478.

Snowball, J. (1996). Asking nurses about advocating for patients:'reactive' and 'proactive' accounts. *Journal of Advanced Nursing, 24*(1), 67–75.

Tang, P. F., Johansson, C., Wadensten, B., Wenneberg, S., & Ahlström, G. (2007). Chinese nurses' ethical concerns in a neurological ward. *Nursing Ethics, 14*(6), 810–824.

The Economist (2013, March 23). Tryst with dynasty: Sonia Gandhi remains a preeminent, troubling politician, p.52.

The National Cancer Institute (2022). *Cancer Disparities*. Available at: https://www.cancer.gov/about-cancer/understanding/disparities

The National Institute of Nursing Research 2022-2026 Strategic Plan. Available at: https://www.ninr.nih.gov/aboutninr/ninr-mission-and-strategic-plan

University of Utah School of Medicine (Fall/Winter 2013/2014). Teaching the ward boys in Gujarat, India. Illuminations, 9(2); 11. Available at: https://medicine.utah.edu/documents/fall-winter-2013-2014linkspdf

University of Utah School of Medicine (2014), global health student research projects. Ward boys in Gujarat, India: Doing much more than meets the eye. Available at: https://medicine.utah.edu/global-health-education/student-research/india

U.S. Food & Drug Administration (FDA). FDA Drug Shortages. Available at: https://www.accessdata.fda.gov/scripts/drugshortages/default.cfm

VeneKlasen, L. & Miller, V. (2007). Power and Empowerment. In: *A new weave of power, people & politics: The action guide for advocacy and citizen participation*, VeneKlasen, L, & Miller, V. (Editors). Practical Action Publishing: Rugby, UK.

Verghese, A. (2012). *Cutting for stone*. Random House India: London.

Willard, C. (1996). The nurse's role as patient advocate: Obligation or imposition? *Journal of Advanced Nursing, 24*(1), 60–66.

Zaman, S. (2009). Ladies without lamps: Nurses in Bangladesh. *Qualitative Health Research, 19*(3), 366–374.

Zaman, S. (2013). Silent saviours: family members in a Bangladeshi hospital. *Anthropology & Medicine, 20*(3), 278–287.

11 Notes on Methods and Recommendations

About This Project

Gaining entrée into the field

In 2004, through a series of serendipitous connections, I was approached by an international cancer nongovernmental organization (here, simply called the NGO) to work collaboratively with local partners in Nepal to strengthen palliative care capacity. At the time I was working as an oncology palliative care nurse practitioner at a large University hospital in Washington, D.C. I had a long-standing interest in global health and working with this particular NGO seemed like a good fit—it was a secular, nonprofit organization, funded in part by the U.S.-based National Cancer Institute[1] and prioritized longitudinal and sustainable partnerships between cancer clinicians in low- and high-resource countries. It also helped that the directors of the program were smart, experienced, energetic, and fun. I joined the palliative care team, a small, but dedicated, group of interdisciplinary palliative care providers who traveled to low- and middle-income countries (LMICs) as requested by the host countries generally for 2–3-week blocks of time. The NGO reimbursed volunteers for travel expenses, but not for our time. (I used accrued vacation time for the majority of my trips.) Most of our efforts were focused on educational initiatives and capacity-building activities related to symptom management, raising awareness about palliative care, and advocating for improved opioid availability. Between the years of 2004 and 2014, most of my work with the NGO occurred in Nepal and India and to a more limited degree in Tanzania, Uganda, and Brazil.

My first trip to Nepal exposed me to the realities of cancer care in a lower income country, especially to what cancer care without pain control looks like. I returned from Nepal haunted by images of children in the pediatric cancer ward crying in agony. I had been an oncology nurse and

---

1 This NGO has since been restructured and does not exist in the same form as it did when I began my work with the organization. Many of the former palliative care-related initiatives have been taken up and continued by a corollary organization based in Canada.

DOI: 10.4324/9781003413158-17

palliative care nurse practitioner long enough by that time to know that most cancer pain can be controlled and the difference between a peaceful death and one of anguish. I was confused and deeply troubled that morphine was unavailable, even for patients days or hours from death. I became increasingly interested in understanding the experience of nurses caring for patients dying of cancer when basic tools to alleviate suffering are unavailable. If it is difficult to control a cancer patient's pain in a resource-rich environment like the U.S. (and too often it is), how do nurses in countries like Nepal or India manage? How do they advocate for patients who are suffering in pain—or do they even try given the limited resources? How do they bear witness to agony day after day when they have little means to help? Exploring these complex questions prompted my subsequent fieldwork in India.

Through my work with the NGO, I knew Dr. Madhu, an indomitable palliative care champion and pioneer at South Indian Cancer Hospital (SICH). I proposed the project to her, and she was enthusiastically supportive and agreed to sponsor my Fulbright application. Although this research could have been conducted at any number of hospitals (I considered sites in Nepal as well), SICH fulfilled the key criteria I was seeking—it was a cancer-focused hospital with a large nursing staff. It was also a government cancer hospital and represented where the majority of patients in India end up receiving care. It was also a hospital with a palliative care team that had achieved progress in ensuring availability of opioids, but that still experienced medication shortages and challenges with access to pain relief. Importantly, I also had a strong ally in Dr. Madhu who was willing to help me navigate critical bureaucratic hurdles, such as obtaining permission from the SICH Ethics Team,[2] the importance of which cannot be overstated.

Although I had been to SICH before, my fieldwork for this project was very different. For one, this time I was solo and not part of, nor representing, the NGO. My role as a researcher was completely separate and different. Second, with the NGO our focus had been the palliative care clinic and staff; for this project the scope was much broader—the entire hospital and beyond—with which I was not nearly as familiar. Third, my trips with the NGO were of much shorter duration and did not involve prolonged engagement and immersion in the field. I never had to figure out, for example, where the grocery store was, or how to do laundry, or what apartment to rent. This time, I wasn't visiting India—I was living in India. So, although the city and SICH were not completely new to me, in important ways this fieldwork represented the need for new strategies of reentry into the field.

2 The SICH Ethics Team is equivalent to an Institutional Review Board (IRB). IRB approval was also obtained from my home research institution.

Study Details and Data Sources[3]

My key data sources involved conversations with those most familiar with the fieldsite and observing people in their day-to-day lives. Conversations were sometimes informal and casual, and other times more structured, formal interviews. Formal interviews were audio-recorded (with permission) and included a translator if needed; casual conversations were recorded as "jottings" (small written notes) in the field and expanded into full field notes as soon as possible. Participants who agreed to be formally interviewed were verbally consented using an approved consent form which explained (in both the local language and English) the purpose of the project, the voluntary nature of their participation, potential risks and benefits, the possible publishing of their thoughts and ideas, and safeguards to protect their identity. No financial compensation was offered to participants, but I did give those who agreed to be formally interviewed a small gift of appreciation (a small first-aid pouch and pen, valued at less than $10) from my home University. At all times, I was transparent about my purpose in the field as a nurse conducting research.

My primary group of participants were nurses, but I was also interested in those who spent a lot of time interacting with nurses—such as physicians, patients, and family members, and so I observed and interviewed them as well. Overall, I formally interviewed 59 individuals (37 nurses, 22 others) and participated in countless more informal conversations. I was surprised at the number of volunteers at SICH during my fieldwork from high-resource countries, and I ended up formally interviewing many of them. One, because I was curious if they were seeing things in a similar way or asking similar questions as I was; and two, because some offered a unique perspective borne of having deep cultural and family roots in both a Western country and in India. Once I recovered from my initial stumbles in the field (such as being mistaken for a spy or naively assuming that the Medical Director had communicated with nursing leadership about my project prior to my arrival), the SICH Nursing Superintendent turned out to be one of my biggest champions and was instrumental in encouraging nurses to speak with me. Almost all of my interviews took place with an independent translator and transcripts of audio-recorded interviews that required translation were independently verified by two native speakers. Observations involved shadowing nurses and others as they went about their work and at times asking clarifying questions or actually participating in events (such as tea breaks, communal meals, or doctors' rounds). I made a concerted effort to observe nurses on different

3 For those interested in additional study details, particularly more granular details regarding data collection and analysis procedures, see Nurse moral distress and cancer pain management: An ethnography of oncology nurses in India. *Cancer Nursing*, 37(5), 331–344; 2014; and An ethnographic study of barriers to cancer pain management and opioid availability in India. *The Oncologist*, 19(5), 515–522; 2014.

wards, at different times of day, during different shifts, and on different days of the week. In total, I spent over 400 hours conducting fieldwork observations at SICH and relevant institutions.

All observational data and informal conversations were recorded in the field as small notes to jog my memory and written up as soon as possible into more detailed and expanded field notes (almost always that same day). Texting myself short messages on my mobile phone served as a discreet and acceptable way to record things as they happened in real time. Key quotes, phrases, and sensory-specific details were recorded in the field so I could recreate full conversations or observations as accurately and thoroughly as possible; not infrequently, I retreated to the hospital bathroom while in the field to write down an entire important conversation verbatim. Conversational passages within the book reflect actual dialogue, either portions of audio-recorded interviews or expanded field notes from informal conversation. All attributed statements at the beginning of chapters are direct quotes from in-depth interviews with participants.

I was an inherent anomaly as an outsider, but the concept of a nurse researcher was especially foreign to most of the hospital staff. Developing rapport is an important part of fieldwork and I utilized some strategies that were more effective than others. Wearing traditional clothing and paying attention to my personal appearance, particularly wearing Indian jewelry, went a long way in establishing connection with the nurses. I also developed rapport by conducting observations on each ward of the hospital on a rotating basis (e.g., a week on the male ward, a week on the female ward, etc.). I observed in all patient care areas of SICH, except for the operating theater. For comparison, and to more fully explore nurse-patient interactions and models of care delivery, I also conducted observations at nearby hospitals, both public and private, as well as with health-related community outreach teams.

Who—and what—to observe and interview were most often identified by a "snowball" technique. Meaning, I would be observing on a ward and a nurse would say, "oh you should talk to so-and-so" or "come to the hospital Diwali celebration." In the beginning, most of these opportunities occurred through the generosity of key informants who clued me in as to where I could, and should, direct my time and energy. As I met more people, developed different questions, and became more familiar with the setting in general, I had a better sense for who I needed to talk with and where I needed to go.

I did my best to understand an issue from multiple angles and perspectives by engaging with a diverse range of individuals, including ward boys and ayahs, patients and nurses, and senior physicians. Another way I did this was to ask similar questions of participants over time, phrased slightly differently, and to compare what I was observing to what people were telling me. I also looked to medical documents and other written artifacts to confirm—or question—what I was discovering. Striking discrepancies often existed between what participants told me and what I observed. For example, nurses would tell me that they saw "serving patients" and "providing moral support" as important parts of their job, but then would interact with patients and family members in ways I interpreted as incongruent with their words. Reconciling this discrepancy between verbal assertions and actions was one of the key challenges of my work (and is discussed further within Chapter 10).

It is also possible that participants simply told me what they thought I wanted to hear as a way to placate me as the researcher or to represent themselves in a certain light.[4] There was also a strong cultural tendency to say something existed, or was happening, in order to be accommodating, but then upon further investigation, discover this was not actually the case. One example of this is reflected in my attempt to obtain a copy of the nurse's job description at Desino Hospital—which at first I was led to believe was available and then was eventually told did not exist. However, this is not a work of journalism, and it was not my goal to corroborate and fact-check every story and experience shared with me. By and large, I took people for their word. Even if events did not happen exactly as people described or the figures were off, their unique perception and viewpoint mattered—as did the simple fact they chose that particular story to share. For example, I did not confirm Ruth's account of the surgical patient who committed suicide on her night shift; even if I wanted to, I'm not sure how I would have, given the limited meaningful patient-focused nursing documentation. It also did not seem wise to run around the hospital asking others if they could verify this sensitive story.

This final book represents a careful integration of interview and observational data that has gone through multiple iterations and revisions. Details were cross-checked with participants, both while I was in the field and after I returned home. Before leaving the fieldsite, I invited all staff to a presentation where I discussed preliminary findings to confirm that I was "on track." This member-checking event is described within Chapter 9.

Generalizability

One may rightfully question whether what they read here applies only to one hospital in India—and if so, why should they care? It is a fair question. My strong belief, based on my personal experiences in other LMIC hospitals, prior research,[5] and what many other global health practitioners and

---

4 My conversations and questions may have changed how nurses talked with me during interviews and acted when I observed on the wards. As Thomas (1993) suggests, "probing for some types of information will create a new awareness by participants. This in turn changes their narratives, their behaviors, and their own 'on-stage performances' in ways that alter the topic" (pp. 67–88). See: Thomas, J. (1993). *Doing critical ethnography*. Newbury Park, CA: Sage Publications.
5 The reader is referred to relevant publications (both journal articles and full-length works) that are referenced within Chapter 10 or listed in the Appendix.

local providers have described to me, is that these findings represent the realities of most government and public-sector hospitals in lower income countries (and likely some higher income countries) around the world. In the field, people often spontaneously volunteered that the challenges faced by SICH, the employees, and the patients were not unique to the specific institution, or India for that matter. Many shared that they viewed SICH as a typical government hospital in a lower income country—an overburdened and under-resourced institution charged with caring for the poorest of the poor.

I would also suggest that issues related to caring for patients with advanced cancer who are socially, economically, or geographically marginalized, how to best support nurses working under difficult circumstances with limited resources, and the complex power dynamics that infuse *all* healthcare interactions—wherever they may occur—are challenges that have applicability around the world and make this research relevant beyond the specifics of India.

Dilemmas, Struggles, and Limitations

Remaining Authentic

My time in the field was a continual dance of trying to blend in and build rapport while striving to remain authentic. I did my best, but I am certain there was room for improvement. I wore a simple ring on my left hand to avoid unwanted advances and did not always correct people who assumed I was engaged or married. I was vague about my age—since being a 38-year-old unmarried woman without children was so outside cultural norms as to make me positively alien. I accepted food when I was about to burst, did not admit to being agnostic so as to not offend the evangelical Christian nurses I hoped to interview, remained silent when I witnessed egregious violations of basic healthcare practice, and feigned patience and humor when repeatedly asked intrusive personal questions.

The truth is there is no getting around the fact that I had an agenda—and one on a timeline. To complete my research, I needed to be accepted and liked—and some things about me were inherently unlikeable, given the cultural context. At times, my anxiety about delays in the field caused me to make decisions that actually cost me more time in the long run. A prime example being when my earnest note-taking—before I had adequately established rapport—triggered the rumor that I was a spy sent from the U.S. government.

I remain conflicted over the reality that completing this project has facilitated professional advancement. I'm not sure I have any clear resolution to this, except to note the importance of being aware of this tension and to be particularly mindful of how we disseminate findings and give back to participants and fieldsites—which I have attempted to do.

My Own Biases and Positionality

Ethnographers are often told "you are the instrument." What they mean is that in other forms of scientific inquiry, researchers may use more "objective" metrics or surveys to record and capture information. With ethnography, it is the human researcher—warts and all—that is absorbing, processing, and repackaging the information. This is a tremendous responsibility. I remember a mentor once describing the importance of being a "well-calibrated instrument." Being a well-calibrated instrument requires you to be self-aware and as transparent as possible about your own position in the world, biases, and assumptions, and how they influenced what you heard and saw in the field, and how you chose to represent it.[6]

I came to this project as a middle-class American White woman trained as a cancer nurse and beginning scientist. My gender, professional background, nationality, socioeconomic status, and skin color all greatly influenced how I was treated in India, the access to information and space I received, and the affordances I was granted—in overt ways and in ways I did not realize at the time and may still remain unaware. As just one example, being out all day with the home care team obviously raised the issue of needing to find restrooms, which is not easy in India as public bathrooms are scarce and often unpleasant. Because of my skin color and status as an American visitor, slipping into a hotel lobby to use a restroom was easy; but for the home care team, it represented a serious logistic issue they had to contend with on a daily basis. Gender, with the exception of being a point of connection with the female-majority nursing staff, was more of a hindrance, often attracting unwanted attention or creating obstacles in terms of how I could conduct the research (e.g., needing to change to a female translator, even though the male translator I initially hired was more proficient). But, overall, being Western and White were clear status advantages that automatically ensured a whole host of unearned privileges, and it is critically important to acknowledge how they influenced my fieldwork. I also brought clinical assumptions to the project based on my background as a cancer nurse. Mainly, that patients with cancer deserve access to pain control, that the benefits of opioids for this patient population outweigh the risks, and that nurses have certain professional and moral obligations to alleviate suffering. These ideas influenced how I interpreted events and interactions and are important for the reader to understand.

---

6 Being reflexive, or turning things back on itself for meaningful reflection, is a vital component of conducting ethnographic research (and qualitative research in general). See Foley, D. E. (2002). Critical ethnography: The reflexive turn. *International Journal of Qualitative Studies in Education, 15*(4), 469–490; Lather, P. (1986). Issues of validity in openly ideological research: Between a rock and a soft place. *Interchange, 17*(4), 63–84; Madison, D. S. (2005). *Critical ethnography: Method, ethics, and performance.* Thousand Oaks, CA: SAGE Publications; Street, A. F. (1992). *Inside nursing: A critical ethnography of clinical nursing practice*: Albany: State University of New York (SUNY) Press.

When to Intervene

Separating me as a "nurse" from me as a "researcher" was not easy, especially when confronted with patients who were clearly suffering or needed assistance. It was particularly difficult for me to watch nurses mix and administer chemotherapy without the proper protection or to see patients suffer when it seemed there was a straightforward way to lessen their pain. I wasn't treading new ground with these types of clinical dilemmas, and many researchers have had to grapple with similar conflicts in the field.[7] I had no set formula for this and approached situations on a case-by-case basis as they arose. In general, I assumed a basic stance of noninterference. Although painful and difficult at times to sit back and "do nothing", I continually reminded myself that I was a researcher who happened to be a nurse and that I had not been invited to the fieldsite to provide clinical support. In fact, I was rarely asked to provide clinical help. In the few instances when I was, I provided general guidance and input but did not provide any direct, hands-on clinical care. In other situations, I felt compelled to gently suggest alternative courses of action to help patients (recall me suggesting to Sister Asha that perhaps she could contact the doctor to verify giving the blood transfusion or me conveying dismay about the patient who had run out of morphine tablets on the night shift, and Sister Agnes realizing that she could get extra morphine tablets for her patient from the pediatric ward). I tried not to do this frequently, but when I did suggest alternatives, some nurses accepted these suggestions easily and would follow through, almost as though the idea had simply not occurred to them; others did not, and I let it drop.

Language

I am not fluent in Hindi or the regional languages of the State where my fieldwork occurred and therefore had to rely on a translator to help conduct most of my formal interviews. My language deficiencies also influenced with whom— and how—I could interact informally, and I tended to gravitate toward those with a greater fluency in English. This is a significant limitation of my fieldwork. However, I was helped by the fact that it was extremely common to pepper Hindi and the local languages with English words and phrases. This, combined with the benefit of strong nonverbal communication cues, and over time, a rudimentary comprehension of Hindi and the primary local language, allowed me to glean the core message of most conversations and interactions in the field.

Protecting Participants

As the project progressed, more and more dilemmas surfaced about how to best present the findings. It is not easy to present members of your own

---

7 See: Morse, J. M. (2007). Ethics in action: Ethical principles for doing qualitative health research. *Qualitative Health Research, 17*(8), 1003–1005.

profession in a less than flattering light, especially those with whom you have shared meals, laughed, and cried. I seriously struggled with questions such as: how do I constructively disseminate findings that may not reflect well on an institution or certain individuals[8]? How do I balance publishing findings to raise awareness of the realities of nursing practice in a setting such as SICH with protecting the confidentiality of my participants?[9] Should I disguise the name of institutions and my geographic location? If so, how could I do that without stripping the book of rich, contextual details? Besides changing names of participants, which identifying details should be altered or removed? Would it be enough? How much is too much? Were there actually some participants who would *want* to be identified? What about my flatmates, who knew I was doing research at the hospital but probably did not expect to show up in a book?

In the end, I—and others with expertise and judgment I trust—read through the book asking: "if the world knew this was me, would I be embarrassed?" If the answer was yes, or a strong maybe, I made an especial effort to disguise or change identifying details; in some cases, when I wasn't sure and the risk seemed too great, I deleted or omitted material to err on the side of protecting participants. I changed all institution and individual names, took pains to de-identify locations to the best of my ability, and strove to alter identifying details to the point where it would be extremely difficult—or ideally impossible—to figure out exactly who was who. The passage of time has also helped, as since my fieldwork was completed, staff have retired, changed positions, moved away, or otherwise ended their affiliation with SICH.

Time in the Field

How much time in the field is enough? I suppose it depends on who you ask and what you are trying to accomplish. By traditional standards, nine months (the amount of time I was in the field) is on the shorter end of the spectrum. Other ethnographies span years or even decades. Ideally, I would have stayed longer, but my Fulbright funding was up, as was my foreigner's residency permit, and I needed to return home. While a longer time in the

---

8 See Kayser-Jones, J. (2003). Continuing to conduct research in nursing homes despite controversial findings: Reflections by a research scientist *Qualitative Health Research*, 13(1), 114–128, for an excellent discussion by a nurse scientist regarding how to disseminate difficult results. This nurse scientist also wrote an ethnography about nursing care of the aged, "Old, Alone & Neglected," which is included in the Appendix.

9 See Harrowing, J., Mill, J., Spiers, J., Kulig, J., & Kipp, W. (2010). Culture, context and community: Ethical considerations for global nursing research. *International Nursing Review*, 57(1), 70–77; and Ellis, C. (1995). Emotional and ethical quagmires in returning to the field. *Journal of Contemporary Ethnography*, 24(1), 68–98. Both articles offer thought-provoking and important discussions related to ethical dilemmas related to ethnographic research.

field would certainly have yielded more data, I am not convinced it would be new data. By around month five, I started to see similar patterns and redundancy within my observations and interviews. In fact, observations started to even get a little boring because I was seeing the same things over and over again. By month seven and eight, this became even more apparent, and I started spending less time observing and interviewing participants and more time reviewing and analyzing field notes and interview transcripts. From a researcher's point of view, this is reassuring—and suggests the most salient themes have been identified.

Giving Back

Good and ethical fieldwork relationships call for reciprocity on the part of the researcher. In keeping with this principle, I taught, and helped a nurse teach, a series of classes for the nurses based on their requests for information related to chemotherapy and cancer care. To my knowledge, these classes were one of the few (only?) professional development opportunities made available to the general ward nurses. Additionally, I created and distributed laminated chemotherapy "cheat sheet" pocket-sized instruction cards to all the nurses[10] (see Appendix). I also taught a number of classes specifically for the palliative care team and those who came to SICH for palliative care training. Organizing and teaching the classes was time-consuming but one of the most rewarding aspects of my time in India. I also donated medical supplies, books, and toys to the pediatric ward. Paul gave a gently used iPod to Hameeda which we programmed with Bollywood music for her to listen to when she was in the hospice. Some of these efforts were of limited benefit and possible harm, which I discuss in the book. At times, I also made carefully considered decisions to help individuals financially; for example, I gave my primary research assistant, who went remarkably above and beyond in supporting this project, additional money at the end of my fieldwork so she could buy a washing machine for her family, something that she desperately wanted to help save her hours of work each day.

Another way I tried to contribute was by preparing a report for the hospital administration about ways to better support the SICH nursing staff.[11] During interviews, I asked nurses, "What could make your job here better?" Most had a surprisingly difficult time answering this question, despite the work-related challenges they shared with me. I believe this was, in part, because the question caught them off-guard; no one had ever asked them this

10 The creation of the chemotherapy cards was the product of careful consultations with pharmacists and nurses both at SICH and other cancer care institutions in the U.S.
11 Describing "what is" but also "what could be" is a core principle of critical ethnography and considered an ethical obligation for qualitative researchers. See Denzin, N. K., & Giardina, M. D. (2010). *Qualitative inquiry and human rights*. Walnut Creek, CA: Left Coast Press; Thomas, J. (1993). *Doing critical ethnography*. Newbury Park, CA: Sage Publications.

before or given voice to their opinions about how to improve their situation in the hospital. In contrast, a few nurses had very specific suggestions and were eager to share their thoughts. After returning to the U.S. I summarized and wrote up these recommendations into both an executive summary and a more detailed full-length report that clearly laid out my key findings and specific ways to support nurses at SICH and those practicing in similar resource-constrained settings. I had both documents translated into the local language and sent English and translated versions electronically and hard copies via Fed-Ex directly to my former research assistant at SICH for distribution to the staff nurses, nursing superintendent, physician leaders, and hospital administrators. I also shared copies with individuals not based full time in India, but that I knew cared deeply about the nurses at SICH—such as some of the Western volunteers I met during my fieldwork. A copy of the executive summary was also shared by Dr. Madhu with the State Health Minister, and these recommendations were also published in the open-access *Indian Journal of Palliative Care*[12]; a number of SICH nurses and other personnel were coauthors on this paper. To my knowledge, these recommendations were well received by SICH staff and leadership, but to what degree, and how successfully, they have, or have not, been implemented is uncertain. An abbreviated version of these recommendations is included in the Appendix.

References

Denzin, N. K., & Giardina, M. D. (2010). *Qualitative inquiry and human rights*. Walnut Creek, CA: Left Coast Press.

Ellis, C. (1995). Emotional and ethical quagmires in returning to the field. *Journal of Contemporary Ethnography*, 24(1), 68–98.

Foley, D. E. (2002). Critical ethnography: The reflexive turn. *International Journal of Qualitative Studies in Education, 15*(4), 469–490.

Harrowing, J., Mill, J., Spiers, J., Kulig, J., & Kipp, W. (2010). Culture, context and community: Ethical considerations for global nursing research. *International Nursing Review, 57*(1), 70–77.

Kayser-Jones, J. (2003). Continuing to conduct research in nursing homes despite controversial findings: Reflections by a research scientist. *Qualitative Health Research, 13*(1), 114–128.

Kayser-Jones, J. (1990). *Old, alone and neglected: Care of the aged in Scotland and the United States*. University of California Press. Oakland, California.

Lather, P. (1986). Issues of validity in openly ideological research: Between a rock and a soft place. *Interchange, 17*(4), 63–84.

LeBaron, V. T., Palat, G., Sinha, S., Chinta Kumari, S., Jamina, B. J., Pilla, U. L., Podduturi, N., Shapuram, Y., Vennela, P., Rapelli, V., Lalani, Z., & Beck, S. L. (2017). Recommendations to support nurses and improve the delivery of oncology and palliative care in India. *Indian Journal of Palliative Care*, 23(2), 188–198.

---

12 See LeBaron et al. (2017). Recommendations to support nurses and improve the delivery of oncology and palliative care in India. *Indian Journal of Palliative Care*, 23(2), 188–198.

LeBaron, V., Beck, S., Black, F., & Palat, G. (2014). Nurse moral distress and cancer pain management: An ethnography of oncology nurses in India. *Cancer Nursing, 37*(5), 331–344.

LeBaron, V., Beck, S., Black, F., Maurer, M., & Palat, G. (2014). An ethnographic study of barriers to cancer pain management and opioid availability in India. *The Oncologist, 19*(5), 515–522.

Madison, D. S. (2005). *Critical ethnography: Method, ethics, and performance.* Thousand Oaks, CA: SAGE Publications.

Morse, J. M. (2007). Ethics in action: Ethical principles for doing qualitative health research. *Qualitative Health Research, 17*(8), 1003–1005.

Street, A. F. (1992). *Inside nursing: A critical ethnography of clinical nursing practice*: Albany: State University of New York (SUNY) Press.

Thomas, J. (1993). *Doing critical ethnography.* Newbury Park, CA: Sage Publications.

Glossary of Medical Terms

Allopurinol: a medication that prevents the toxic accumulation of uric acid, which can be caused by the cancer itself or released by cells when they are destroyed by chemotherapy.

Asepsis: practices and techniques, such as handwashing and wearing gloves, used to reduce contamination and the risk of infection.

Brachytherapy: a form of localized radiation treatment used to treat cancer where a source of radiation is placed/implanted near the tumor.

Buccal: pertaining to the cheek or oral cavity.

Butterfly needle: a small, metal needle with "winged" tips commonly used for drawing blood, but sometimes also used for administrating fluids or medications intravenously.

Cachexia: a complex metabolic disorder associated with serious illness that results in significant muscle wasting and weight loss. Patients suffering from cachexia are described as "cachectic."

Cannula: a thin tube inserted into a vein or body cavity to administer medicine or drain off fluid.

Central line or catheter: a more permanent type of intravenous (IV) access that allows frequently given drugs, like chemotherapy, to be administered into larger veins (as opposed to a peripheral IV inserted temporarily into smaller veins). Central lines are more secure and help reduce the discomfort of repeated needle sticks. They also reduce the likelihood that drugs can leak from the vein into surrounding soft tissue, which can be extremely damaging.

Chest physiotherapy: a technique involving percussion (a specific type of tapping/clapping) of a patient's chest and/or back to loosen and expel mucus from the lungs to help them breathe more efficiently.

Colposcopy: a procedure where the cervix is examined with a special magnifying device to check for evidence of cervical cancer.

Computerized Axial Tomography (CAT or CT) scan: a type of X-ray imaging commonly used to diagnose, stage, and monitor cancer.

Edematous: medical term for swollen. Edema results from excess fluid trapped in the soft tissue of the body and can occur due to a variety of reasons, including underlying medical conditions or infiltrated IVs.

Hydrocortisone: a corticosteroid, in this context given to mitigate the effects of a potential allergic reaction to chemotherapy.

Infiltrated: an IV whose fluid has leaked out of the vein and into the surrounding soft tissue.

IV: an abbreviation for "intravenous" or "into the vein." A very common medical procedure where a small needle or catheter (tube) is inserted into a patient's vein, allowing medication or fluid to be given directly into the patient's bloodstream where it is quickly absorbed by the body.

Karaya powder: a hydrocolloid powder used in stoma care to absorb moisture and help protect the skin.

Magnetic Resonance Imaging (MRI):   an imaging test that uses large magnet and radio waves to create detailed pictures. MRIs are especially helpful in providing structural information about organs and soft tissues not captured by X-ray exams. MRI scans can be useful to help diagnose and monitor certain types of cancers.

Metrogel: an antibiotic which can be used topically to help control infection and odor. Also known by the trade name Flagyl or the generic name metronidazole.

Multiple myeloma: a type of blood cancer that involves plasma cells (a type of white blood cell).

Mucositis: inflamed mucus membranes of the mouth (and/or gut) that can result in pain and difficulty swallowing and talking. Mucositis is a common side effect of chemotherapy and radiation treatments and can be a source of significant pain and distress for patients with cancer.

Nasogastric tube: A tube inserted into a patient's nostril that is passed through the esophagus and into the stomach. A nasogastric tube can be used to provide short-term supplemental feeding for patients with difficulty eating and drinking or as a way to decompress the gut or drain stomach contents.

Neutropenia: a common problem for patients with cancer due to the side effects of therapy or due to the cancer itself. Neutropenia occurs when the number of neutrophils (white blood cells that fight infection) drop to dangerously low levels, putting patients at high risk for serious bacterial or fungal infections. One way to protect patients with neutropenia is to isolate them and reduce their exposure to potential pathogens. **Febrile neutropenia** is a life-threatening emergency when patients who are neutropenic develop a fever, indicating potential infection.

Non-rebreather oxygen mask: a special face mask that can deliver a higher concentration of oxygen to patients experiencing respiratory difficulty.

Ostomy: an opening (stoma) connecting an internal organ to the surface of the body (for example, a colostomy). Ostomies can be surgically created for therapeutic reasons, or they may be caused by the cancer itself. An ostomy bag is a device put over the opening to manage odor and capture fluid to prevent it from leaking onto the patient's skin.

Paracentesis: a procedure to remove excess fluid from the abdomen by draining it with a small flexible tube. Tumors can cause excess fluid to be produced or block fluid from proper drainage by the lymph system, resulting in a build-up of fluid in the lining of the abdomen (peritoneal cavity), which can be extremely uncomfortable for patients. The discomfort can be temporarily relieved by periodically draining the fluid.

Parenteral: medications that are given via infusion or injection, not by mouth.

Positron Emission Tomography (PET): an imaging test that measures metabolic activity and provides information about the functioning of organs and tissues. PET scans can be useful to help diagnose and monitor certain types of cancers.

Retinoblastoma: cancer that originates in the retina of the eye; it most commonly affects young children and can cause blindness if left untreated.

Rhabdomyosarcoma: a type of sarcoma, or cancer that forms from the muscle and soft tissue.

Saline: sterile salt-water fluid that is given intravenously to patients who have low blood pressure, are dehydrated, or need additional medical support.

Sentinel event: a serious adverse patient care related event that results in death or permanent disability. Depending on the context, healthcare organizations may be required to track and report sentinel events to regulatory authorities.

Septic: a patient who is experiencing sepsis, a life-threatening systemic infection characterized, in part, by low blood pressure.

Sharps: any medical device/instrument with sharp edges or points (e.g., needles, syringes, scalpels) that can cut or pierce the skin when handled. Sharps that have been used for patient care are considered contaminated and a biohazard as they can transmit bloodborne pathogens if they puncture someone else. Ideally, used sharps are disposed of in secure, specially designated containers and destroyed as biomedical waste.

Spinal cord compression: a serious complication of cancer where the tumor presses on the spinal cord, causing severe pain, and if left untreated, incontinence and eventual paralysis.

Subcutaneously: administering medication (or sometimes other fluids) into the fatty tissue under the skin (e.g., an insulin shot for a diabetic patient). It has a slower route of absorption compared to intravenous administration.

Sucralfate: an antiseptic ulcer drug, which can be used topically to help prevent bleeding. Also known by the trade name Carafate.

Tracheostomy: a surgical opening made from a patient's windpipe (trachea) to the front of the neck. It is often done to help patients breathe who have head and neck cancers.

Tramadol: an opioid pain medication. Generally considered a "weaker" opioid by palliative care specialists and often inadequate to treat severe cancer pain.

Tumor lysis syndrome: a life-threatening metabolic complication that can occur after the initiation of chemotherapy. It is caused by large numbers of cells dying rapidly and releasing their intracellular contents into the bloodstream, resulting in potentially fatal levels of potassium, calcium, etc.

Universal precautions: an approach to infection control that involves using protective equipment (e.g., gloves) to avoid contact with bodily fluids for all patients, regardless of known pathogens.

Uric acid: a natural cellular waste product that can accumulate to toxic levels due to cancer and cancer therapy.

Vesicant: a class of chemotherapy agents that are especially damaging if they infiltrate (leak) into the soft tissue; when vesicants infiltrate it is called extravasation. In the worst cases, extravasation can lead to extensive soft tissue damage or the functional loss of an extremity.

Voveran: a non-steroidal anti-inflammatory drug (NSAID) used to treat pain; in the same class of medications as ibuprofen/Motrin in the U.S. Also known as Diclofenac.

Appendix 1

Abbreviated policy and practice recommendations based on the research are summarized below[1]

Recommendation 1: Make Safety a Priority

- Create a statewide, standardized chemotherapy training and certification course that is mandatory for all personnel who may handle, mix, or administer chemotherapy (nurses, ward boys, ayahs). This course should include basic information about cancer biology, safe ways to handle, mix, and administer chemotherapy, and prevention and management of side effects related to chemotherapy. Particular attention should be given to preventing extravasations (chemotherapy leaking from the vein into the soft tissue).
- Provide equipment to protect nurses from unnecessary inhalation and skin exposure when handling, mixing, and administering chemotherapy. This includes masks, gloves, and aprons and appropriate ventilation systems ("hoods") to safely mix chemotherapy.
- Pharmaceutical companies who distribute chemotherapy agents should be required to include adequate amounts of protective supplies for nurses along with their shipments, and senior and head nurses should be responsible for ensuring they are used.
- Larger concerns about safe disposal of biohazardous waste is a crucial environmental and safety issue that needs to be addressed by the local and state governments, but most urgently hospital staff, patients, and family members must be protected from unnecessary exposure to chemotherapy and needlesticks while in the hospital.

---

1   For a full discussion of these recommendations, see Recommendations to support nurses and improve the delivery of oncology and palliative care in India. *Indian Journal of Palliative Care*, 23(2), 188–198; 2017.

- Ensure running water, soap, and disposable towels are available to promote handwashing to prevent infection and chemotherapy contamination.
- Educate nurses and other hospital personnel (ward boys, ayahs) about the importance of safe needle practices. Provide tools such as plastic point-of-use trays and appropriate disposal bins to protect everyone from accidental needlesticks.

Recommendation 2: Support Individualized Patient Care

- Ratios on general wards of one nurse to sometimes over 50 patients make it impossible for the nurse to provide individualized patient care. It is important to hire more nurses to have better nurse-to-patient ratios, and at the same time to encourage nurses to practice to the full extent of their training.
- Reduce nonessential clerical work performed by nurses.

Recommendation 3: Invest in Nurse Education and Professional Development

- All nursing educational curricula (both BSc and GNM level) should include cancer and palliative care content. Nurses should be taught the basics of cancer care, pain assessment and management, opioid use, wound care, and how to provide compassionate care to dying patients.
- Provide incentives for healthcare institutions to organize and fund continuing education programs and training for nurses.
- Support nurses in community outreach efforts, particularly related to cancer prevention and screening.
- Hold senior nurses and nurse administrators accountable for patient-related outcomes.

Recommendation 4: Reduce Barriers to Opioid Availability and Pain Management

- Ensure that all health institutions in the State have an adequate supply of opioids especially oral and intravenous morphine to treat pain.
- Support State and Central Government health policies and initiatives that facilitate access to opioids for medicinal purposes.
- Support education related to palliative care and use of opioids to manage pain.
- Increase nurse accountability for assessing and managing pain in the hospital setting.
- Consider creation of a specially trained team of nurses to improve access to opioids in rural areas, as has been successfully done in countries such as Uganda.

Recommendation 5: Engage in Future Training and Research Opportunities

- Actively encourage and support training and research that

  - involves nurses in finding solutions to challenges they encounter on the job;
  - improves access to cancer care, especially screening/prevention and palliative care;
  - enhances pain and symptom management for patients;
  - improves working conditions of nurses, especially related to needle and chemotherapy safety;
  - educates nurses, assistant personnel (ward boys, ayahs), family attendants, and the general public about cancer care, chemotherapy, palliative care, and pain management;
  - improves health policies related to access to opioids for patients

For Further Reading:

Publications in Peer-Reviewed Journals Related to this Fieldwork

LeBaron, V., Palat, G., Sinha, S., Chinta Kumari, S., Jamina, B. J., Pilla, U. L., Podduturi, N., Shapuram, Y., Vennela, P., Rapelli, V., Lalani, Z., & Beck, S. L. (2017). Recommendations to support nurses and improve the delivery of oncology and palliative care in India. *Indian Journal of Palliative Care, 23*(2), 188–198.

LeBaron, V., Iribarren, S., Perri, S., & Beck, S. (2015). A practical fieldguide to conducting nursing research in low and middle-income countries. *Nursing Outlook, 63*(4), 462–473.

LeBaron, V., Beck, S., Black, F., & Palat, G. (2014). Nurse moral distress and cancer pain management: An ethnography of oncology nurses in India. *Cancer Nursing, 37*(5), 331–344.

LeBaron, V., Beck, S., Black, F., Maurer, M., & Palat, G. (2014). An ethnographic study of barriers to cancer pain management and opioid availability in India. *The Oncologist, 19*(5), 515–522.

Related Scholarly Works (India; Cancer; Nursing; Ethnography)

Enduring Cancer: Life, Death, and Diagnosis in Delhi.
Dwaipayan Banerjee, Duke University Press, 2020.
Indian Sisters: A History of Nursing and the State, 1907–2007.
Madelaine Healey, Routledge Press, 2013.
Improvising Medicine: An African Oncology Ward in an Emerging Cancer Epidemic.
Julie Livingston, Duke University Press, 2012.
Old, Alone, and Neglected: Care of the Aged in Scotland and the United States.
Jeannie Schmit Kayser-Jones, University of California Press, 1981.

Inside Nursing: A Critical Ethnography of Clinical Nursing Practice.
Annette Fay Street, State University of New York (SUNY) Press, 1992.
The Cancer Unit: An Ethnography.
Carol P. Hanley Germain, Nursing Resources, 1979.

General Readership (Non-Fiction)

Caste: The Origins of Our Discontents.
Isabel Wilkerson, Random House, 2020, 2023.
Beyond the Beautiful Forevers: Life, Death, and Hope in a Mumbai Undercity.
Katherine Boo, Random House, 2014.
May You Be the Mother of a Hundred Sons.
Elisabeth Bumiller, Penguin Books India, 1991.

General Readership (Fiction and memoir that provide additional context about India)

Mohsin Hamid, Riverhead Books, 2012.
Henna for the Broken-Hearted
Sharell Cook, Macmillan, 2011.
A Fine Balance
Rohinton Mistry, Vintage, 2010.
The God of Small Things
Arundhati Roy, Random House, 2008.
White Tiger
Aravind Adiga, Simon & Schuster, 2008.
Home
Manju Kapur, Random House India, 2007.
The Space Between Us
Thrity Umrigar, HarperPerennial, 2005.

Appendix 2

Chemotherapy information card created for nurses at SICH

Drug Name/ Diluent	Class/Primary Cancer Indications	Adverse Reactions/Common Side Effects	Nursing Considerations
Bleomycin NS	• Anti-tumor antibiotic; lymphomas, squamous cell, testicular	• Pulmonary toxicities (pneumonitis, pulmonary fibrosis), allergic reaction, skin problems (rash, redness, tender skin), fever	• Monitor for difficulty breathing; allergic reactions
Carboplatin NS or D5W	• Alkylating agent; cervical, ovarian, lung cancer	• Peripheral neuropathies, kidney damage (at high doses), nausea/vomiting, myelosuppression, allergic reactions with ≥ six infusions	High risk nausea/vomiting; give anti-emetics; if ≥ six infusions, give premedication to avoid allergic reaction
Cisplatin NS	• Alkylating agent; cervical, testicular, ovarian, bladder	• Kidney damage, hearing loss, peripheral neuropathies, nausea/vomiting, myelosuppression	Pre- and post-hydration (1–2 L 0.9% NS) is crucial; taste changes (metallic taste of food); decreased blood levels of Mg++, K+, Ca+; high risk nausea/vomiting; give anti-emetics
Cyclophosphamide NS or D5W	• Alkylating agent; cervical, lymphomas, leukemia, breast, neuroblastoma	Nausea/vomiting, hemorrhagic cystitis, (bleeding from bladder), myelosuppression	Pre- and post-hydration (1–2 L 0.9% NS) is crucial; give bladder protectant (Mesna), monitor for hematuria; high risk nausea/ vomiting; give anti-emetics
Cytarabine (ara-C) NS or D5W	• Antimetabolite; leukemia	• Myelosuppression, nausea/vomiting	Conjunctivitis with doses >1,000 mg/m2 requires steroid eye drops; cerebellar toxicity with doses >1,000 mg/m2
Dacarbazine (DTIC) NS or D5W	• Alkylating agent; metastatic melanoma, Hodgkin's lymphoma	• Myelosuppression, nausea/vomiting; thrombophlebitis (reduce by hot compress to arm, slow infusion rate, dilute drug appropriately, may need 500 ml diluent)	• High risk nausea/vomiting, be sure to give anti-emetics; thrombophlebitis **protect drug from light**

(Continued)

Drug Name/Diluent	Class/Primary Cancer Indications	Adverse Reactions/Common Side Effects	Nursing Considerations
Daunorubicin NS	• Anthracycline antibiotic; leukemia	• Cardiomyopathy when lifetime dose exceeds 550 mg/m2, myelosuppression, hair loss	• Vesicant
Doxorubicin (Adriamycin) NS	• Anthracycline antibiotic; leukemia	• Cardiomyopathy when lifetime dose exceeds 450 mg/m2, myelosuppression	• Vesicant
Etoposide NS or D5W	• Plant alkaloid/topoisomerase II inhibitor; leukemia, testicular CA, small cell lung CA	• Myelosuppression, hair loss	• Give as slow IV infusion (30–60 minutes) to avoid hypotension; dilute to final concentration of 0.2–0.4mg/ml
5-Fluorouracil (5-FU) NS or D5W	• Anti-metabolite; colon, rectum, breast, stomach, and pancreatic CA	• Mouth ulcers, myelosuppression, nausea/vomiting, diarrhea	• GI toxicities can be severe with dysphagia, nausea/vomiting, diarrhea; hand-foot syndrome
Ifosfamide NS or D5W	• Alkylating agent; ovarian, testicular, sarcomas, breast, lymphoma	• Nausea/vomiting (medium), hair loss, myelosuppression, hemorrhagic cystitis; neurotoxicities	Hydration (with 1–2 L 0.9% NS) is crucial; give bladder protectant (Mesna), monitor for hematuria
L-asparaginase NS	• Anti-cancer enzyme; leukemia	• Allergic reactions, pancreatitis (rare)	• Can affect the way methotrexate works, allergic reactions
Methotrexate NS (preservative free for IT)	• Anti-metabolite; leukemia, breast, head and neck, lymphomas, lung cancer, osteosarcomas	• Mouth ulcers, myelosuppression, nausea/vomiting	Rescue doses of leucovorin (folic acid) are required for doses > 500 mg/m2
Paclitaxel NS or D5W	• Plant alkaloid or taxane; breast, ovarian, lung	• Peripheral neuropathies, muscle/joint pain; myelosuppression, hair loss, allergic reactions	• Potentially fatal allergic reactions Vesicant; give before Cisplatin or Carboplatin
Vinblastine NS	• Vinca alkaloid; breast, testicular, lymphomas	• Peripheral neuropathies, myelosuppression, constipation, mouth ulcers, IV USE ONLY	• Vesicant, IV USE ONLY; Intrathecal (IT) use is fatal
Vincristine NS	• Vinca alkaloid; leukemia, lymphomas, neuroblastoma, Wilms' Tumor	• Constipation, peripheral neuropathies, neurological toxicities, hair loss, IV USE ONLY	• Vesicant, IV USE ONLY; Intrathecal (IT) use is fatal

*Note: All chemotherapies have the potential to cause an allergic reaction; those specifically listed have a higher risk of causing an anaphylactic reaction; Vesicant (definition): chemotherapy that will cause serious tissue damage if it leaks out of the vein; requires additional, careful monitoring during infusion.

Cancer Nurse Reference Card

[SICH]

Blood Test	Normal Value
WBC (white blood count)	• 4.1–10.9/µL
Hemoglobin	• 13.2–16.2 gm/dL (male)
	12.0–15.2 gm/dL (female)
Hematocrit	• 40–52% (male)
	37–46% (female)
Platelet	• 150,000–450,000/mcL

Remember...

Keep yourself and others SAFE by handling chemotherapy with CARE.

C ontain drugs and drips, Create ventilation
H andwashing before and after handling chemotherapy
E at away from chemotherapy
M asks and gloves must be worn
O nly for trained staff

Blood Test	Normal Value
Sodium	• 137–145 mEq/L
Potassium	• 3.6–5.0 mEq/L
Chloride	• 98–110 mEq/L
Glucose	• 65–110 mg/dL
BUN (blood urea nitrogen)	• 7–21 mg/dL
Creatinine	• 0.5–1.4 mg/dL
Magnesium	• 1.7–2.2 mg/dL
Phosphorus	• 3.0–4.5 mg/dL
Calcium	• 8.9–10.4 mg/dL

ANC (absolute neutrophil count)	Interpretation
1500 cells/mm³	• Normal
1000–<1500/mm³	• Mild neutropenia
500–<1000/mm³	• Moderate neutropenia
<500/mm³	• Severe neutropenia, high risk of infection

Nursing is an art: and if it is to be made an art, it requires an exclusive devotion as hard a preparation, as any painter's or sculptor's work; for what is the having to do with dead canvas or dead marble, compared with having to do with the living body, the temple of God's spirit? It is one of the Fine Arts: I had almost said, the finest of Fine Arts.

Florence Nightingale

Index

Note: Page numbers followed by "n" denote endnotes.

For Product Safety Concerns and Information please contact our EU
representative GPSR@taylorandfrancis.com
Taylor & Francis Verlag GmbH, Kaufingerstraße 24, 80331 München, Germany

www.ingramcontent.com/pod-product-compliance
Lightning Source LLC
Chambersburg PA
CBHW060239220326
41598CB00027B/3983

* 9 7 8 1 0 3 2 5 3 8 6 0 0 *